Personalized Health Systems for Cardiovascular Disease

Personalized Health Systems for Cardiovascular Disease

Edited by

ANNA MARIA BIANCHI
Department of Electronics, Information, and Bioengineering, Politecnico di Milano, Milan, Italy

JORGE HENRIQUES
Center for Informatics and Systems of the University of Coimbra (CISUC), Department of Informatics Engineering, University of Coimbra, Coimbra, Portugal

VICENTE TRAVER SALCEDO
Department of Electronic Engineering, Universitat Politècnica de València, Valencia, Spain

ELSEVIER

ACADEMIC PRESS
An imprint of Elsevier

Academic Press is an imprint of Elsevier
125 London Wall, London EC2Y 5AS, United Kingdom
525 B Street, Suite 1650, San Diego, CA 92101, United States
50 Hampshire Street, 5th Floor, Cambridge, MA 02139, United States
The Boulevard, Langford Lane, Kidlington, Oxford OX5 1GB, United Kingdom

Notices
Knowledge and best practice in this field are constantly changing. As new research and experience broaden our understanding, changes in research methods, professional practices, or medical treatment may become necessary.

Practitioners and researchers must always rely on their own experience and knowledge in evaluating and using any information, methods, compounds, or experiments described herein. In using such information or methods they should be mindful of their own safety and the safety of others, including parties for whom they have a professional responsibility.

To the fullest extent of the law, neither the Publisher nor the authors, contributors, or editors, assume any liability for any injury and/or damage to persons or property as a matter of products liability, negligence or otherwise, or from any use or operation of any methods, products, instructions, or ideas contained in the material herein.

British Library Cataloguing-in-Publication Data
A catalogue record for this book is available from the British Library

Library of Congress Cataloging-in-Publication Data
A catalog record for this book is available from the Library of Congress

ISBN: 978-0-12-818950-4

Publisher: Mara Conner
Acquisitions Editor: Carrie Bolger
Editorial Project Manager: Chiara Giglio
Production Project Manager: Kamesh Ramajogi
Cover Designer: Christian J. Bilbow

Typeset by MPS Limited, Chennai, India

Dedication

To our families

Contents

List of contributors

Giuseppe Baselli
Department of Electronics, Information, and Bioengineering, Politecnico di Milano, Milan, Italy

Jozef Beňačka
Faculty of Health Care and Social Work, University of Trnava, Trnava, Slovakia

Anna Maria Bianchi
Department of Electronics, Information, and Bioengineering, Politecnico di Milano, Milan, Italy

Alberto Bonomi
Philips Research, Eindhoven, The Netherlands

Francisco Castells
Institut ITACA, Universitat Politècnica de València, Valencia, Spain

Sergio Cervera-Torres
Adhera Heath Inc, Seville, Spain

Raquel Cervigón
Escuela Politécnica, UCLM, Cuenca, Spain

Ioanna Chouvarda
Lab of Computing, Medical Informatics, and Biomedical Imaging Technologies, School of Medicine, Aristotle University of Thessaloniki, Thessaloniki, Greece

Stefania Coelli
Department of Electronics, Information, and Bioengineering, Politecnico di Milano, Milan, Italy

Paulo de Carvalho
Center for Informatics and Systems of the University of Coimbra, Department of Informatics Engineering, University of Coimbra, Coimbra, Portugal

Enrique Dorronzoro-Zubiete
Participatory Health Informatics and Personalization Research Group, Universidad de Sevilla, Seville, Spain

Lino Gonçalves
Department of Cardiology, Coimbra University Hospital Centre, Coimbra, Portugal; ICBR Coimbra Institute for Clinical and Biomedical Research (iCBR), Faculty of Medicine, Universidade de Coimbra, Coimbra, Portugal

Illapha Cuba Gyllensten
Philips Research, Eindhoven, The Netherlands

Gunnar Hartvigsen
Department of Computer Science, Arctic University of Tromsø, Tromsø, Norway

Jorge Henriques
Center for Informatics and Systems of the University of Coimbra, Department of Informatics Engineering, University of Coimbra, Coimbra, Portugal

Alexandra Krištúfková
Faculty of Medicine, Comenius University in Bratislava, Bratislava, Slovakia

Fedor Lehocki
Slovak University of Technology in Bratislava, Bratislava, Slovakia; National Center of Telemedicine Services, Bratislava, Slovakia

Riccardo Lolatto
Department of Electronics, Information, and Bioengineering, Politecnico di Milano, Milan, Italy

Antonio Martinez-Millana
Institut ITACA, Universitat Politècnica de València, Valencia, Spain

Timotej Matak
Slovak University of Technology in Bratislava, Bratislava, Slovakia

José Millet
Institut ITACA, Universitat Politècnica de València, Valencia, Spain

James Milner
Department of Cardiology, Coimbra University Hospital Centre, Coimbra, Portugal

Jens Mühlsteff
Philips Research, Eindhoven, The Netherlands

Marek Mydliar
National Center of Telemedicine Services, Bratislava, Slovakia; Faculty of Health Care and Social Work, University of Trnava, Trnava, Slovakia

Francisco J. Nuñez-Benjumea
Adhera Heath Inc, Seville, Spain

Reinhold Orglmeister
Electronics and Medical Signal Processing, Technische Universität Berlin, Berlin, Germany

Simão Paredes
Department of Informatics and Systems, Polytechnic Institute of Engineering; Center for Informatics and Systems of the University of Coimbra, Department of Informatics Engineering, University of Coimbra, Coimbra, Portugal

Alexandru Pielmus
Electronics and Medical Signal Processing, Technische Universität Berlin, Berlin, Germany

Dario Pirovano
Pirovano Management, Waterloo, Belgium

Silvia Putekova
Faculty of Health Care and Social Work, University of Trnava, Trnava, Slovakia

Pierluigi Reali
Department of Electronics, Information, and Bioengineering, Politecnico di Milano, Milan, Italy

Octavio Rivera-Romero
Participatory Health Informatics and Personalization Research Group, Universidad de Sevilla, Seville, Spain

Teresa Rocha
Department of Informatics and Systems, Polytechnic Institute of Engineering; Center for Informatics and Systems of the University of Coimbra, Department of Informatics Engineering, University of Coimbra, Coimbra, Portugal

Vicente Traver Salcedo
Department of Electronic Engineering, Universitat Politècnica de València, Valencia, Spain

Erez Shalom
Medical Informatics Research Center, Ben-Gurion University of the Negev, Beer-Sheva, Israel

Warner ten Kate
Philips Research, Eindhoven, The Netherlands

About the editors

Anna Maria Bianchi is a Full Professor in Biomedical Engineering, with teaching responsibility in Biomedical Signal Processing and Medical Informatics, in BS, MS, and PhD Bioengineering programs. Her research interests are mainly related to the processing of biomedical signals and images and to the development of innovative methodologies for feature extraction, information enhancement, and model development. Applications are both in physiological studies and in clinics through design of interpretative and diagnostic models. In recent years, applications have been in the field of medical informatics and artificial intelligence. Prof. Bianchi is the scientific coordinator of the Medical Informatics Lab at DEIB and is a member of the management committee of two interdepartmental labs at Politecnico di Milano (i.e., the BrainLab@Polimi and PHEEL). She has authored 20 book chapters and more than 110 peer-reviewed papers in ISI international journals. She has been a fellow of EAMBES (European Alliance for Medical and Biological Engineering and Science) since 2012. Dr. Bianchi serves as a scientific expert in the EMBS Technical Committee on Neuroengineering and the Technical Committee on Cardiopulmonary Systems. She is an Associate Editor of *IEEE Transactions on Neural System and Rehabilitation Engineering* and a member of the editorial board of the *Journal of Biomedical Signals Processing and Control* and of *Electronics—Open Access Journal*. She has participated in many EU-funded (from VI framework program to H2020) and Italian-funded research projects with scientific responsibility and has active collaborations with companies operating in the field of biomedical instrumentation and systems.

Jorge Henriques is an Associate Professor, with teaching responsibility in Informatics Engineering and Biomedical Engineering in BS, MS, and PhD programs. His main research interests are computational intelligence methodologies with application to modeling, prediction, diagnosis, and decision making, in particular in the clinical context. He has been particularly active in the development of innovative solutions in p-health scenarios, with particular application to situations in preventive medicine and chronic diseases management, namely in the research and implementation of advanced algorithms for biosignals' analysis and processing (in particular, electrocardiogram, photoplethysmogram, heart sounds, and blood pressure). He is a senior researcher in the Adaptive Computation Group at the Center for Informatics and Systems of the University of Coimbra (CISUC). His publications include seven book chapters and over 200 papers in refereed international journals and conferences. He is a reviewer for many biomedical engineering journals and has been involved in numerous program committees of major international conferences. He has coordinated and participated in several projects at national and international levels (European FP6, FP7, and H2020). He is a licensed professional engineer, was the executive coordinator of the Informatics Laboratory of Instituto Pedro Nunes, and has provided consulting services to various companies and national institutions in the clinical informatics and e-health areas.

Vicente Traver Salcedo has a bachelor's degree (1998) and a PhD (2004) in Telecommunications Engineering from the Universitat Politècnica de València. He is a member of the academic board for the interuniversity master's degree in Biomedical Engineering at the Universitat Politècnica de València. He is also the coordinator of the *Healthy Living* cluster, which combines six different R&D university groups working in the field. Since 1998, his research focus has been on telemedicine, e-health, and e-inclusion, especially on the provision of home healthcare services through telematic media and the concepts of patient empowerment and the citizen as health coproducer. He has participated in more than 50 EU-funded projects (from IV framework program to H2020) and Spanish-funded projects, and has taken part in multiple research agreements with companies in healthcare and social services that make use of information communication technologies. He has published more than 120 technical papers in national and international journals and has participated in several seminars and conferences as an invited speaker. He is a member of international scientific congress committees and a member of the editorial board of *IET Networks*. He was the keynote lecturer at BIOSTEC 2010. He was the chairman and organizer of pHealth 2008 and the four editions of the International Workshop on Technology for Healthcare and Healthy Lifestyle (2008, 2010, 2011, 2012). He was conference cochair of IEEE Biomedical Health Informatics 2014. He is cofounder of two SME IT health-related companies, currently employing more than 40 people. A full list of his publications is available at goo.gl/Wg2JZR.

Preface

Noncommunicable diseases (NCDs) or chronic diseases are of long duration and usually slow in progressing health conditions with a determinant impact on the quality of life of the patient and the sustainability of health systems. According to the WHO, chronic diseases are responsible for 63% of all deaths worldwide, and they force many people into poverty as a result of catastrophic expenditures for treatment while undercutting productivity. Although high-income countries are the dominant contributors to the global economic burden of NCDs, the developing countries is expected to assume an ever larger share as their economies and populations grow.

Among all NCDs, cardiovascular diseases (CVDs), such as stroke, arrhythmia, heart failure, and myocardial infarction, are the most dominant contributors to the global economic burden of NCDs. Most CVDs are preventable and manageable; that is, they might benefit from adopting a preventive health management paradigm that could avoid or delay their development or help in keeping patients already experiencing CVD dysfunctions on the right path to avoid acute episodes of the disease.

The current health provision paradigm is acute illness driven, that is, it is focused on handling acute situations. This focus has brought high-impact innovations in the management of acute illness, but it has disregarded the growth in chronic advanced illness, which requires a paradigm shift. In light of the increases in NCDs, the focus should be redirected toward (1) preventive healthcare, mainly by promoting healthy lifestyle changes, and (2) shifting from acute disease treatment to management of NCDs. This requires a completely new approach to health organization, putting the patient in the center, developing a continuous process of care, and shifting care from a hospital-driven approach to a home-driven (or, more generally, a pervasive) approach. This shift poses significant challenges at different levels: political, financial, legal, and technological. Significant and promising steps are being made to promote change. For instance, the United States has implemented a readmission reduction program in which patient 30-day readmissions are highly penalized financially, and in Germany, health apps are now available by prescription.

From a technological point of view, new low-cost and intelligent solutions for remote patient management are required. These solutions pose significant engineering challenges, since besides the accuracy and low-cost requirements, these systems should be designed to be operated by patients who are not highly trained and sometimes by patients who have significant cognitive or functional impairments. They should also be as unintrusive as possible. Strategies to promote long-term adherence present another relevant challenge in implementing this type of system.

The idea for this book started during the H2020 EU Project (H2020–692023) LINK: Linking Excellence in Biomedical Knowledge and Computational Intelligence Research for Personalized Management of CVD Within PHC, in which we developed a reference curricula for advanced training programs for intelligent algorithms for personal healthcare in CVD management. This book corresponds to the reference material required to implement this course and might be applied entirely or partially in this context as a single-volume reference text by instructors and students. It could also be a valuable source of information for researchers and engineers active in the field who want to learn more about current approaches and open issues in the field, since this book presents a structured overview of current challenges, gaps, and developments in p-health for CVD. The book starts in Chapter 1, Telemonitoring applications in cardiology, with clinical foundations and needs related to patient monitoring for CVD management. Chapter 2, Data and signals for the assessment of the cardiovascular system, introduces a medical perspective on the available data and signals for CVD assessment, and Chapter 3, Systems, sensors, and devices in personal healthcare applications, lays out the fundamental sensor technologies that are available to deploy personal healthcare solutions for CVD.

Chapters 4–7 lay out the processing steps required for p-health solution deployment. In particular, Chapter 4, Signal processing for cardiovascular applications in p-health, introduces a holistic view related to signal processing, whereas Chapter 5, Models for risk assessment and stratification, and Chapter 6, Connected health technologies for knowledge extraction and knowledge-based medicine in cardiac care, introduce an overview of patient risk assessment and stratification as well as connected health. Chapter 7, Increasing and standardizing quality of care using computerized guidelines for clinical decision support, describes application frameworks and the life cycle of the creation of computerized guidelines to facilitate clinical decision-making support.

One of the main challenges facing p-health systems is patient compliance. Chapter 8, Digital coaching for personalized healthcare of cardiovascular diseases, is dedicated to coaching strategies to improve patient feedback and patient engagement. Finally, Chapters 9–11 are dedicated to the development of health apps for p-health. Chapter 9, Methods for app development in p-health, addresses aspects related to the development and design, testing and evaluation, and certification of such apps. Chapter 10, Devices for p-health: Which regulations in Europe?, discusses relevant regulations and standards for deployment of the devices. Chapter 11, Remote management of heart failure patients: A p-health example, introduces an integrated system example.

Paulo de Carvalho

Introduction

What is the meaning of the term p-health? It could be "personal" health or "personalized" health. Other interpretations are also possible. The aspects of p-health discussed in this book are mainly related to people and patients, especially their active role in the management of their own health, but also to physicians who make use of technology for a more efficient management of their patients and engineers who collaborate to address technological issues in the challenges of p-health.

The purpose of this book is to provide, from a technical point of view, a complete description of most of the elements that are part of such systems, including the current state of the art and new directions for innovative solutions. Therefore, the reader will find in this book the fundamental elements that need to be taken into account in developing devices and systems in the field of p-health.

The viewpoint of the physician is fundamental. Which pieces of information are needed for effective monitoring of the patient? Which are the relevant parameters that allow assessment of the status of the patient? To address these problems, Chapter 1, Telemonitoring applications in cardiology, coordinated by Dr. Lino Gonçalves, shows the state of the art and how telemonitoring is already being used in cardiology. Chapter 2, Data and signals for the assessment of the cardiovascular system, led by Dr. Castells, provides the basis of the data and the different signals that allow proper and personalized handling of a cardiovascular disease.

The second important aspect of p-health is how to get the relevant information when the patient is not in a clinical environment but is living at home and clinical devices and expert personnel are not available. Jens Mühlsteff introduces in Chapter 3, Systems, sensors, and devices in personal healthcare applications, an overview of the hardware and middleware to be used for personal healthcare applications, covering systems, sensors, and devices. In Chapter 4, Signal processing for cardiovascular applications in p-health, Prof. Bianchi presents the key concepts in the use of proper signal processing in order to extract clinical information for cardiovascular applications in p-health.

Once data have been collected and preprocessed from the point of care, it is vital to manage and prioritize patients on the basis of models for risk assessment and stratification, which are addressed in Chapter 5, Models for risk assessment and stratification, coordinated by Dr. Teresa Rocha. Chapter 6, Connected health technologies for knowledge extraction and knowledge-based medicine in cardiac care, led by Prof. Chouvarda, covers the issue of connected health technologies for knowledge management and knowledge-based medicine in cardiac care. How to reduce variability and increase the quality of care using computerized guidelines for clinical decision support is the focus of Chapter 7, Increasing and standardizing quality of care using computerized guidelines for clinical decision support, led by Prof. Lehocki.

Dr. Dorronzoro takes the perspective of patient empowerment in Chapter 8, Digital coaching for personalized healthcare of cardiovascular diseases, and remarks on the importance of coaching for behavior and lifestyle change to improve personalized management of diseases. Chapter 9, Methods for app development in p-health, coordinated by Dr. Martinez-Millana, shows how to develop apps that cover all the key issues in p-health.

The legal aspects of p-health are outlined in Chapter 10, Devices for p-health: Which regulations in Europe?, in which Dr. Pirovano shows how regulations in Europe are affecting the development of devices for p-health.

In Chapter 11, Remote management of heart failure patients: A p-health example, the editors conclude the book with a p-health example that collects key messages from the different chapters, showing how they can be implemented in practice in the remote management of patients with heart failure.

Students and researchers in biomedical engineering will find in this book an integrated and practical view of many subjects that are part of their courses and how the different topics covered in the book can contribute to the development of actual solutions in the field of biomedical engineering.

Anna Maria Bianchi, Jorge Henriques, and Vicente Traver Salcedo

CHAPTER 1

Telemonitoring applications in cardiology

James Milner[1] and Lino Gonçalves[1,2]
[1]Department of Cardiology, Coimbra University Hospital Centre, Coimbra, Portugal
[2]ICBR Coimbra Institute for Clinical and Biomedical Research (iCBR), Faculty of Medicine, Universidade de Coimbra, Coimbra, Portugal

1.1 Background

Healthcare systems are facing increasing difficulties and challenges. Population aging is a global reality, particularly in Western nations, where lower birth rates have progressively led to an inversion of the age pyramid, in such a way that for the first time in history the number of people over 65 years old will be higher than the number of children under 5 years of age (Why Population Aging Matters: A Global Perspective, 2017). Globally, the number of people over 60 years is expected to triple by 2100 (World Population Prospects: Key findings & advance tables, 2017). The increase in life expectancy is also determinant in these changes, and advances of public health, medicine, and economic development over diseases that limit life expectancy mean that many pathological conditions are now chronic, manageable diseases. The increasing number of older patients with more comorbidities presents a tremendous challenge to governments and healthcare systems. These patients require regular and continuous monitoring by different healthcare providers, in many cases for the duration of their lives. Healthcare systems that are organized around a model focused on the management of acute episodes are clearly insufficient to satisfy the needs of these patients. A suggested new model involves the decentralization of healthcare to the patient's home, with a progressively bigger involvement of the patient, the family, and community structures in the management of the patient's conditions, as part of the solution to this problem. In this setting, the use of technologies, devices, and telemedicine systems that help the patient and healthcare providers in monitoring and managing the patient's health state are becoming essential. The use of these technologies may also play a significant role in reducing healthcare-associated expenses, which are becoming

Personalized Health Systems for Cardiovascular Disease
DOI: https://doi.org/10.1016/B978-0-12-818950-4.00002-1

a significant burden in modern societies. This is particularly significant regarding cardiovascular diseases, since these account for close to one-third of all deaths in the United States and are responsible for more deaths than all forms of cancer (Benjamin et al., 2019).

Broadly, telemedicine is a unique entity that involves patient management based on telecommunications. Telemedicine applications in cardiology have witnessed a significant growth in the past few years and are expected to become a staple in clinical practice. The need for and implementation of telemedicine strategies was further escalated by the 2020 COVID-19 pandemic, which placed a significant strain on healthcare structures and forced physicians and organizations to reorganize and to implement new strategies in order to continue to deliver high-quality healthcare in outpatient settings without compromising patient and healthcare provider safety.

Uses of telemedicine in cardiovascular medicine are varied and encompass an array of different applications, including remote interactions between patient and healthcare provider by telephone or videoconference, remote transmission of information derived from home measurements (which can include self-reported symptoms and measures of simple parameters such as blood pressure, heart rate, or weight), the use of web-based or smartphone apps, and activity-tracking devices that have gained significant popularity in the past few years, which has even led the U.S. Food and Drug Administration to approve the Apple Watch as a medical device for atrial fibrillation diagnosis, following publication from the Apple Heart Study investigators in 2019 (Perez et al., 2019). Other telemedicine applications include remote monitoring of cardiac implantable electronic devices, such as implantable loop recorders, pacemakers, and implantable defibrillator-cardioverters. Telemedicine applications aim to improve the healthcare provided to patients, their quality of life, and even hard outcomes such as hospitalization rates and all-cause mortality. We will address some of these applications in this chapter.

1.2 Telemonitoring applications in cardiology

1.2.1 Remote Monitoring for CIED

Remote home monitoring of cardiac implantable electronic devices (CIED) began over a decade ago. Since then, extensive evidence has been collected regarding their usefulness in early detection of significant arrhythmias, as well as maintaining a continuous surveillance of the system's performance, allowing for early detection of generator battery depletion and lead dysfunction. Beyond their obvious clinical significance, the implementation of remote monitoring of CIED into everyday clinical practice has contributed to a better optimization of healthcare resources.

Atrial fibrillation (AF), the most common arrhythmia in clinical practice (Nieuwlaat et al., 2005), is often asymptomatic and may remain undetected by patients. Early diagnosis of AF is of utmost importance, since it is the most common arrhythmia in clinical practice, with an incidence that increases with age (Zulkifly, Lip, & Lane, 2018). This is particularly significant because AF patients are frequently hospitalized and have a five-fold increase in the risk of stroke (Nieuwlaat et al., 2005; Zulkifly et al., 2018). European Registries showed that up to 50% of patients with AF are not actually treated (Nieuwlaat et al., 2005), which is unsurprising, since most patients with AF are asymptomatic and may receive a diagnosis only following a thrombotic complication. Early detection is particularly important in patients carrying CIED, since they have an even higher prevalence of AF than the rest of the population.

Several studies have concluded on the usefulness of CIED for the documentation of episodes of AF. CIED may emit alerts of many natures, and AF accounts for over 50% of the alerts emitted by remote home-monitoring systems (Lazarus, 2007). The Asymptomatic Atrial Fibrillation and Stroke Evaluation in Pacemaker Patients and the Atrial Fibrillation Reduction Atrial Pacing Trial concluded that detection by CIED of these arrhythmias was associated with an increased risk of thromboembolic events (including ischemic stroke) (Hohnloser et al., 2006). Consequently, it is easy to understand that remote, automatic monitoring may help in detecting these arrhythmias at an earlier stage, allowing for a timely therapeutic adjustment (including oral anticoagulation) in order to prevent long-term complications. In fact, home monitoring has been showed to reduce stroke risk by 9%–18% when compared to conventional regular, presential scheduled visiting (Ricci, Morichelli, Gargaro, Laudadio, & Santini, 2009). Furthermore, the Cardiovascular Outcome for People Using Anticoagulation Strategies trial showed that remote monitoring of CIED reduced hospital admissions due to stroke or atrial arrhythmias (Mabo et al., 2012).

There is sufficient evidence to support generalized use of remote monitoring for AF development in patients with CIED. These recommendations are echoed by European Society of Cardiology guidelines, which recommend remote monitoring for the detection of arrhythmias or device-related problems (Brignole et al., 2013), a class IIa indication.

1.2.2 Remote monitoring for heart failure

Heart failure (HF) is a common condition, affecting 1.5% of the world population (Saner & van der Velde, 2016). HF is becoming progressively more prevalent as populations age and as treatment of comorbidities such as coronary artery disease or type 2 diabetes mellitus improves. HF is associated with substantial clinical and financial burdens (Lin et al., 2017) and requires close management by healthcare providers, family, community networks, and patients, who have a crucial role in their medical condition in terms of adherence to therapy, lifestyle modifications, and symptom monitoring, among others. Several different trials and a metaanalysis have reported a benefit from telemedicine applications in the management of HF. The role of telemedicine in HF is varied but focuses mostly on early detection of signs and symptoms of decompensation, presenting the physician with an opportunity to intervene before the patient requires hospitalization. Initial applications of telemonitoring in HF consisted of telephone contacts between healthcare providers and patients to monitor for symptoms and disease progression. Currently, telemonitoring strategies in HF are several and much more complex, including the implantation of CIED that may be triggered by the development of arrhythmias and the implantation of hemodynamic sensors and other devices that can collect different vital signs and parameters and transmit them to healthcare providers.

Hospitalizations due to decompensated HF become increasingly common as the disease progresses, and each episode of hospitalization carries significant risks of morbidity and mortality, increases the risk of further readmissions due to HF, and is a powerful predictor of poor outcomes. In fact, the last 2 years of life for HF patients are estimated to cost over $156,000, and more than 75% of that amount corresponds to costs related to hospital admissions due to decompensated HF (Russo et al., 2008). Applications of telemedicine in HF have focused on reducing the likelihood of hospitalizations due to HF, most of which are related to the worsening of congestion (Mabo et al., 2012). However, it is known that cardiac filling pressures may be significantly increased even weeks before congestion is clinically apparent (Abraham et al., 2011), and clinical evaluation of congestion (through physical examination, symptom evaluation, and the use of biomarkers such as natriuretic peptides) is often difficult before it becomes significant, since congestion may be subtle and masked by other pathologies and because signs and symptoms of congestion are not entirely specific for HF.

Imaging tools such as chest X-ray and echocardiography may help to improve congestion detection. Remote monitoring of natriuretic peptides as surrogate markers for congestion also seemed like a desirable approach. However, results from the GUIDE-IT trial, which aimed to compare a strategy of natriuretic peptide-level therapy with usual care, were negative in relation to the primary outcome of cardiovascular death or time to first HF admission (Felker et al., 2017). Whether or not these biomarkers could be incorporated into models that also take into consideration other clinical or imaging parameters remains to be evaluated.

In 2011 results were published from the CHAMPION trial, a randomized, controlled trial of patients with advanced HF who were blindly randomized to either a standard of care strategy or implantation of a wireless hemodynamic monitoring system (the CardioMEMS device, a wireless, radiofrequency pulmonary artery pressure sensor that can be safely implanted percutaneously). Patients in the intervention group were submitted to daily measurements of pulmonary artery pressure, and the authors concluded that wireless hemodynamic monitoring significantly reduced the risk of readmission due to decompensated HF, with a 30% reduction in the first 6 months (Abraham et al., 2011). These findings were further validated following a 2017 prespecified subgroup analysis that concluded that patients with HF with reduced ejection fraction benefited from remote, invasive pulmonary artery pressure monitoring. Readmission due to decompensated HF was also reduced by about 28% in the intervention group, a result that strengthens the potential impact of pulmonary artery–based therapy (Givertz et al., 2017).

Beyond invasive hemodynamic monitoring, simpler applications of telemedicine in HF can contribute towards better outcomes. Weight monitoring, which may act as a surrogate for clinical congestion and elevated filling pressures (Abraham et al., 2011), is an accessible yet powerful parameter in HF evaluation, since an unexplained weight increase may signify worsening of congestion and impending HF decompensation. Monitoring of simple parameters such as blood pressure and heart rate can provide significant insight into the hemodynamic status of the patient and contribute toward a more tailored pharmacological therapy. Trained healthcare practitioners can make clinical decisions based on objectively monitored HF-related parameters, and variations of these parameters beyond predefined limits can even trigger alerts for the patient or the physician

However, not every trial for telemonitoring in HF has yielded positive results. In 2016 the better effectiveness after transition-heart failure trial randomized patients following hospitalization due to decompensated HF to a either a standard of care strategy or an intervention group that included regular telephone coaching and home monitoring of symptoms and parameters such as blood pressure, heart rate, and weight. Results found that patients in the intervention arm had a significant improvement in self-reported quality of life, despite the lack of difference regarding readmissions due to HF in the first 30 or 180 days (Ong et al., 2016).

In the recently published Telemedical Interventional Management in patients with Heart Failure (TIM-HF2) trial, it was shown that a structured remote patient management intervention, when used in a selected HF population, is able to reduce the percentage of days lost due to unplanned cardiovascular hospital admissions and all-cause mortality. Friedrich Koehler et al. (2018).

Despite conflicting evidence regarding the effectiveness of telemedicine in HF, implementation of these strategies into the management of HF is likely to have a significant impact in patient outcomes.

1.3 Challenges and future perspectives

In multiple areas of cardiovascular sciences it seems that telemedicine can at the very least improve patient engagement and involvement in their condition, facilitate communication between patients and healthcare providers, and possibly even modify the natural history of the diseases. However, we remain without unequivocal evidence to extensively integrate telemedicine into daily clinical practice. This is echoed by the lack of clear guidelines from international cardiovascular societies for the use of telemedicine. This lack of evidence refers not only to the strictly clinical aspect, but also to the question of economic viability. Furthermore, cost effectiveness is still a major setback for broad implementation of these strategies. It is likely that these approaches may be more economically viable if implemented in high-risk groups (who also correspond to the population evaluated in most trials), who are likely to derive the most benefit.

Health literacy is also a major factor affecting adherence to remote monitoring strategies (whenever these require user input). In fact, it has been demonstrated that patient adherence to remote monitoring is directly correlated with survival. These issues, which already constitute a barrier between physician and patient under conventional circumstances, are vastly amplified when it comes to virtual contacts and to resorting to medical apps or to devices to measure different parameters. This may be even more true for older and more fragile patients, who would probably derive the most benefit from these measures.

Portability and ease of use of these devices is another concern, since these factors may also significantly affect patient adherence to remote monitoring strategies. These tools not only need to be easy to use but also should be adequately integrated and connected to other systems that are widely used (such as smartphones and computers). This bridge between user interfaces and healthcare services [also known as mHealth (Saner & van der Velde, 2016)] is absolutely essential nor only to ensure patient adherence but also to promote patients' engagement in the process, increasing their motivation to achieve better outcomes. These platforms may also help to establish a shorter bridge between patients and healthcare providers, increasing patient confidence and giving them a way to contact care providers in case of doubt or medical emergency. Progressively, mHealth seems also to be improving the way in which physicians and other providers interact with each other, ensuring that adequate connections between hospitals and community care are in play, working in synergy to achieve better results, despite concerns about privacy and data protection.

Telemedicine is progressing at a stupendous rate, and artificial intelligence will certainly come into play, given the overwhelming amount of information generated by remote monitoring devices. Big data can obviously lead to an improvement in the way in which we deal with chronic conditions, but adequate tools to analyze and integrate such a high volume of data are clearly necessary. However, this also raises the important question of liability. Once artificial intelligence and algorithms for big data management fully take over remote monitoring, the relative responsibilities of the patient, the physician, and the healthcare center are unclear.

Regardless of the type of intervention, it is becoming increasingly clear that telemedicine applications are becoming part of the standard of care for many different pathologies. These interventions have increased patient engagement and involvement in their own condition and management, increasing therapeutic compliance, increasing patients' knowledge and confidence, and reducing the incidence of acute episodes requiring hospitalization. Therefore implementing these strategies into clinical practice is necessary and should be incentivized.

References

Abraham, W. T., Adamson, P. B., Bourge, R. C., Aaron, M. F., Constanzo, M. R., Stevenson, L. W., ... Yadav, J. S. (2011). Wireless pulmonary artery haemodynamic monitoring in chronic heart failure: A randomised controlled trial. *Lancet*, *377*(9766), 658–666. Available from https://doi.org/10.1016/S0140-6736(11)60101-3.

Benjamin, E. J., Muntner, P., Alonso, A., Bittencourt, M. S., Callaway, C. W., Carson, A. P., ... Virani, S. S. (2019). Heart disease and stroke statistics-2019 update: A report from the American Heart Association. *Circulation*, *139*(10), e56–e528. Available from https://doi.org/10.1161/CIR.0000000000000659.

Brignole, M., Auricchio, A., Baron-Esquivias, G., Bordachar, P., Boriani, G., Breithardt, O., ... Vardas, P. (2013). 2013 ESC guidelines on cardiac pacing and cardiac resynchronization therapy. *European Heart Journal*, *34*, 2281–2329. Available from https://doi.org/10.1093/eurheartj/eht150, https://doi.org/10.1016/j.rec.2013.11.003.

Felker, G. M., Anstrom, K. J., Adams, K. F., Ezekowitz, J. A., Fiuzat, M., Houston-Miller, N., ... O'Connor, C. M. (2017). Effect of natriuretic peptide-guided therapy on hospitalization or cardiovascular mortality in high-risk patients with heart failure and reduced ejection fraction: A randomized clinical trial. *JAMA: The Journal of the American Medical Association*, *318*(8), 713–720. Available from https://doi.org/10.1001/jama.2017.10565.

Friedrich Koehler, K., Koehler, O., Deckwart, S., Prescher, K., Wegscheider, B.-A., Kirwan, S., ... Stangl, K. (2018). Efficacy of telemedical interventional management in patients with heart failure (TIM-HF2): A randomised, controlled, parallel-group, unmasked trial. *Lancet*, *392*(10152), 1047–1057. Available from https://doi.org/10.1016/S0140-6736(18)31880-4, Epub August 25, 2018.

Givertz, M. M., Stevenson, L. W., Costanzo, M. R., Bourge, R. C., Bauman, J. G., Ginn, G., ... CHAMPION Trial Investigators. (2017). Pulmonary artery pressure-guided management of patients with heart failure and reduced ejection fraction. *Journal of the American College of Cardiology*, *70*(15), 1875–1886. Available from https://doi.org/10.1016/j.jacc.2017.08.010.

Hohnloser, S. H., Capucci, A., Fain, E., Gold, M. R., van Gelder, I. C., Healey, J., & Israel, C. W. (2006). ASymptomatic atrial fibrillation and Stroke Evaluation in pacemaker patients and the atrial fibrillation Reduction atrial pacing Trial (ASSERT). *American Heart Journal*, *152*(3), 442–447. Available from https://doi.org/10.1016/j.ahj.2006.020.016.

Lazarus, A. (2007). Remote, wireless, ambulatory monitoring of implantable pacemakers, cardioverter defibrillators, and cardiac resynchronization therapy systems: Analysis of a worldwide database. *Pacing and Clinical Electrophysiology: PACE*, *30*(Suppl. 1), S2–S12. Available from https://doi.org/10.1111/j.1540-8159.2007.00595.x.

Lin, M. H., Yuan, W. L., Huang, T. C., Zhang, H. F., Mai, J. T., & Wang, J. F. (2017). Clinical effectiveness of telemedicine for chronic heart failure: A systematic review and *meta*-analysis. *Journal of Investigative Medicine: The Official Publication of the American Federation for Clinical Research*, *65*(5), 899–911. Available from https://doi.org/10.1136/jim-2016-000199.

Mabo, P., Victor, F., Bazin, P., Ahres, S., Babuty, D., Da Costa, A., ... Daubert, J. (2012). A randomized trial of long-term remote monitoring of pacemaker recipients (the COMPAS trial). *European Heart Journal*, *33*(9), 1105–1111. Available from https://doi.org/10.1093/eurheartj/ehr419.

Nieuwlaat, R., Capucci, A., Camm, A. J., Olsson, S. B., Andresen, D., Davies, D. W., . . . Crijns, H. J. G. M. (2005). Atrial fibrillation management: A prospective survey in ESC member countries: The Euro Heart Survey on Atrial Fibrillation. *European Heart Journal*, *26*(22), 2422–2434. Available from https://doi.org/10.1093/eurheartj/ehi505.

Ong, M. K., Romano, P. S., Edgington, S., Aronow, H., Auerbach, A. D., Black, J. T., . . . Fonarow, G. C. (2016). Effectiveness of remote patient monitoring after discharge of hospitalized patients with heart failure: The better effectiveness after transition – Heart failure (BEAT-HF) randomized clinical trial. *JAMA Internal Medicine*, *176*(3), 310–318. Available from https://doi.org/10.1001/jamainternmed.2015.7712.

Perez, M. V., Mahaffey, K. W., Hedlin, H., Rumsfeld, J. S., Garcia, A., Ferris, T., . . . Turakhia, M. P. (2019). Large-scale assessment of a smartwatch to identify atrial fibrillation. *The New England Journal of Medicine*, *381*(20), 1909–1917. Available from https://doi.org/10.1056/NEJMoa1901183.

Ricci, R. P., Morichelli, L., Gargaro, A., Laudadio, M. T., & Santini, M. (2009). Home monitoring in patients with implantable cardiac devices: Is there a potential reduction of stroke risk? Results from a computer model tested through monte carlo simulations. *Journal of Cardiovascular Electrophysiology*, *20*(11), 1244–1251. Available from https://doi.org/10.1111/j.1540-8167.2009.01543.x.

Russo, M. J., Gelijns, A. C., Stevenson, L. W., Sampat, B., Aaronson, K. D., Renlund, D. G., . . . Willer, L. W. (2008). The cost of medical management in advanced heart failure during the final two years of life. *Journal of Cardiac Failure*, *14*(8), 651–658. Available from https://doi.org/10.1016/j.cardfail.2008.06.005.

Saner, H., & van der Velde, E. (2016). eHealth in cardiovascular medicine: A clinical update. *European Journal of Preventive Cardiology*, *23*(2 suppl), 5–12. Available from https://doi.org/10.1177/2047487316670256.

Why Population Aging Matters: A Global Perspective. (2017). United States Department of State.

World Population Prospects: Key findings & advance tables. (2017). Department of Economic and Social Affairs, United Nations.

Zulkifly, H., Lip, G. Y. H., & Lane, D. A. (2018). Epidemiology of atrial fibrillation. *International Journal of Clinical Practice*, *72*(3), e13070. Available from https://doi.org/10.1111/ijcp.13070.

CHAPTER 2

Data and signals for the assessment of the cardiovascular system

Francisco Castells[1], Raquel Cervigón[2], and José Millet[1]
[1]Institut ITACA, Universitat Politècnica de València, Valencia, Spain
[2]Escuela Politécnica, UCLM, Cuenca, Spain

2.1 Introduction

Diagnosis of a patient's cardiovascular condition starts with a visit to the doctor, which may be triggered by either a symptomatic episode of the patient or a routine inspection. An accurate diagnosis relies on specific tests that will be endorsed by the doctor according to his or her professional criteria, meeting in any case the standards described in management guidelines and following hospital protocol. The most common tests for the assessment of the cardiovascular system involve, among others, blood pressure, electrocardiography, phonocardiography, echocardiography, electrophysiological study, computerized tomography scan, and cardiac magnetic resonance imaging. Each of these involves a different principle, as follows:

- *Electrical potential*: The electrocardiogram (ECG) is the surface observation of the electrical activation of the heart as a result of the transmembrane ionic currents of the myocytes (muscle cells). It is obtained as the potential difference between two sites on the body surface, so the resulting waveform depends on their location. Despite its simplicity, the ECG is a powerful test to diagnose electrical disorders such as cardiac arrhythmias. Moreover, the electrical activation of the heart can be more precisely characterized during an electrophysiological study by inserting a catheter into the heart chambers. With this technique, localized electrograms can be registered and anatomically mapped to detect the sites causing the arrhythmia.
- *Ultrasound*: Echocardiography is an image technique based on the reflections (or echoes) of ultrasound beams. Specifically, Doppler

Personalized Health Systems for Cardiovascular Disease
DOI: https://doi.org/10.1016/B978-0-12-818950-4.00009-4

approaches are able to provide images from everything that moves, while the static parts are filtered out. By placing the ultrasound transducer on the chest, this technique is able to provide an echocardiogram showing heart walls, chambers, valves, and blood flow. From these images, the doctor can obtain measurements related to the heart's structure and function. Apart from the echocardiogram, ultrasounds can also be employed to diagnose important vascular information, such as carotid artery stenosis.

- *Sound*: The phonocardiogram (PCG) is the result of the sound wave generated by the mechanical movement of the heart. This involves mainly the contraction and relaxation of the heart (systole and diastole, respectively), but also the sound produced by the blood flow through the heart chambers and the opening and closing of the heart valves. The acoustic signal is captured by placing an acoustic chamber on the patient's chest.
- *X-rays*: X-rays are electromagnetic radiation with wavelengths ranging from 10 pm to 10 nm. The use of this principle in cardiovascular applications involves computed tomography (CT) scan and fluoroscopy. For instance, cardiac CT makes use of computer-based reconstruction from a number of X-ray measurements from different angles to obtain cross-sectional images of the thorax. These images are then combined and segmented to create a three-dimensional model of the whole heart. New-generation CT scanners provide improved images with lower radiation exposure. X-rays can also be employed in angiography studies. This is an imaging test to visualize the lumen of blood vessels and can be obtained from CT or fluoroscopy.
- *Magnetic resonance (MR)*: Cardiac MR imaging is able to obtain pictures of the heart from the interaction of the body with a magnetic field. A number of different MR sequences and techniques are defined to retrieve specific information about the structure, tissue characterization, and ventricular function, among others.
- *Blood pressure*: Blood pressure (BP) gives the physician information about the patient's hemodynamic condition. This signal is the result of the mechanical pumping of the heart and the fluid dynamics of the complex arterial system. The cardiovascular system as a whole smoothes the pulsatile source of the heart into a more continuous blood flow.
- *Optics*: By means of a light-emitting diode (LED) and a photodetector, it is possible to measure changes in light absorption that are associated

with changes in blood flow. This technique can also measure the peripheral oxygen saturation (SpO_2).

Moreover, some tests are intended to lead the patient to a certain physical condition in order to bring up the cardiac anomalies (if any) and make them more visible and evident:

- *Stress test*: The patient is asked to do some exercise while the cardiac activity is being monitored, for example, by means of an ECG. The aim of this test is to raise the cardiac frequency and check how the heart responds under these conditions.
- *Tilt table test*: The patient is initially lying on a table. After a resting period, the table is tilted upright, while the ECG and BP are continuously monitored. This test is intended to check how the body reacts to the action of gravity upon standing up, which makes more difficult blood flow to the brain. This is a useful diagnostic tool for patients with syncope of unknown origin.
- *Six minute walk test*: The patient is asked to walk, as fast as possible, for a period of 6 minutes. This test is used to evaluate the cardiopulmonary response to exercise.
- *Drug administration*: Some heart diseases, such as Brugada syndrome, can be unmasked by the administration of drugs.

These techniques are obviously done in a clinical environment. However, if the patient is unaware of any abnormality that he or she may be suffering, the visit to the doctor may never occur. Some cardiovascular pathologies can have sudden and dramatic consequences. The important question here is what the technology can increase the probability of early detection. With the development of wearables, the so-called Internet of things, and artificial intelligence, some of these sensors (e.g., the ECG) can be embedded in personal smart devices that are able to monitor a person's cardiovascular condition on a daily basis (Dias & Cunha, 2018). This is important not only for the first diagnosis. The above-mentioned techniques can also be used for full and complete assessment of the patient's conditions after the diagnosis, and wearable devices and p-health solutions may help in detecting any changes with respect to the assessed baseline and thus in the early identification of a worsening situation. When this strategy becomes used on a wide scale, enormous benefits will be brought to society. This chapter explores which of these signals and features are able to be included in personal devices, the information that can be extracted from them, and in which the situations in which an alert should occur.

2.2 The electrocardiogram

The ECG is the most frequently used clinical system in cardiology for several reasons. First, it is very easy and quick to obtain an ECG from a patient, since it is a noninvasive technique; that is, it is not necessary to explore inside the body as occurs with other invasive techniques such as catheters. Second, it provides as much as 90% of the information about the electrical activity of the heart. Indeed, most cardiac arrhythmias and other heart diseases can be diagnosed after observation and interpretation of the ECG. In this section we describe how the electric activity of the heart can be measured and explained from the signals recorded by a set of sensors located at the human body surface.

2.2.1 The electrical nature of cardiac activation

From the bioelectromagnetism theory it is well known that any mechanical activity of a muscle cell is preceded by an electric excitation. This is mainly caused by the exchange of diverse ions through the membrane, from inside the cell toward the extracellular liquid and vice versa. If we were able to measure the intracellular potential with a voltmeter, the cathode measuring the potential inside the cell and the anode measuring outside, it could be observed that during a nonactivity period the membrane voltage would remain constant around -85 mV. In this state, it is said that the cell is polarized; that is, the cell is at its resting potential. When a cardiac cell is electrically stimulated, that is, the membrane potential exceeds the threshold potential, an action potential is triggered. This is a result of a sequence of inward and outward ionic currents that occur in cascade flows (mainly involving Na^+, Ca^{++}, and K^+), which result in the typical action potential curve shown in Fig. 2.1. At the end of the process, the voltage returns to its original value (repolarization).

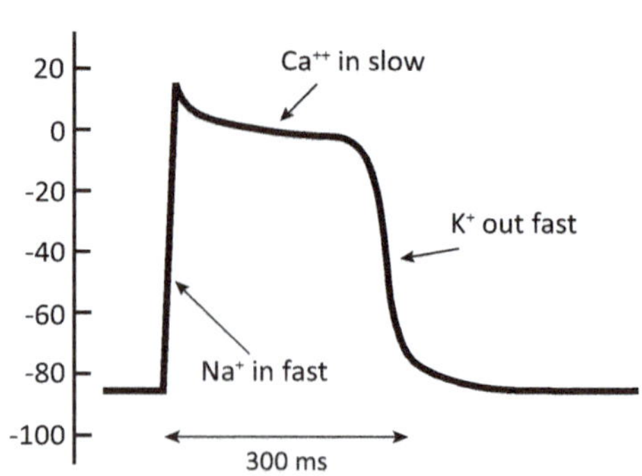

Figure 2.1 Typical action potential of ventricular myocytes.

The cardiac cycle starts at the natural pacemaker, the sinus node, which consist of specialized self-activating cells located in the superior right atrium. Then their surrounding myocytes are activated. As the activation of a myocyte is triggered, it triggers its neighbor myocytes as well, owing to an elaborate system of intercellular junctions. As a result, the electrical activation is propagated along the right atrium. The electrical activation rapidly arrives at the left atrium because of a highway that interconnects the two atria (called the Bachmann bundle or the interatrial tract). The atria and the ventricles are connected through the atrioventricular node, which captures the activation at the atria. The propagation through the atrioventricular junction is very slow, which introduces a delay in the progress of activation; this is a desirable pause that allows completion of ventricular filling. The electrical activation of the ventricles is achieved through the Hiss bundle and the terminations of the Purkinje fibers. According to the action potential curve, after the refractory period has passed, the myocytes are repolarized again to be ready for the next beat.

The heart as a whole, as seen externally, acts as a syncytium, with a vast number of myocytes being activated in a coordinated manner. As a consequence, the joint effect of the action potentials of the myocytes can be summarized by a resultant electrical dipole, whose direction and amplitude changes along the cardiac cycle (Fig. 2.2). The basis of electrocardiography is placing two electrodes at different sites of the body surface to capture the potential difference between them and interpreting the signal by associating the expected waveform described by the dipole model with cardiac electrophysiology.

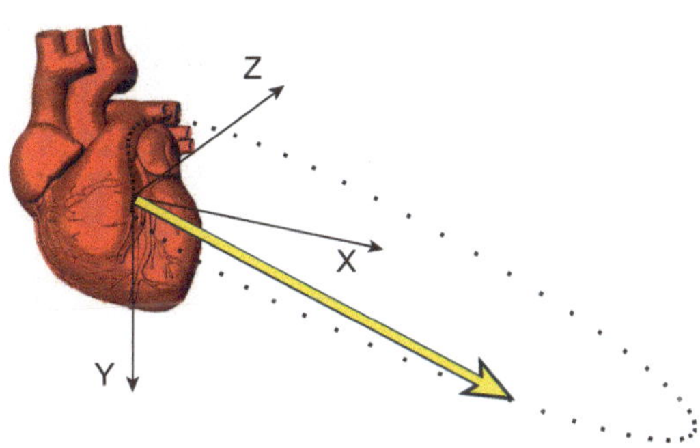

Figure 2.2 The dipole model represents the electrical activation of the heart working as a syncytium.

Owing to the vectorial nature of the dipole, changing the placement of the electrodes will change the morphology of the signal. Einthoven determined the first clinically important ECG system by locating three electrodes at the right arm, left arm, and left foot, defining the Einthoven standard leads in the following way (Einthoven, 1906):

$$\begin{aligned} \text{Lead } I\text{: } V_{\mathrm{I}} &= \phi_{\mathrm{L}} - \phi_{\mathrm{R}} \\ \text{Lead II: } V_{\mathrm{II}} &= \phi_{\mathrm{F}} - \phi_{\mathrm{R}} \\ \text{Lead III: } V_{\mathrm{III}} &= \phi_{\mathrm{F}} - \phi_{\mathrm{L}} \end{aligned} \tag{2.1}$$

where

V_{I} = voltage of lead I
V_{II} = voltage of lead II
V_{III} = voltage of lead III
ϕ_{L} = potential at the left arm
ϕ_{R} = potential at the right arm
ϕ_{F} = potential at the left foot

According to Kirchhoff's second law, the voltages of the Einthoven limb leads have the following relationship:

$$V_{\mathrm{II}} = V_{\mathrm{I}} + V_{\mathrm{III}} \tag{2.2}$$

Three additional limb leads were obtained by Goldberger by measuring the potential between a single limb electrode and the midpotential of the two remaining electrodes, chosen as reference. These additional leads are called augmented leads because of the augmentation of the signal. The central point of the two electrodes is achieved by means of connecting two resistances of 5 kΩ. Notice that the Goldberger augmented leads are fully redundant with respect to the Einthoven leads I, II, and III, with the following relationship:

$$\begin{aligned} aV_{\mathrm{R}} &= \phi_{\mathrm{R}} - \frac{\phi_{\mathrm{L}} + \phi_{\mathrm{F}}}{2} = -V_{I} + \frac{V_{\mathrm{III}}}{2} \\ \mathrm{aV_L} &= \phi_{L} - \frac{\phi_{R} + \phi_{F}}{2} = -\mathrm{V_I} + \frac{\mathrm{V_{II}}}{2} \\ aV_{\mathrm{F}} &= \phi_{\mathrm{F}} - \frac{\phi_{\mathrm{R}} + \phi_{\mathrm{L}}}{2} = -V_{\mathrm{III}} + \frac{V_{\mathrm{I}}}{2} \end{aligned} \tag{2.3}$$

The scheme of the limb leads of the ECG is shown on the right in Fig. 2.3.

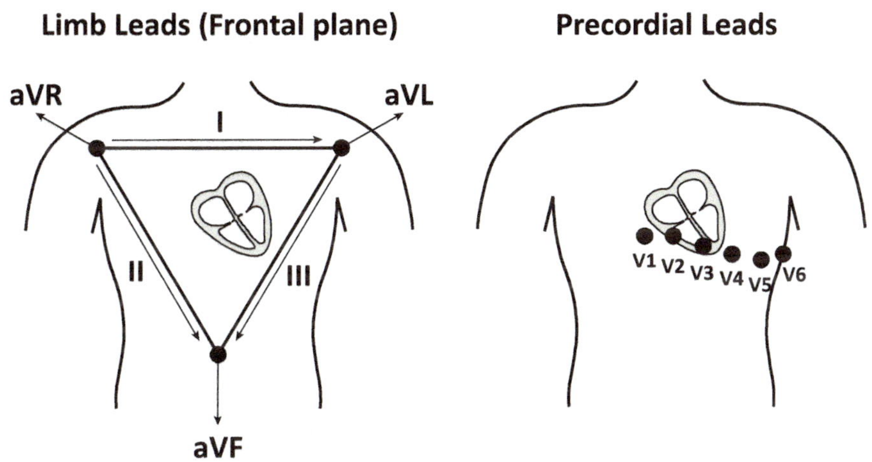

Figure 2.3 Scheme of the limb leads (*left*) and precordial leads (*right*).

In 1944 Wilson introduced the precordial leads to measure the potential close to the heart. These leads, V1—V6, are located over the left chest (Fig. 2.3). In contrast to the bipolar limb leads, precordial leads are unipolar. Therefore a reference electrode with zero potential is needed. Wilson ingeniously proposed a practical solution consisting of the average potential of the three limbs by connecting them to a central point through a resistor network (Wilson, Johnston, Macleod, & Barker, 1934). This reference is now known as Wilson's central terminal.

The 12-lead standard ECG is the one with the greatest clinical use and consists of the 12 leads that have been explained above:

I, II, III

aVR, aVL, aVF

V1, V2, V3, V4, V5, V6

The first six leads are derived from just three electrodes. Therefore any two of them contain the same information as the other four. Overall, the 12-lead ECG contain eight independent leads. Nevertheless, all 12 leads are usually visualized by the clinician, as this provides a simultaneous representation with different projections of the resultant dipole.

2.2.2 The ECG signal

From electrocardiographic theory it is possible to examine the generation of the ECG by taking into account the progression of activation within a cardiac cycle. As was mentioned earlier, after the electric activation of the heart has begun at the sinus node, it spreads along the atrial walls. The resultant vector of the atrial electric activity is reflected on the P wave of the ECG. This is followed by a short isoelectric line with no electrical activity, which corresponds to the delay within the atrioventricular junction. Subsequently, there is a sharp pulse with a much higher amplitude than the P wave, known as the QRS complex, which is associated to the depolarization of the ventricles. The fiducial points Q, R, and S are defined as consecutive negative–positive–negative peaks of the pulse. Depending on the leads, we may observe different patterns of the QRS complex. Subsequently, a short silent segment can be observed, which is associated to the plateau of the action potential. The cardiac cycle ends with the ventricular repolarization phase. In the ECG this is reflected in the T wave, which is smoother and with lower amplitude than the QRS complex. (The deflections of the ECG signal are denoted in alphabetical order, starting with P and followed by Q, R, S, and T.) The reason for this is the smoother slope of the AP at the repolarization phase with respect to the sharp response at the beginning of the activation. Notice that the repolarization of the atria is not visible, as it is masked by the QRS complex. A new cardiac cycle will start with the self-activation of the sinus node. A normal ECG is shown in Fig. 2.4, which also includes definitions for various segments and intervals in the ECG. For example, the RR interval is the common measure of the time between consecutive beats and is employed to compute the heart rate.

The ECG exhibits a high redundancy degree in the morphology of successive beats (Castells, Laguna, Sörnmo, Bollmann, & Millet, 2007). Fig. 2.5 illustrates how a sequence of beats can be mostly explained with a single component after principal component analysis. This property can be exploited for different purposes, which could be of interest in

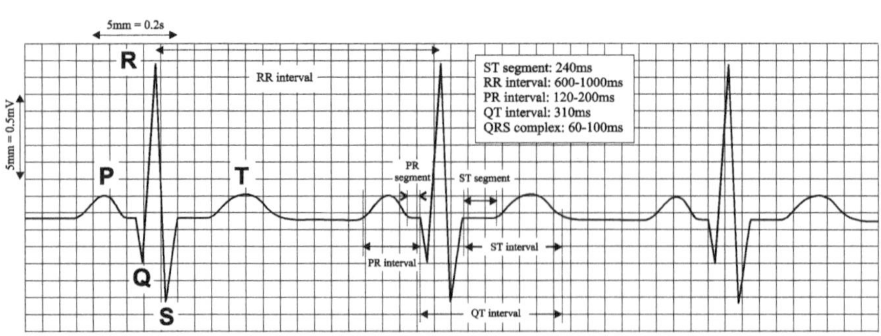

Figure 2.4 A normal electrocardiogram.

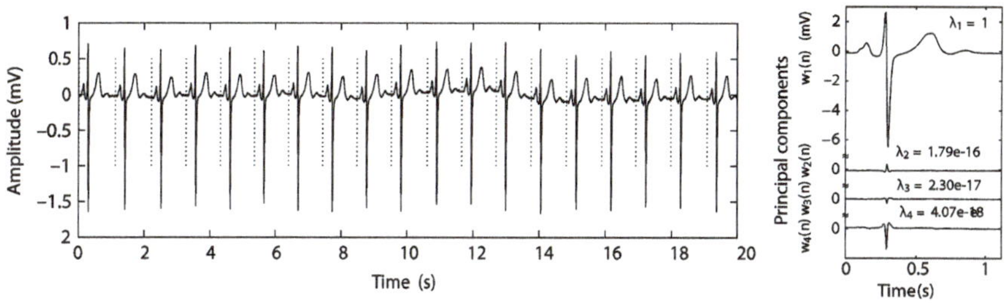

Figure 2.5 Illustration of how the morphology of the beat can be explained with a single component after principle component analysis decomposition. *Adapted from Castells, F., Laguna, P., Sörnmo, L., Bollmann, A., & Millet, J. (2007). Principal component analysis in ECG signal processing.* EURASIP Journal on Applied Signal Processing, *5(1), 49–58.*

wearables. One of them is noise reduction, which can be notably improved by averaging several beats (Turitto, Benson, Wong, & El-Sherif, 2013). Moreover, removing redundancy allows for lossless data compression, which could be of high interest in wearables for data storage and telemetry (Li, Pan, Chen, Cheng, & Huan, 2014).

2.2.3 The ECG in p-health devices

Several differences arise in comparing the ECG setup in a clinical environment respect to the ECG recording with a smart p-health device. In a clinical scenario the patient lies on a table in a resting position. There are few restrictions about space, power requirements, number of leads, or data storage, and the ECG acquisition system (including electronic instrumentation and disposable electrodes) must be compliant with the corresponding standards and approved by the administration. The case with personal devices is completely different, as will be described.

For the acquisition of the ECG, two separated locations of the body surface should be in contact with a couple of electrodes, placed directly on the skin. Here we can find the first differences between clinical practice and p-health devices. In the former, disposable Ag/AgCl electrodes covered with electrolyte gel are usually employed, following ANSI/AAMI EC12:2000/(R)2015 standard. However, reusable dry electrodes (Meziane, Webster, Attari, & Nimunkar, 2013) are more likely to be used in a p-health device, such as stiff metal plate electrodes, other flexible materials, or fabric electrodes to be integrated into smart textiles (Chi, Jung, & Cauwenberghs, 2010; Park & Jayaraman, 2010). In this context, new electrode materials are constantly being researched to develop wireless wearable sensors with improved comfort and signal quality (Pani, Achilli, & Bonfiglio, 2018).

To make electrode attachment easier and less costly, the ECG signal is usually captured from just two electrodes, which allow recording a single lead. For example, the ECG can be obtained from the potential difference between the fingers of the two hands (in this case, lead I would be obtained). These features are already integrated in some smart watches such as the Apple Watch Series 4 (Fig. 2.6). Other third-party companies such as AliveCor have also developed accessories for smart watches and smartphones. Other devices may record the potential difference between two sites on the chest flanking the heart, for example, by means of a chest band, such as the wearable vest developed by Nuubo (Fig. 2.7). Bansal and Joshi reviewed current technologies for out-of-hospital electrocardiography (Bansal & Joshi, 2018).

Although recording the ECG from two leads has the advantage of safety, as the ground electrode is no longer used, the system will be more sensitive to electromagnetic interference. Moreover, baseline fluctuations due to muscular activity are expected to be higher in wearables, especially if the subject is moving (Alkhidir, Sluzek, & Yapici, 2015). Under these circumstances a significant portion of these interferences and artifacts could be part of the differential signal, which could not be rejected even with an instrumentation amplifier; instrumentation amplifiers are the core of most ECG amplifiers, as they provide high input impedance, differential amplification and common-mode rejection ratio over 80 dB. Actually, the main problem with high-amplitude interference is to reach amplifier saturation (see Fig. 2.8), and additional electronics may be required to avoid it (Hwang & Webster, 2008).

The amplified signal is then digitized according to a sampling frequency and bit depth. The temporal resolution depends on the sampling rate, which should fulfill the Nyquist theorem, that is, being at least twice

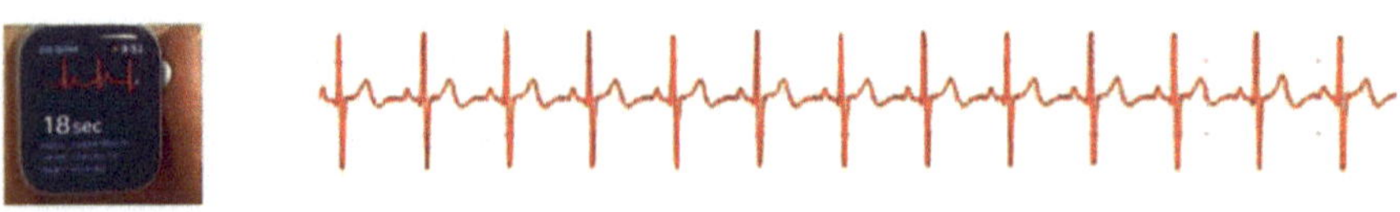

Figure 2.6 The Apple Watch Series 4 can record the electrocardiogram by touching the Digital Crown with a finger of the opposite hand. *Adapted from Isakadze, N., & Martin, S. S. (2019). How useful is the smartwatch ECG?* Trends in Cardiovascular Medicine, 30*(7), 442–448.*

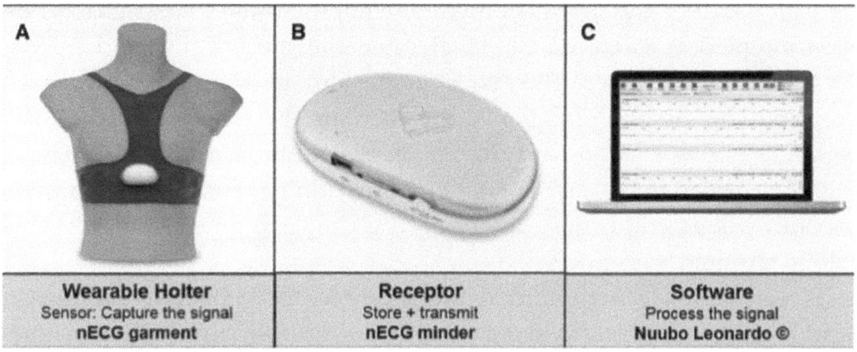

Figure 2.7 Nuubo wearable electrocardiogram, which consists of a vest with a sensor (A), a receptor that stores and transmits the signals (B) and a software that process the signals (C). *Adapted from Campal, J. M. R., Torres, M. A. G., Borque, P. S., Vinagre, I. N., Capdepón, I. Z., Blanco, A. M., . . . Fernández, J. M. S. (2020). Detecting atrial fibrillation in patients with an embolic stroke of undetermined source (from the daf-esus registry).* The American Journal of Cardiology, 125*(3), 409–414.*

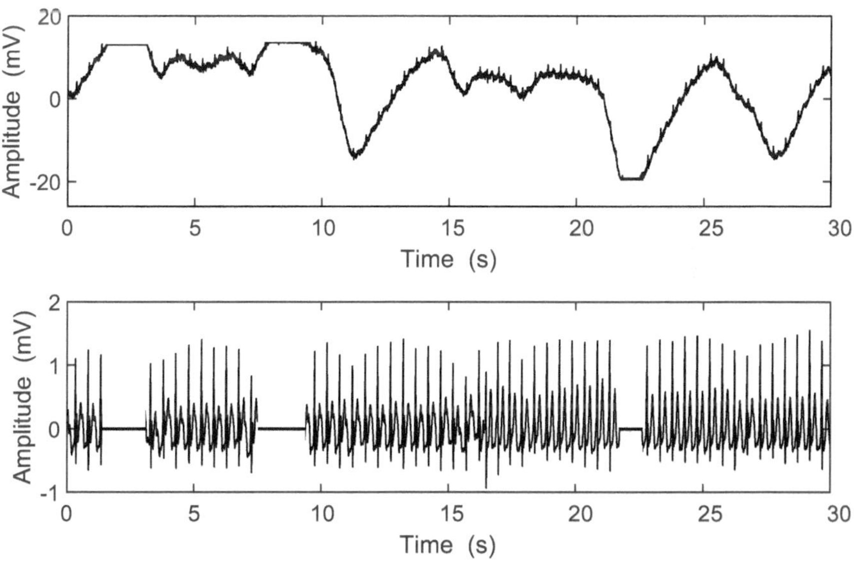

Figure 2.8 Electrocardiogram (ECG) acquisition may be contaminated by muscular electrical activity due to movement or electromagnetic interference (*top*). An extended amplitude range is required to prevent clipping, as the ECG signal cannot be retrieved if saturation occurs (*bottom*).

the bandwidth of the signal. In medical equipment the ECG signal is very often sampled at a rate of 1 kHz. Because the spectral power density of the ECG signal above 100 Hz is negligible, it is unnecessarily oversampled. The sampling frequency can therefore be reduced to 250 Hz or even 125 Hz with almost no impact on diagnostic features. This has the following benefits: Because energy consumption depends on the sampling rate, this will extend battery autonomy. At the same time, less data storage will be required.

Regarding quantization, there are some technical concerns about ECG recording in wearables to consider, especially those regarding amplitude range, bit depth, and signal resolution:

- *Amplitude range*: The typical amplitude of QRS peaks is a few mV (e.g., 0.5–2 mV). However, if artifacts due to movement and electromagnetic interference are not filtered out before the analog-to-digital conversion, an extended amplitude range is required to prevent clipping.
- *Signal resolution*: Despite the high amplitude of QRS complexes, important diagnostic information may be lost with poor amplitude resolution. Consider the lower amplitude of P and T waves as illustrated in Fig. 2.9.
- *Bit depth*: The bit depth (e.g., 8, 12, or 16 bits) at which the analog signal is quantified and digitized determines the dynamic range. A higher number of bits provides better performance at the expense of higher electronic complexity.

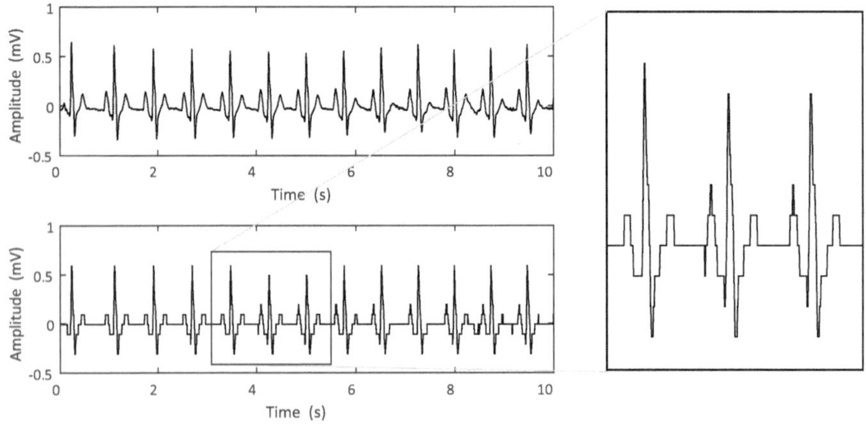

Figure 2.9 Degradation of the electrocardiogram with poor amplitude resolution.

There is an obvious tradeoff between these three items, as it is not possible to achieve a high-amplitude range and fine resolution with a low number of bits. Higher amplitude ranges can be achieved at the expense of either poorer resolution or increasing the bit depth. For instance, let us consider the quantification of a signal with 8 bits and an amplitude resolution of 10 μV. This stands for an amplitude range of ± 1.28 mV, which is insufficient to capture the raw ECG. Just by extending the bit depth to 12 bits, the amplitude range can be increased to ± 20.5 mV, which could be acceptable.

The digital ECG can be finally processed and analyzed in the device itself, or it can be sent to an external unit (e.g., PC, smartphone, server). As the ECG signal may be heavily corrupted by motion artifacts, it would be a smart decision to process it with a noise reduction algorithm (Sehamby & Singh, 2016; Thakor & Zhu, 1991). Indeed, the noise could still persist afterwards. Accordingly, a real-time assessment of the signal quality (Satija, Ramkumar, & Manikandan, 2017) may be required to discard noisy signals in order to avoid a wrong diagnosis.

In addition to all these requirements, p-health devices may include other sensors, such as accelerometers and global positioning system (GPS), as well as connectivity features for data transfer and software updates. Overall, the recording of ECG in p-health devices is challenging, as users demand high signal quality in a tiny, light, and inexpensive product. Furthermore, the system is expected to be efficient in terms of battery consumption and data storage, particularly those intended for long-term monitoring.

An overview of the system is illustrated in Fig. 2.10. The data signal obtained from a couple of electrodes is amplified and digitized. From this point there are several options: (1) The signal can be analyzed by the device itself (stand-alone monitoring), (2) data can be stored for offline analysis, or (3) data can be transferred for remote monitoring.

2.2.4 Potential of p-health devices

Personal devices can never replace the diagnostic skills of a cardiologist. However, an expert clinician cannot supervise a patient's cardiovascular condition on a daily basis. Personal devices can do that and can show or send an alert if something worsens. Besides the devices shown in the Section 2.2.3, innovative smart products can be developed to monitor the ECG. Imagine, for instance, placing two electrodes on the arms of a smart

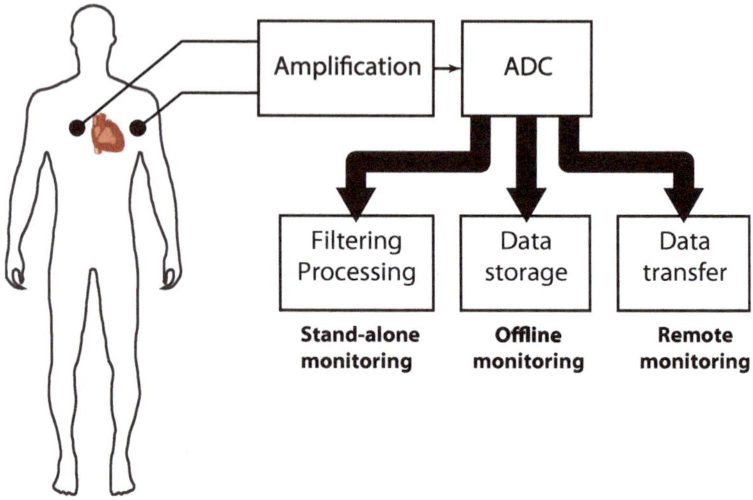

Figure 2.10 Overview of different strategies for electrocardiogram monitoring with a p-health device: stand-alone, offline, or remote monitoring.

armchair, on the steering wheel of a car at the place where the driver holds it, into any other object that can be handled with both hands, or incorporated into a smart T-shirt that is worn during sports training sessions. Personal devices will be definitely be a breakthrough, as they could monitor cardiac activity without the user having to do anything on purpose—or even having to be aware of it.

2.2.4.1 Early detection of atrial fibrillation

Early detection of atrial fibrillation (AF) is one of the most promising applications of ECG monitoring in p-health devices (Bumgarner et al., 2018). Atrial fibrillation is the most common cardiac arrhythmia, being especially prevalent in older adults (Chugh et al., 2013; Go et al., 2001; Schnabel et al., 2015). During the first stage, known as paroxysmal AF, onset and termination occur spontaneously. In many patients, AF episodes become progressively more frequent, and it can evolve into persistent AF (Vos et al., 2010). AF is characterized by an uncoordinated electrical activation of the atria, which prevents them from carrying out an effective contraction and pumping function. As a consequence, the stagnant blood within the atria can lead to dangerous clot formation. Undiagnosed AF is a major cause of stroke (Friberg, Hammar, & Rosenqvist, 2009; Petersen & Godtfredsen, 1986), so anticoagulation therapies are the first steps in AF management (Wann, Calkins, Chen, & Cigarroa, 2019).

AF can be diagnosed from the analysis of the ECG (Ros, Mota, Fernández, Toro, & Bernier, 2005). Owing to the irregular activation of the atria, no P waves are observable in the ECG signal; they are replaced by a continuous and chaotic wave. The absence of a periodic atrial pace results in an irregular ventricular rate, with RR intervals that change from beat to beat. The mean heart rate becomes significantly higher than in normal conditions even if no exercise is being performed. Fig. 2.11 shows an example of an AF ECG signal.

Although the atrial wave can be estimated by means of QRST cancellation (Castells, Mora, Rieta, & Millet, 2005), the irregularity of the RR interval is probably the most useful information to be exploited for AF diagnosis in wearables, for the following reasons:

- The potential difference between both hands or both wrists allows us to record lead I. With this ECG projection the atrial fibrillatory wave is scarcely visible, in contrast with other precordial leads such as V1 or V2, which capture higher voltage from the atrial electrical activity.
- The poor signal-to-noise ratio makes it difficult to detect the absence of P waves robustly.

Nevertheless, AF is not a unique arrhythmia with an irregular ventricular pace. Therefore different features can be exploited to improve performance in terms of sensitivity and specificity (Hagiwara et al., 2018). In 2017 the PhysioNet platform launched its annual Challenge for AF classification from short single leads recorded with personal devices (Clifford et al., 2017). Over 12,000 ECGs donated by AliveCor were used for the challenge. According to competition rules, winners achieved a score of 0.83. A more recent study compared the automated AF detection from single-lead ECGs obtained with Kardia Mobile Cardiac Monitor with physician-interpreted simultaneous 12-lead ECG recordings (William

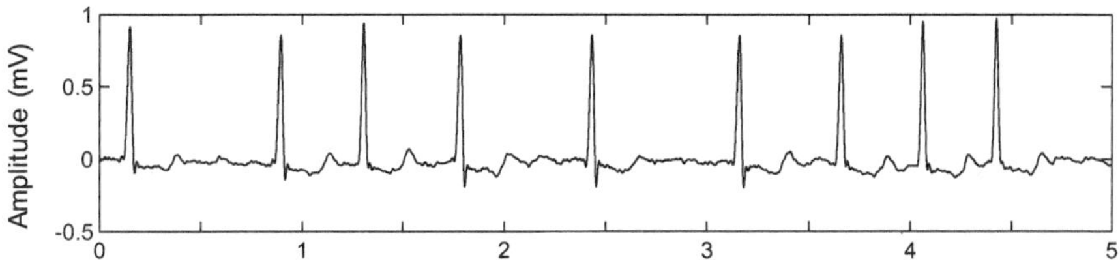

Figure 2.11 Example of an atrial fibrillation signal. Notice the irregularity of the RR intervals and the absence of P waves. The continuous atrial fibrillatory wave is especially noticeable in TQ intervals.

et al., 2018). Despite the excellent attainment in terms of specificity and sensitivity, the study concluded that direct physician review can enhance AF diagnosis. Rather than being a robust and sophisticated diagnostic tool, what personal devices might bring is an alert or recommendation for a visit to the doctor.

2.2.4.2 ECG monitoring during exercise

Some inherited cardiomyopathies, such as hypertrophic cardiomyopathy or arrhythmogenic cardiomyopathy, are major causes of sudden cardiac death during sports practice (Burke, Farb, Virmani, Goodin, & Smialek, 1991; Zorzi, Pelliccia, & Corrado, 2018). Unfortunately, they remain very often undiagnosed, as they are asymptomatic in many cases. Consequently, it would be very dangerous if someone who, for example, is unaware of suffering from hypertrophic cardiomyopathy, decided to participate in competitive sports. As illustration of how exercise may induce increasing frequency of ventricular arrhythmias is shown in Fig. 2.12, in this case in a patient with catecholaminergic polymorphic ventricular tachycardia.

Moreover, there are some more evidences of sport-related risk of sudden cardiac death. In fact, despite athletes enjoy excellent health outcomes of training, an increase of ventricular arrhythmias is associated to endurance athletic conditioning (Maron & Pelliccia, 2006). As the aspiration of participating in sports competitions is massively increasing in population, including ultra-long-distance races, the probabilities of serious ventricular arrhythmias and cardiac arrest events.

Monitor ECG devices may play an important role in sport sessions to alert the subject in case of increasing frequency of ventricular arrhythmias, as they are superior to simpler heart rate monitor devices (Gajda, Biernacka, & Drygas, 2017). Furthermore, they could be a valuable aid to suggest decreasing activity intensity or even the end of the session if necessary to prevent the initiation of a malignant arrhythmia.

2.2.4.3 Remote alerting of life-threatening conditions

A breakthrough in ECG monitoring would be the possibility of detecting life-threatening conditions, including the possibility of sending alerts to a remote emergency center. Ventricular fibrillation (VF) and pulseless ventricular tachycardia (VT) are life-threatening arrhythmias that can lead to sudden death (Liberthson et al., 1974), as they are associated with no effective cardiac output. Therapy to prevent a fatal end involves electrical

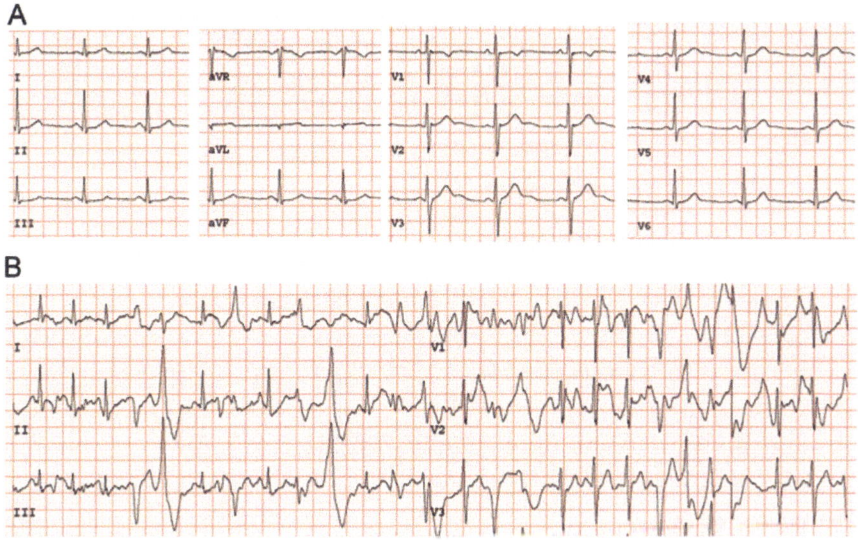

Figure 2.12 Exercise stress testing of catecholaminergic polymorphic ventricular tachycardia (CPVT). (A) A baseline electrocardiogram (ECG) and (B) an ECG during exercise stress testing in a patient with CPVT are shown. The ECG during exercise testing shows ventricular extrasystoles and nonsustained ventricular tachycardia. *Reproduced from Mizusawa Y. (2016). Recent advances in genetic testing and counseling for inherited arrhythmias.* Journal of Arrhythmia, 32, *389–397.*

shock with an automated external defibrillation (AED), in combination with cardiopulmonary resuscitation (Cobb et al., 1999). Time to defibrillation is crucial for patient outcome, as longer periods from arrhythmia onset until blood circulation can be restored are associated with lower survival rates (Delayed time to defibrillation after in-hospital cardiac arrest, 2008). The idea of detecting these malignant arrhythmias in wearables has recently been proposed (Manikandan & Prabhakararao, 2016), although commercial devices may not have been developed yet.

Because VF and VT are pulseless rhythms, detection cannot rely on a beat-to-beat assessment. On the other hand, the ECG signal of VF and VT episodes have distinctive spectral properties with respect to other cardiac rhythms, as shown in Fig. 2.13. Indeed, beyond detection of malignant arrhythmias, spectral-based analysis has been also proposed as a predictor of mortality and cerebral outcome in patients undergoing hypothermia therapy (Filgueiras-Rama et al., 2015). Algorithms for detection of shockable rhythms are implemented in AEDs (Clifford, 1996) for robust decision making about shock delivery. Wearable cardioverter

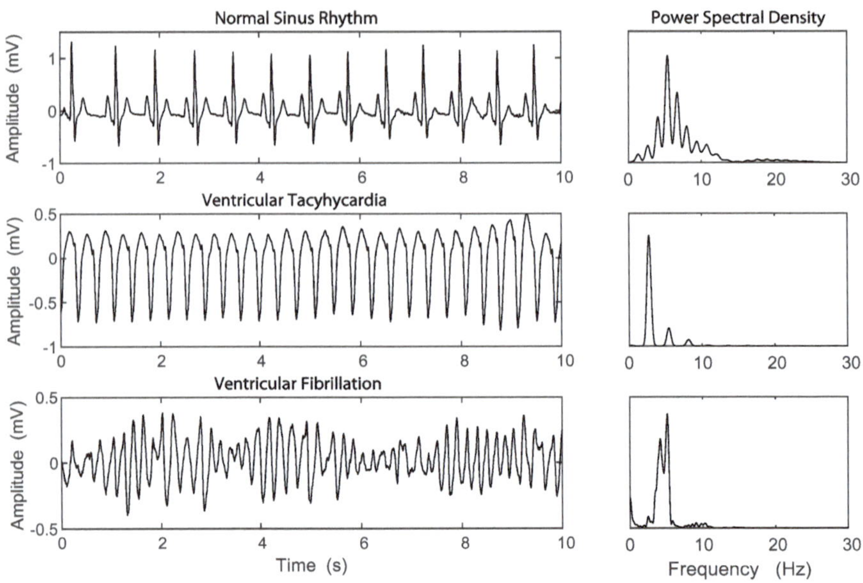

Figure 2.13 Example of life-threatening arrhythmias: ventricular tachycardia (*center*) and ventricular fibrillation (*bottom*). Their spectral content, shown in the right panel, are compared with normal sinus rhythm (*top*).

defibrillators (WCDs) have also shown their potential to protect patients during a period of risk stratification (Kutyifa et al., 2015).

In a manner similar to the way in which AEDs and WCDs are able to detect life-threatening arrhythmias, p-health wearables could also do it and send an alarm to an emergency center indicating the need for immediate rescue, including in the message the automatic diagnosis, an excerpt of the ECG signal, and the user's GPS location.

ST-elevation myocardial infarction (STEMI) is another life-threatening condition, caused by coronary artery occlusion (O'Gara et al., 2013). On the ECG, STEMI is characterized by persistent ST segment elevation, mainly in the precordial leads. A recent pilot study evaluated the performance of STEMI detection with a smartphone-based ECG with promising results (Muhlestein et al., 2014).

2.3 RR series

Timing of cardiac beats can be detected from ECG analysis as well from alternative techniques, such as photoplethysmography (PPG). This allows for long-term tracking of the cardiac rhythm. Fig. 2.14 shows an example

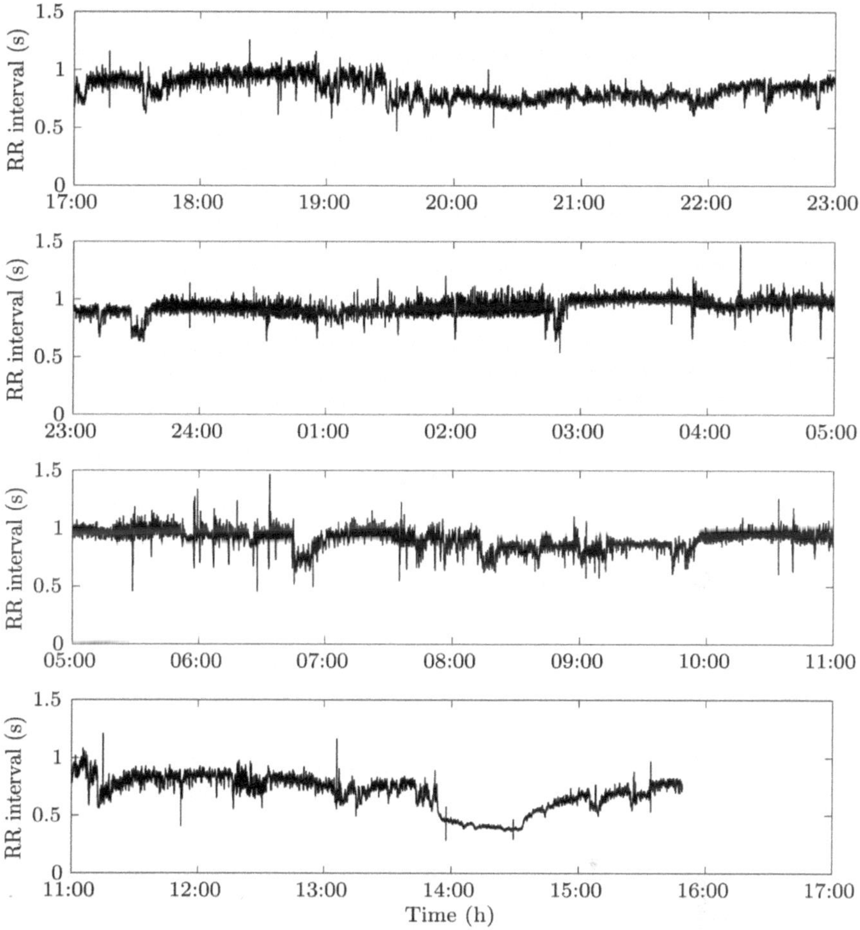

Figure 2.14 Example of an RR series recorded extracted from a 24-h recording. *Reproduced from Sörnmo, L., & Laguna, P. (2005).* ECG signal processing: Heart rate variability. *Elsevier Academic Press.*

of an RR series during a 1-day recording. As can be observed, the heart rhythm is not constant but exhibits variations and fluctuations. For example, the RR interval is higher (i.e., the heart rate is slower) during sleeping, and it can be lower (i.e., a more rapid heart rhythm) during exercise. If the cardiac activity is tracked over several days, circadian rhythms can be observed and analyzed (Watanabe et al., 2007). In addition to long-term changes in the heart rate (HR), short-term variations of the RR interval can be observed on a beat-to-beat basis. Moreover, specific tests such as the table tilt test or the orthostatic test can be used to emphasize abnormal features related to HR response. Fig. 2.15 shows the continuous HR monitoring of a patient with asymptomatic orthostatic intolerance during a 6-minute walk test.

2.3.1 Heart rate variability

The HR is determined by the activation of the sinus node, which in turn is regulated by the sympathetic (activation) and parasympathetic (rest) branches of the autonomous nervous system (ANS) (Task Force of the European Society of Cardiology the North American Society of Pacing Electrophysiology, 1996). Parasympathetic regulation (also known as vagal regulation) lowers the HR below the intrinsic HR (considered to be about 100 beats per minute, although it is subject dependent) and has a short-term effect, returning quickly to the intrinsic rate if it is no longer

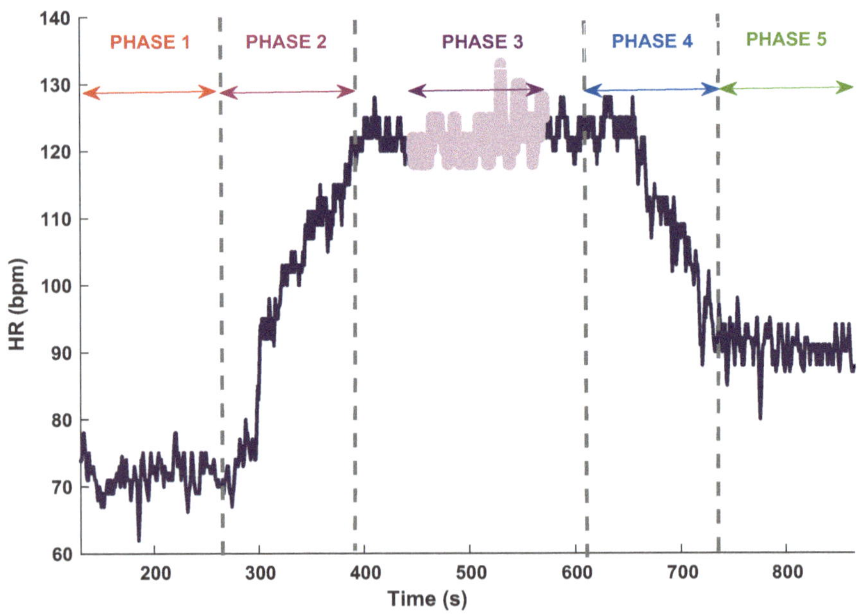

Figure 2.15 Continuous heart rate (HR) monitoring during the 6-min walk test corresponding to a patient with asymptomatic orthostatic intolerance. Phase 1: basal conditions; phase 2: the patient starts walking (HR increases); phase 3: HR gets stable at an intense rate; phase 4: the patient stops walking (HR starts decreasing after some seconds); phase 5: HR becomes stable (though still higher than in basal conditions). *Reproduced from Hortelano, M., Reilly, R., Castells, F., & Cervigón, R. (2018). Refined multiscale fuzzy entropy to analyse post-exercise cardiovascular response in older adults with orthostatic intolerance.* Entropy, 20*(11), 860.*

present. Therefore when the parasympathetic activity dominates, the HR is lower (longer RR intervals) and more variable (see in Fig. 2.14 the period between 2 and 3 hours). On the other hand, sympathetic regulation increases the HR above the intrinsic HR. The effect of parasympathetic activation is longer, affecting a larger number of consecutive beats. Accordingly, when the sympathetic activity dominates, the HR is higher (shorter RR intervals) and more constant (see in Fig. 2.14 the period between 14 and 15 hours). In this context, HR variability has been defined as an important biomarker to assess the condition of the ANS (Task Force of the European Society of Cardiology the North American Society of Pacing Electrophysiology, 1996). This can be also an indicator of well-being, as regular exercise strengthens the heart muscle and so lowers the HR while increasing the HR variability.

RR series may be corrupted by artifacts, due to false R detections, which should be corrected (Clifford, Mcsharry, & Tarassenko, 2002). Moreover, there may be several ectopic beat occurrences in long-term monitoring. These should be also corrected, as they are not related to sinus node activation (Sörnmo & Laguna, 2005). Fig. 2.16 shows a 10-minute monitorization of an ECG with a couple of ectopic beats. When an ectopic beat occurs, an RR is shortened with respect to the regular RR. This is then followed by a longer RR interval. This phenomenon is usually referred as a compensatory pause. As can be appreciated, the sum of both RR intervals approximately doubles the duration of the regular RR interval.

The RR series of this ECG is displayed in the top part of Fig. 2.17. Actually, the best way to deal with ectopic beats is to take them out and interpolate RR values from previous and posterior beats. The center part of Fig. 2.17 shows the RR series after ectopic beat correction. If desired,

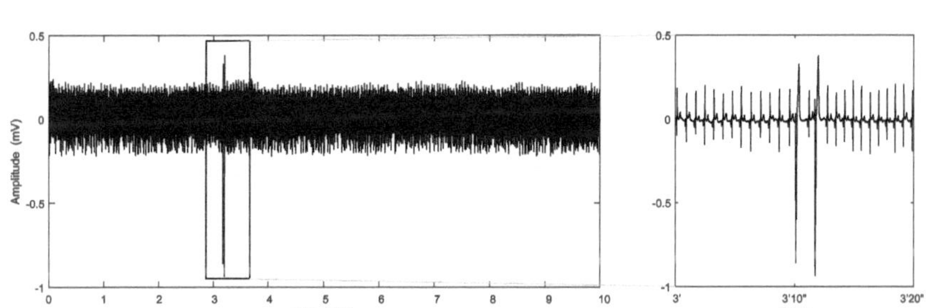

Figure 2.16 Example of a 10-minute electrocardiogram recording with ectopic beats.

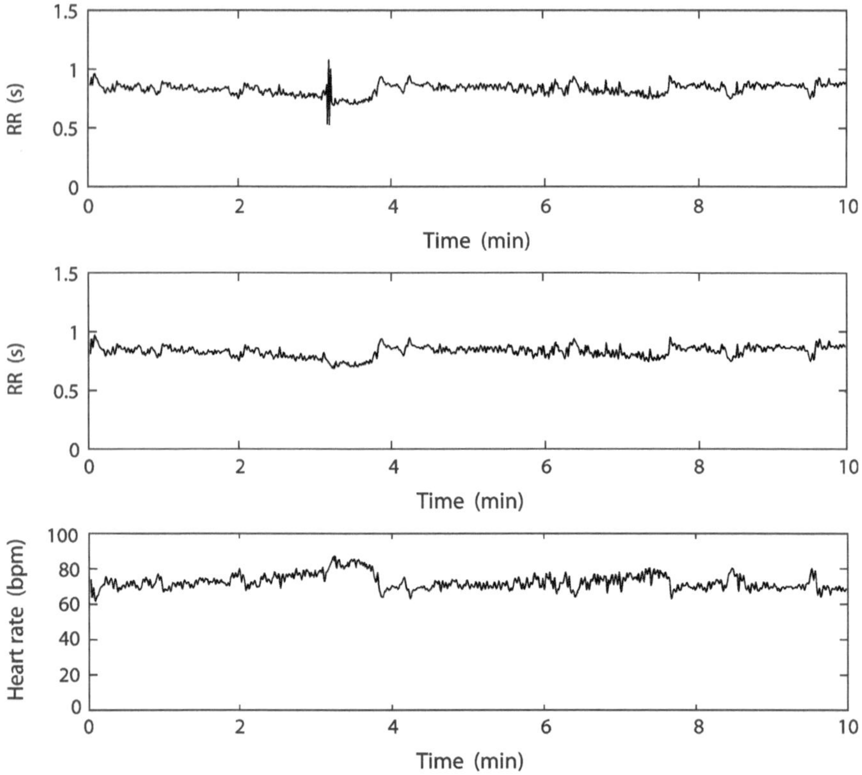

Figure 2.17 RR series with ectopic RR intervals (*top*), corrected RR series (*center*), and transformation of the RR series to heart rate expressed in bpm (*bottom*).

the RR series can be transformed to its inverse and expressed in beats per minute (bpm) to better describe the HR (bottom part of Fig. 2.17).

The spectral analysis of the RR series has been proposed as a useful tool to reflect sympathetic and vagal responses. The former is associated with the lower part of the spectrum, whereas the latter is associated with the upper part. Before proceeding with the Fourier transformation, one issue needs to be solved. As the samples of the RR series are taken at each beat, time occurrences are not uniformly distributed. Accordingly, the RR series needs to be uniformly resampled, for example, by spline interpolation. The maximum frequency that we can expect to retrieve is about half the average HR. For example, for an average HR of 60 bpm, that is, 1 Hz, the spectral content would reach 0.5 Hz at most. Fig. 2.18 shows the spectrum of the RR series from Fig. 2.17. The interpretation

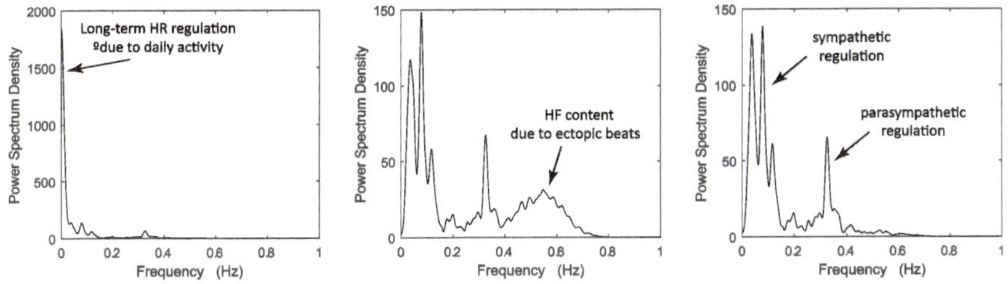

Figure 2.18 Spectrum of the RR series from the raw data (*left*), after filtering out long-term heart rate regulation (*center*), and after removing ectopic beats (*right*).

of this figure is as follows: In the raw spectrum we can find a dominant component that is associated with the long-term HR regulation (Fig. 2.18 left). After filtering these ultra-low-frequency components, we obtain the spectral distribution shown in the center part Fig. 2.18. Here, we can observe the effect of the ectopic beats and other possible artifacts, which are reflected as some spectral content above 0.4 Hz. Fig. 2.18 (right) shows the spectrum of the RR after removal of ectopic beats. Here, we can find two distinct frequency bands, the lower corresponding to sympathetic regulation and the upper to vagal regulation.

2.3.2 Detection of atrial fibrillation

Because AF is characterized by irregular RR intervals, this can be employed for detection of AF episodes. Fig. 2.19 shows an example of AF onset after a period during which the patient is in normal sinus rhythm. As can be observed in the instantaneous HR series (bottom part of Fig. 2.19), the regular HR suddenly changes to a more chaotic pattern and higher average HR.

Another way to represent the regularity of consecutive RR intervals is from what some authors refer as the Poincaré plot, which consists of a scatterplot of consecutive RR intervals, that is, RR_n, RR_{n+1}, and so on, for each n from 1 to $N-1$, N being the number of RR intervals (Piskorski & Guzik, 2007). This kind of representation could be useful to identify AF episodes (Climent et al., 2009). Fig. 2.20 shows two examples of this representation for normal sinus rhythm (left) and AF (right). As can be observed, in normal sinus rhythm the pairs are concentrated closely along the main diagonal, whereas in AF episodes they are much more dispersed.

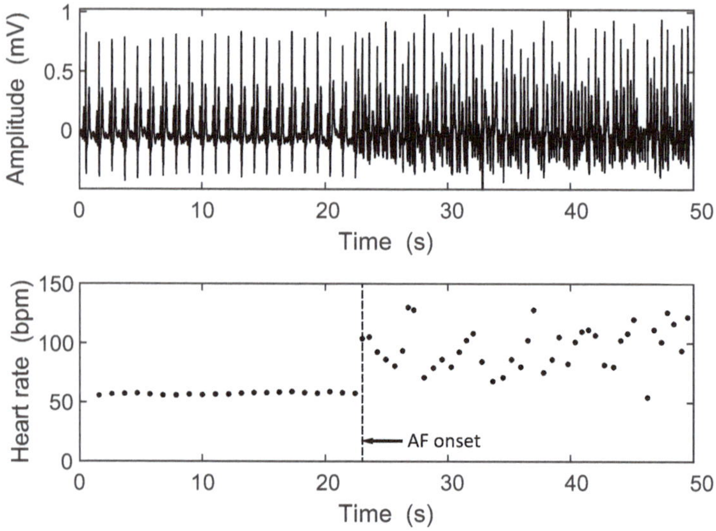

Figure 2.19 Example of atrial fibrillation onset. Electrocardiogram (*top*) and instantaneous HR (*bottom*).

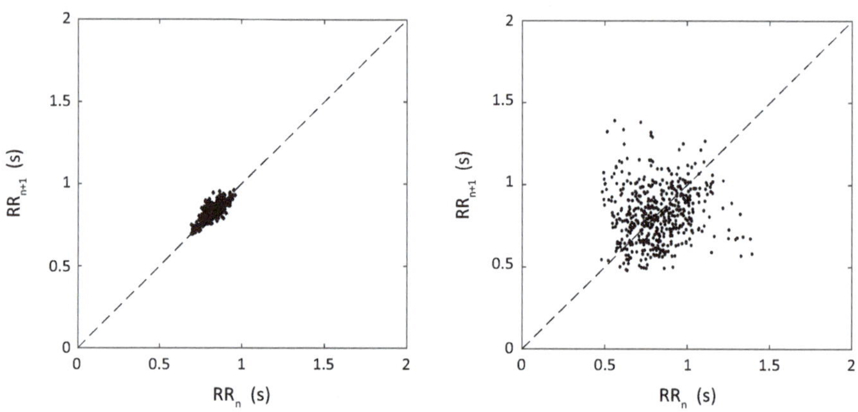

Figure 2.20 Example of a Poincaré plot of normal sinus rhythm (*left*) and atrial fibrillation (*right*).

2.4 Arterial blood pressure

The pumping action of the heart is what makes the blood flow through the circulatory system. When the ventricles contract, the pressure in their cavities is higher than that in the aorta and pulmonary arteries, so the blood is pushed forward. At the same time, the closing of the tricuspid and mitral valves prevents the blood from returning to the atria. After this, when the heart is once again in diastole, the pressure within the heart chambers is lower than that in the venae cavae and pulmonary veins arriving at the atria, which causes the suction of blood coming from the veins and hence the filling of the heart chambers. This time, the aortic and pulmonary valves prevent the blood from returning to the ventricles from the main arteries.

Blood pressure is not constant along the circulatory system, as shown in Fig. 2.21. In general, the internal pressure of the left ventricle has a high pressure in systole and a very low pressure in diastole. The fluctuations between systole and diastole modulate the blood pressure through the circulatory system. Initially, in the large arteries (e.g., the aorta), the mean blood pressure is maximal and is progressively decreasing as it passes through arterioles, capillaries, and veins. In fact, the venae cavae arriving at the right atria have very low BP. Also, the systolic/diastolic modulation is scarcely perceptible after fluid exchange through the thin walls of the capillaries. Several factors are responsible for BP fluctuations, including vessel elasticity, peripheral resistance, cardiac output, and blood volume (Nakashima & Tanikawa, 1971).

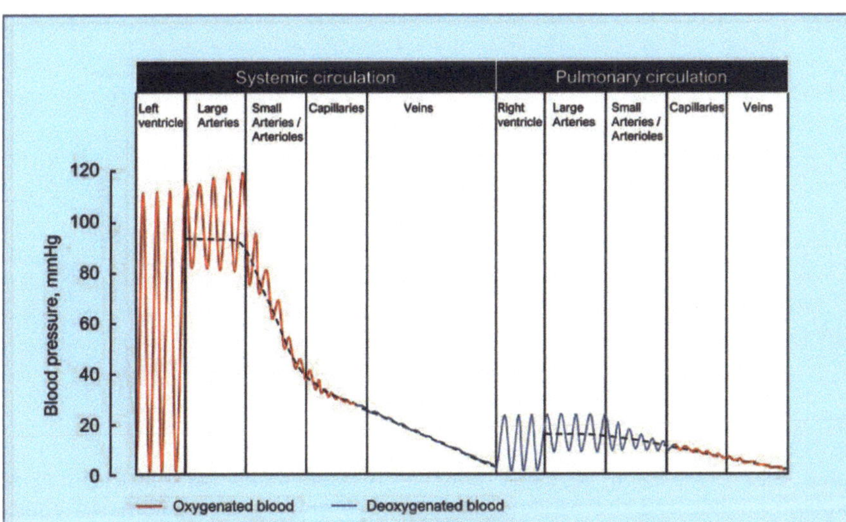

Figure 2.21 Blood pressure along the circulatory system. *Reproduced from Wikimedia Commons under Creative Commons Attribution-Share Alike 3.0 Unreported license.*

Arterial BP is an important measurement to assess the status of the circulatory system. Although BP can be accurately measured through invasive methods, such measurement is impractical in daily life as it requires insertion of a catheter. Noninvasive blood pressure measurement methods are indirect and based mainly on measuring counterpressure. Thereby, the most common noninvasive BP measurement methods for routine examination of BP at clinics, relies on a inflatable cuff, including the auscultation method and oscillometric technique.

Fig. 2.22 (top and center) illustrates the method proposed by Nikolai Korotkoff in 1905. The top part of the figure shows the BP signal (in gray) with real systolic and diastolic pressures (systolic and diastolic, respectively). A cuff is initially inflated to achieve cuff pressure above SYS. As the cuff is slowly deflated, it reaches a point at which sounds corresponding to arterial palpitations can be heard by means of a stethoscope (also known as Korotkoff sounds). The cuff pressure at this point is

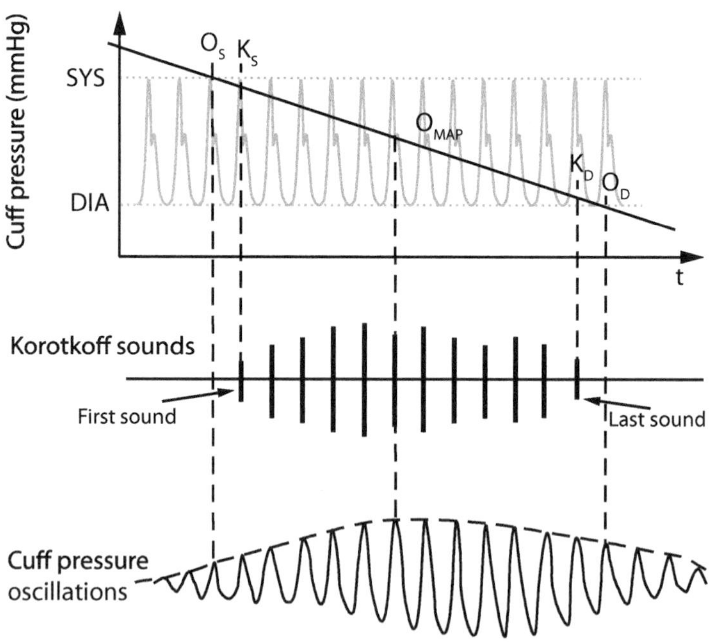

Figure 2.22 Comparison of blood pressure measurements from auscultation of Korotkoff sounds and the oscillometric technique employed in automated equipment. K_S and K_D refer to systolic and diastolic pressure according to the Korotkoff method, whereas O_S and O_D refer to systolic and diastolic pressure measurements using an oscillometric technique.

estimated as the systolic pressure (K_S in Fig. 2.22). As cuff pressure drops below DIA, Korotkoff sounds are no longer audible (Geddes & Badylak, 1991). This reference is used to estimate the diastolic pressure (K_D in Fig. 2.22). The bottom part of Fig. 2.22 shows the oscillometric method, which was first introduced by Marey in 1876. This method is able to estimate systolic and diastolic pressures from cuff pressure oscillations. Taking the envelope of the signal, SYS and DIA can be determined from specific fractions of the maximum oscillation amplitude, also known as characteristic ratios. The characteristic ratios for systolic and diastolic blood pressures are 50% and 80%, respectively. Nevertheless, this type of oscillometric blood pressure measurement fails to achieve an adequate accuracy level with critically ill patients (Bur et al., 2003).

In 1987 Boehmer (of Ohmeda Monitoring Systems) developed a device for continuous BP monitoring, later known as Finapres (from FINger Arterial PRESsure), based on the vascular unloading method, in which a cuff on the finger is pressurized to the same pressure as the artery. It was designed principally as a noninvasive hemodynamics monitor for research, displaying arterial pressure, rate, and flow.

Finger cuffs can be combined with photoplethysmography sensors (see Section 2.5) to control and adjust dynamically the cuff pressure, as shown in Fig. 2.23. With this technique, also referred as the volume clamp method, the pressure controller balances the pressure in the vessel under the cuff. As the blood flow becomes practically constant, the PPG signal

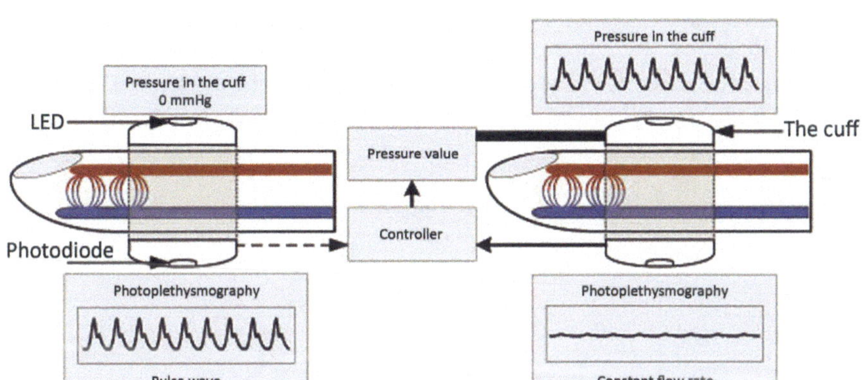

Figure 2.23 Volume clamp method principle. *Reproduced from Peter, L., Noury, N., & Cerny M. (2014). A review of methods for non-invasive and continuous blood pressure monitoring: Pulse transit time method is promising?* IRBM, *35(5), 271–282.*

turns almost flat. In contrast to other totally occlusive methods, this technique is only partially occlusive.

2.4.1 The arterial pulse wave

The arterial pulse wave (PW) contains important information about the cardiovascular system. It is widely used for physiological assessment in both consumer devices and clinical devices. With the help of new information technology, a range of physiological parameters can be estimated from the PW analysis, which are very useful for monitoring and to detect many aspects of heart diseases, especially the ones involving arterial stiffness and clinical decision making. Fig. 2.24 shows one cycle of the arterial pulse wave with its main parameters:

- SYS: systolic pressure, as the maximum arterial pressure in systole
- DIA: diastolic pressure, as the minimum arterial pressure before the next upstroke
- MAP: mean arterial pressure, as the true integrated mean pressure
- IBI: interbeat interval
- LVET: left ventricular ejection time, as the time between the current upstroke and the dicrotic notch.

Short-term and long-term fluctuations of BP parameters are shown in Fig. 2.25 (left and right, respectively). As can be observed, BP increases significantly during physical and digestive activity, whereas it drops below daily mean in the nighttime, while sleeping. In the latter case, not only the body is at rest, but as it is in supine position, blood circulation does not have to overcome the gravity force to irrigate the brain.

The shape of the pressure wave on its way to the periphery changes along the arterial tree, owing to wave reflections and a pressure gradient. For instance, finger blood pressure pulsations are tens of milliseconds

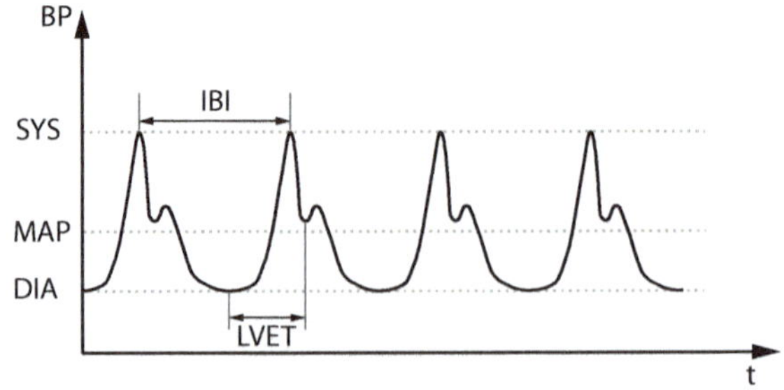

Figure 2.24 Pulse waveform.

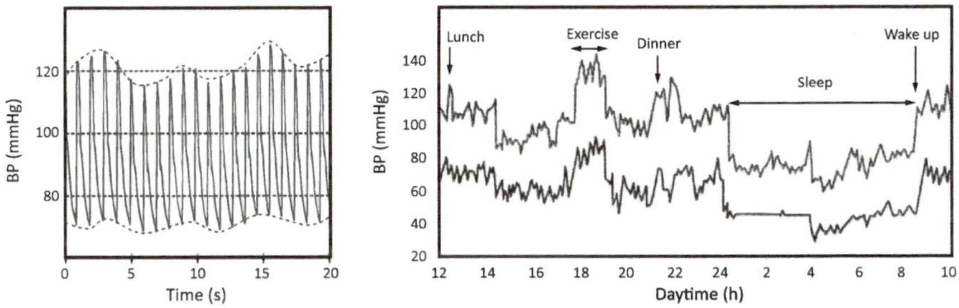

Figure 2.25 Short-term (*left*) and long-term (*right*) blood pressure monitoring.

delayed with respect to intrabrachial ones, since they travel farther. Moreover, their levels are generally lower, and the waveforms appear more distorted. This requires further processing of the measurements to accurately estimate BP. For example, PW from Finapress is processed to reconstruct brachial artery pressure from finger pressure measurements, which requires an initial calibration for each patient.

Nowadays, a variety of cuffless methods for BP and PW estimation have been explored. Among them, the finger-pressing method, which is based on oscillometric pressure at the fingertip (Chandrasekhar et al., 2018); pulse transit time (PTT), where PTT refers to the time for a pulse wave to travel between two arterial points (e.g., from the heart to the fingertip) (Mukkamala et al., 2015); ultrasound techniques, which have also showed promising results for BP monitoring at the expense of higher complexity (Zakrzewski, Huang, Zubajlo, & Anthony, 2018); and PPG, which consists of an optical technique with a light emitter and a photodetector to detect volumetric changes in peripheral circulation (Millasseau et al., 2000). With this amalgam of technologies and methods and with the aim to establish universal criteria for the validation of BP measuring devices, the Association for the Advancement of Medical Instrumentation, the European Society of Hypertension, and the International Organization for Standardization have recently agreed to develop a joint standard in the near future (Stergiou et al., 2018).

2.5 Photoplethysmography

In recent years, PPG has arisen as one of the most popular techniques for HR and PW assessment, as it is embedded in most fitness monitors and smart watches, among other wearables. This simple and inexpensive technology allows continuous monitoring of the cardiovascular status, not only for clinical use but also for personal use. An interesting site for the optical measurement of arterial blood volume changes is provided by the radial artery in the wrist, since it is located near the skin surface and the wrist serves as a good attachment point for the measuring device. In addition, patients and healthy consumers are unlikely to object to this place of measurement.

Essentially, PPG technology is composed of a light emitter (e.g., an LED) to illuminate the tissue and a photodetector to measure the small variations in light intensity via reflection from or transmission through the tissue. In reflectance mode, the photodetector detects the light that is backscattered or reflected from tissue, bone, or blood vessels (Tamura, Maeda, Sekine, & Yoshida, 2014). By contrast, in transmission-mode PPG, the light is transmitted through the medium and detected by a photodetector at the opposite side. What the PPG signal captures is the pulsatile component related to changes in blood volume inside the arteries. As more blood volume absorbs more light, this has a direct effect in the photodetector. After cardiac systole, local blood volume increases acutely, hence reducing the received light intensity. By contrast, light reflection (or transmission) increases during diastole, when the blood volume decreases (Castaneda, Esparza, Ghamari, Soltanpur, & Nazeran, 2018). In clinical practice, PPG is routinely used to monitor cardiac-induced blood volume changes in microvascular beds at peripheral body sites, such as the finger, forehead, earlobe, and toe (Zheng, Poon, Yan, & Lau, 2016). The most recognized waveform feature from the PPG signal is the peripheral pulse, which is synchronized to each heartbeat. From this signal, the heart rate can be estimated from the IBI sequence, as can other hemodynamic parameters such as blood pressure, pulse velocity, or pulse oximetry (Elgendi, Liang, & Ward, 2018; Hsu, Wu, & Sun, 2018; Rajala, Lindholm, & Taipalus, 2018).

2.5.1 Potential of PPG devices

Compared to the ECG, PPG devices do not have a complex hardware implementation. PPG also does not have the requirement of a reference signal; hence PPG sensors can be easily embedded in wrist bands. A smartphone camera could also be used as a photoplethysmographic sensor to obtain a PPG waveform (Pelegris, Banitsas, Orbach, & Marias, 2010). Consequently, PPG becomes an interesting technology for massive HR tracking as an alternative to the ECG. Because the cardiac rhythm can be extracted, all the applications mentioned in Section 2.3 could potentially be dealt with. Of special interest is AF detection. Fig. 2.26 shows an example of a PPG signal during AF, in which fluctuations of SYS and DIA envelopes are caused by the irregular RR interval.

Based on the current literature, there is clear evidence that the fluctuations in BP are reflected in the PPG signals. Given that the exact relationships between PPG waveforms and BP are not yet clear, BP estimates are difficult to achieve by the simple fitting of models or equations. Moreover, high-frequency components are largely attenuated in the PPG PW, which may hinder the estimation of LVET, as it is defined from the dicrotic notch. Nevertheless, recent advances in signal processing show a reasonable agreement for LVET estimation from PPG signals (Mathieu, Charlton, & Alastruey, 2018).

The iCare Health Monitor makes use of the smartphone's camera to acquire a finger PPG signal and estimate the BP (iCare Health Monitor). Although iCareFit does not disclose its exact method for deriving BP from the PPG signal, the mobile app instructions require the user to press one finger on the mobile phone camera and simultaneously press the thumb of the other hand on the front touch screen of the phone, which balances the force of the finger pressing against the back-side camera.

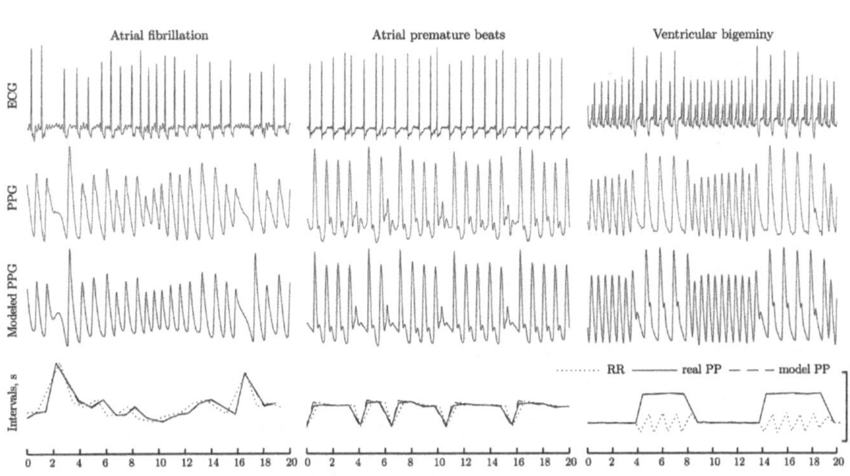

Figure 2.26 Electrocardiogram (*top*) and photoplethysmography (*bottom*) waveforms during an atrial fibrillation episode. *Adapted from Sološenko, A., Petrėnas, A., Marozas, V., & Sörnmo, L. (2016). Modeling of the photoplethysmogram during atrial fibrillation.* Computers in Biology and Medicine, 81, *130–138.*

Using the touch screen sensor to estimate the finger pressure, it is possible to implement the oscillometric measurement method for BP estimation. A variety of estimation methods continue to be explored, including those that exclusively utilize wearable PPG devices for applications in healthcare (Castaneda et al., 2018).

2.6 The phonocardiogram

The heart is an organ that is in constant movement. The mechanical action of rapid contraction and relaxation generates sounds, which are propagated through the internal tissue and structure of the torso. Heart sounds have traditionally been evaluated by auscultation with acoustic stethoscopes (Hamer, 1971). Besides the pumping activity of the heart, these sounds include friction sounds due to the opening and closing of the cardiac valves, blood regurgitation, and sounds of the respiratory system. Originally, heart sounds were evaluated only by direct interpretation of the clinician when listening to them. Neither printed copies of the signal waveform nor digitized signals were available. This hindered the possibility of signal processing, storage, playback, and visual display. This also hindered teaching, as there were no means to share sounds between several listeners and discuss their clinical interpretation. With time, cardiac auscultation became a test associated with the past. But now, with the development of inexpensive and portable devices that can digitize and record heart sounds, new perspectives are opening up (Tavel, 2006). Fig. 2.27 shows two examples of such devices: EKuore Pro, which is a whole system including the acoustic resonator, and SONEhealth SONE Pro, which consists of electronic olives compatible with Littmann

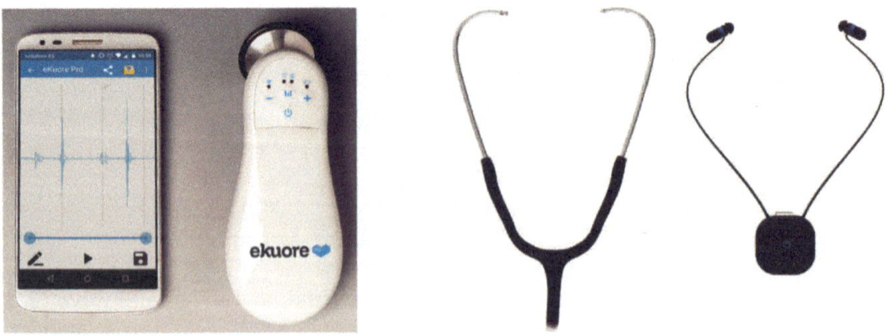

Figure 2.27 Example of electronic devices for recording heart sounds: EKuore Pro (*left*) and SONEhealth SONE Pro (*right*). *Courtesy eKuore and SONEhealth, respectively.*

stethoscopes that are able to provide acoustic and digital signals simultaneously. Because of this technological development, there is an increased interest in the evaluation of heart sounds.

The audio signal provided by means of cardiac auscultation is known as the phonocardiogram (PCG). In the PCG, normal cardiac function is characterized by a first sound burst due to ventricular contraction or diastole (also known as S1), followed by a short silent segment until a second sound burst is produced, due to ventricular relaxation or diastole (S2). Other weaker sounds, such as the third heart sound (S3) and the sound due to atrial contraction, may be also present. This sequence is repeated at each cardiac cycle (see Fig. 2.28A). Murmurs during supposedly silent periods may be a sign of cardiovascular disease (Fig. 2.28B–F). These murmurs should be reproducible in subsequent cardiac cycles. This property could be used to distinguished them from sounds caused by respiration and other nonphysiological events.

The diseases that can be detected by means of PCG listening, visualization, and/or analysis are mainly associated with the mechanical action of the heart and blood flow. This involves problems with the action of

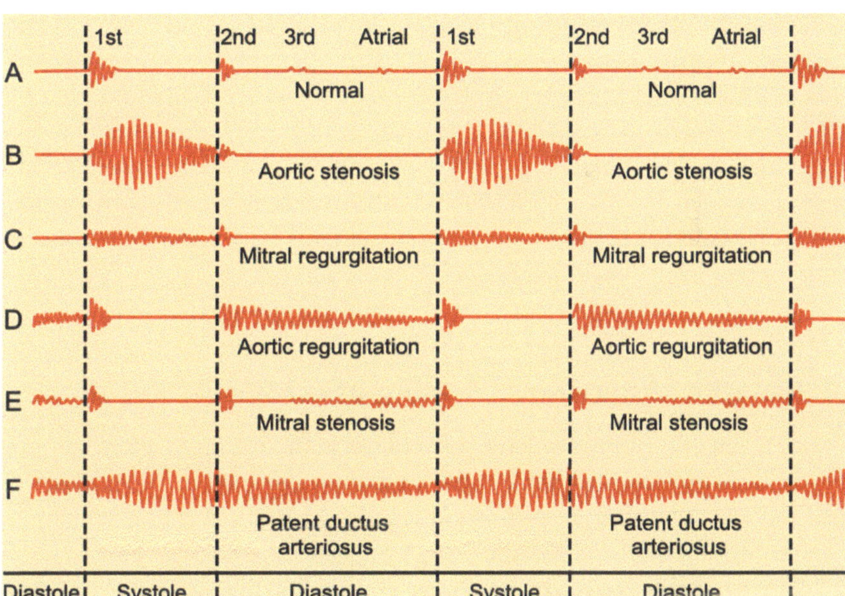

Figure 2.28 Typical phonocardiogram for normal cardiac function and several cardiac disease. *Adapted from Wikimedia Commons under Creative Commons Attribution-Share Alike 3.0 Unreported license.*

cardiac valves, as they may not open and close properly. There are four heart valves, and there might be problems associated with any of them: the tricuspid valve, located between the right atrium and right ventricle; the mitral valve, located between the left atrium and the left ventricle; the pulmonary valve, located between the right ventricle and the pulmonary artery, and the aortic valve, located between the left ventricle and the aortic artery. Accordingly, four standard locations are commonly used to emphasize their respective sounds. Appropriate opening and closing allow for effective blood pumping as the ventricles contract and return back to their rest position. Otherwise, valve diseases may severely affect blood flow and lead to serious complications. As an example, the narrowing of the aortic valve (known as aortic stenosis) restricts the blood flow from the left ventricle to the aorta and is characterized by a prolongation of S1 (Leatham, 1951). On the other hand, aortic regurgitation occurs when the aortic valve does not close tightly. In this case, a fraction of the blood pumped out of the heart returns back to the left ventricle, which generates a murmur following S2. As a result, effective blood flow is reduced. Patients suffering from valve diseases may feel fatigued and short of breath. In many cases, surgery is required to repair or replace the damaged valve.

Automated diagnosis using the PCG involves signal filtering and preprocessing, feature extraction (signal envelope, energy operators, spectrogram analysis), and a classifier. In 2016 an open access database with 2435 PCGs was created to facilitate the evaluation of heart sound classifiers (Liu et al., 2016). This extensive dataset has allowed the development and training of deep learning algorithms, with promising classification performance. Definitely, beyond the notable past of cardiac auscultation, we augur a great future to PCG devices.

2.7 Benefits of massive screening of cardiovascular signals

Wearable health monitors have experienced increasing market growth, with millions of devices being sold annually. The present and future of these devices offer unique opportunities for massive screening, which can bring enormous benefits for the detection of cardiovascular problems. In this context a massive study involving almost 200,000 subjects for home monitoring with smart device–based PPG was able to identify cases of suspected AF, with a positive predicting value over 90% (Guo et al., 2019). A recent study suggested AF screening at pharmacies by means of smartphone-based ECG as a way to reduce risks of stroke and other AF-related complications (Zaprutko et al., 2019).

Obviously, suspected cases should be further evaluated and confirmed by a clinician, as misdiagnosis can occur. Particularly, it has been questioned whether this technology is too sensitive and is prone to high levels of false positives, hence increasing substantially supervision costs in healthcare units (Afzal et al., 2019). This is a topic that has gained increased research interest, and many studies regarding detection performance with smart devices are expected to be published in the next years. One of the latest studies compared the performance of smart devices with implantable cardiac monitors (ICMs). This work concluded that smart devices showed a high agreement with respect to ICMs (Jeremiah et al., 2019).

Overall, smart devices are promising technologies for the assessment of cardiovascular conditions. In the near future we will see important advances as sensors are improved, diagnosis performance is refined by means of artificial intelligence, and use of the devices becomes widespread as prices decrease, with the potential to revolutionize the way we manage healthcare.

References

Afzal, M., Mease, J., Koppert, T., Okabe, T., Tyler, J., Houmsse, M., ... Daoud, E. (2019). Incidence of false-positive transmissions during remote rhythm monitoring with implantable loop recorders. *Heart Rhythm*, *17*(1), 75–80.

Alkhidir, T., Sluzek, A., & Yapici, M. K. (2015, August). Simple method for adaptive filtering of motion artifacts in e-textile wearable ECG sensors. In *2015 37th Annual International Conference of the IEEE Engineering in Medicine and Biology Society (EMBC)* (pp. 3807–3810).

Bansal, A., & Joshi, R. (2018). Portable out-of-hospital electrocardiography: A review of current technologies. *Journal of Arrhythmia*, *34*.

Bumgarner, J., Lambert, C., Hussein, A., Cantillon, D., Baranowski, B., Wolski, K., ... Tarakji, K. (2018). Automated atrial fibrillation detection algorithm using smartwatch technology. *Journal of the American College of Cardiology*, *71*.

Bur, A., Herkner, H., Vlcek, M., Woisetschläger, C., Derhaschnig, U., Karth, G. D., ... Hirschl, M. M. (2003). Factors influencing the accuracy of oscillometric blood pressure measurement in critically ill patients. *Critical Care Medicine*, *31*(3), 793–799.

Burke, A., Farb, A., Virmani, R., Goodin, J., & Smialek, J. (1991). Sports-related and non-sports-related sudden cardiac death in young adults. *American Heart Journal*, *121*, 568–575.

Campal, J. M. R., Torres, M. A. G., Borque, P. S., Vinagre, I. N., Capdepón, I. Z., Blanco, A. M., ... Fernández, J. M. S. (2020). Detecting atrial fibrillation in patients with an embolic stroke of undetermined source (from the DAF-ESUS registry). *The American Journal of Cardiology*, *125*(3), 409–414.

Castaneda, D., Esparza, A., Ghamari, M., Soltanpur, C., & Nazeran, H. (2018). A review on wearable photoplethysmography sensors and their potential future applications in health care. *International Journal of Biosensors & Bioelectronics*, *4*(4), 195–202.

Castells, F., Laguna, P., Sörnmo, L., Bollmann, A., & Millet, J. (2007). Principal component analysis in ECG signal processing. *EURASIP Journal on Applied Signal Processing*, *5* (1), 49–58.

Castells, F., Mora, C., Rieta, J. J., & Millet, J. (2005). Estimation of atrial fibrillatory wave from single-lead atrial fibrillation electrocardiograms using principal component analysis concepts. *Medical & Biological Engineering & Computing*, *43*, 557–560.

Chandrasekhar, A., Kim, C.-S., Naji, M., Natarajan, K., Hahn, J.-O., & Mukkamala, R. (2018). Smartphone-based blood pressure monitoring via the oscillometric finger-pressing method. *Science Translational Medicine*, *10*(431).

Chi, Y., Jung, T., & Cauwenberghs, G. (2010). Dry-contact and noncontact biopotential electrodes: Methodological review. *IEEE Reviews in Biomedical Engineering*, *3*, 106–119.

Chugh, S., Havmoeller, R., Narayanan, K., Singh, D., Rienstra, M., Benjamin, E., ... Murray, C. (2013). Worldwide epidemiology of atrial fibrillation: A Global Burden of Disease 2010 Study. *Circulation*, *129*, 837–847.

Clifford, A. C. (1996). Comparative assessment of shockable ecg rhythm detection algorithms in automated external defibrillators. *Resuscitation*, *32*, 217–225.

Clifford, G., Liu, C., Moody, B., Lehman, L. W., Silva, I., Li, Q., ... Mark, R. (2017, September). *AF classification from a short single lead ECG recording: The PhysioNet/Computing in Cardiology Challenge 2017.*

Clifford, G. D., Mcsharry, P., & Tarassenko, L. (2002). Characterizing artefact in the normal human 24-hour RR time series to aid identification and artificial replication of circadian variations in human beat to beat heart rate using a simple threshold. *Computers in Cardiology*, *29*, 129–132.

Climent, A. M., Guillem, M. S., Husser, D., Castells, F., Millet, J., & Bollmann, A. (2009). Poincaré surface profiles of rr intervals: A novel noninvasive method for the evaluation of preferential av nodal conduction during atrial fibrillation. *IEEE Transactions on Biomedical Engineering*, *56*(2), 433–442.

Cobb, L., Fahrenbruch, C., Walsh, T., Copass, M., Olsufka, M., Breskin, M., & Hallstrom, A. (1999). Influence of cardiopulmonary resuscitation prior to defibrillation in patients with out-of-hospital ventricular fibrillation. *JAMA: The Journal of the American Medical Association*, *281*, 1182–1188.

Delayed time to defibrillation after in-hospital cardiac arrest. (2008). *Survey of Anesthesiology*, *52*(12), 322–324.

Dias, D., & Cunha, J. P. (2018). Wearable health devices—Vital sign monitoring, systems and technologies. *Sensors*, *18*, 2414, 1–28, 07.

Einthoven, W. (1906). Le télécardiogramme. *Arch International Physiology*, *4*, 132–164.

Elgendi, M., Liang, Y., & Ward, R. (2018). Toward generating more diagnostic features from photoplethysmogram waveforms. *Diseases*, *6*(1).

Filgueiras-Rama, D., Calvo, C., Montañés, O., Cádenas, R., Ruiz-Cantador, J., Armada, E., ... Millet, J. (2015). Spectral analysis-based risk score enables early prediction of mortality and cerebral performance in patients undergoing therapeutic hypothermia for ventricular fibrillation and comatose status. *International Journal of Cardiology*, *186*, 250–258.

Friberg, L., Hammar, N., & Rosenqvist, M. (2009). Stroke in paroxysmal atrial fibrillation: Report from the Stockholm Cohort of Atrial Fibrillation. *European Heart Journal*, *31* (8), 967–975.

Gajda, R., Biernacka, K., & Drygas, W. (2017). Are heart rate monitors valuable tools for diagnosing arrhythmias in endurance athletes? *Scandinavian Journal of Medicine Science in Sports, 28*, 05.

Geddes, L. A., & Badylak, S. F. (1991). Power capability of skeletal muscle to pump blood. *ASAIO Transactions/American Society for Artificial Internal Organs, 37*(1), 19–23.

Go, A. S., Hylek, E. M., Phillips, K. A., Chang, Y. C., Henault, L., Selby, J., & Singer, D. (2001). Prevalence of diagnosed atrial fibrillation in adults: National implications for rhythm management and stroke prevention: The Anticoagulation and Risk Factors in Atrial Fibrillation (ATRIA) study. *JAMA: The Journal of the American Medical Association, 285*, 2370–2375.

Guo, Y., Wang, H., Zhang, H., Liu, T., Liang, Z., Xia, Y., … Lip, G. Y. H. (2019). Mobile health technology for atrial fibrillation screening using photoplethysmography-based smart devices: The Huawei Heart Study. *Journal of the American College of Cardiology*.

Hagiwara, Y., Fujita, H., Oh, S. L., Tan, J. H., Tan, R. S., Ciaccio, E., & Acharya, U. R. (2018). Computer-aided diagnosis of atrial fibrillation based on ECG signals: A review. *Information Sciences, 467*, 99–114.

Hamer, J. (1971). Auscultation of the heart and phonocardiography. *Proceedings of the Royal Society of Medicine, 64*.

Hortelano, M., Reilly, R., Castells, F., & Cervigón, R. (2018). Refined multiscale fuzzy entropy to analyse post-exercise cardiovascular response in older adults with orthostatic intolerance. *Entropy, 20*(11), 860.

Hsu, P.-C., Wu, H.-T., & Sun, C.-K. (2018). Assessment of subtle changes in diabetes-associated arteriosclerosis using photoplethysmographic pulse wave from index finger. *Journal of Medical Systems, 42*(3), 43.

Hwang, I. D., & Webster, J. (2008). Direct interference canceling for two-electrode biopotential amplifier. *IEEE Transactions on Bio-Medical Engineering, 55*, 2620–2627.

iCare Health Monitor. http://www.icarefit.com.

Isakadze, N., & Martin, S. S. (2019). How useful is the smartwatch ECG? *Trends in Cardiovascular Medicine, 30*(7), 442–448.

Jeremiah, W., Cindy, Y., Ruchi, P., Alexander, V., David, A., & Rod, P. (2019). Smartwatch performance for the detection and quantification of atrial fibrillation. *Circulation: Arrhythmia and Electrophysiology, 12*(6), e006834.

Kutyifa, V., Moss, A., Klein, H., Biton, Y., McNitt, S., MacKecknie, B., … Goldenberg, I. (2015). Use of the wearable cardioverter defibrillator in high-risk cardiac patients: Data from the prospective registry of patients using the wearable cardioverter defibrillator (WEARIT-II Registry). *Circulation, 132*.

Leatham, A. (1951). The phonocardiogram of aortic stenosis. *British Heart Journal, 13*, 153–158.

Li, K., Pan, Y., Chen, F., Cheng, K., & Huan, R. (2014). Real-time lossless ECG compression for low-power wearable medical devices based on adaptive region prediction. *Electronics Letters, 50*(25), 1904–1906.

Liberthson, R., Nagel, E., Hirschman, J., Nussenfeld, S., Blackbourne, B., & Davis, J. (1974). Pathophysiologic observations in prehospital ventricular fibrillation and sudden cardiac death. *Circulation, 49*, 790–798.

Liu, C., Springer, D., Li, Q., Moody, B., Juan, R., Chorro, F. J., … Clifford, G. (2016). An open access database for the evaluation of heart sound algorithms. *Physiological Measurement, 37*, 2181–2213.

Manikandan, M., & Prabhakararao, E. (2016). Efficient and robust ventricular tachycardia and fibrillation detection method for wearable cardiac health monitoring devices. *Healthcare Technology Letters, 3*, 239–246.

Maron, B., & Pelliccia, A. (2006). The heart of trained athletes: Cardiac remodeling and the risks of sports, including sudden death. *Circulation*, *114*, 1633–1644.
Mathieu, A., Charlton, P. H., & Alastruey, J. (2018). Using smart wearables to monitor cardiac ejection. *Multidisciplinary Digital Publishing Institute Proceedings*, *4*, 48.
Meziane, N., Webster, J., Attari, M., & Nimunkar, A. J. (2013). Dry electrodes for electrocardiography. *Physiological Measurement*, *34*, R47–R69.
Millasseau, S. C., Guigui, F. G., Kelly, R. P., Prasad, K., Cockcroft, J. R., Ritter, J. M., & Chowienczyk, P. J. (2000). Noninvasive assessment of the digital volume pulse. Comparison with the peripheral pressure pulse. *Hypertension*, *36*(6), 952–956.
Mizusawa, Y. (2016). Recent advances in genetic testing and counseling for inherited arrhythmias. *Journal of Arrhythmia*, *32*, 389–397.
Muhlestein, J. B., Le, V., Albert, D., Moreno, F. L., Anderson, J., Yanowitz, F., ... Muhlestein, J. B. (2014). Smartphone ECG for evaluation of STEMI: Results of the ST LEUIS Pilot Study. *Journal of Electrocardiology*, *48*, 260–264.
Mukkamala, R., Hahn, J.-O., Inan, O. T., Mestha, L. K., Kim, C.-S., Töreyin, H., & Kyal, S. (2015). Toward ubiquitous blood pressure monitoring via pulse transit time: Theory and practice. *IEEE Transactions on Bio-Medical Engineering*, *62*(8), 1879–1901.
Nakashima, T., & Tanikawa, J. (1971). A study of human aortic distensibility with relation to atherosclerosis and aging. *Angiology*, *22*(8), 477–490.
O'Gara, P. T., Kushner, F. G., Ascheim, D. D., Casey, D. E., Chung, M. K., de Lemos, J. A., ... Zhao, D. X. (2013). 2013 accf/aha guideline for the management of st-elevation myocardial infarction: Executive summary. *Circulation*, *127*(4), 529–555.
Pani, D., Achilli, A., & Bonfiglio, A. (2018). Survey on textile electrode technologies for electrocardiographic (ecg) monitoring, from metal wires to polymers. *Advanced Materials Technologies*, *3*, 1800008.
Park, S., & Jayaraman, S. (2010). Smart textile-based wearable biomedical systems: A transition plan for research to reality. *IEEE Transactions on Information Technology in Biomedicine*, *14*, 86–92.
Pelegris, P., Banitsas, K., Orbach, T., & Marias, K. (2010). A novel method to detect heart beat rate using a mobile phone. In *2010 Annual International Conference of the IEEE Engineering in Medicine and Biology* (pp. 5488–5491). IEEE.
Peter, L., Noury, N., & Cerny, M. (2014). A review of methods for non-invasive and continuous blood pressure monitoring: Pulse transit time method is promising? *IRBM*, *35*(5), 271–282.
Petersen, P. F., & Godtfredsen, J. (1986). Embolic complications in paroxysmal atrial fibrillation. *Stroke; A Journal of Cerebral Circulation*, *17*, 622–626.
Piskorski, J., & Guzik, P. (2007). Geometry of the poincaré plot of RR intervals and its asymmetry in healthy adults. *Physiological Measurement*, *28*, 287–300.
Rajala, S., Lindholm, H., & Taipalus, T. (2018). Comparison of photoplethysmogram measured from wrist and finger and the effect of measurement location on pulse arrival time. *Physiological Measurement*, *39*(7), 075010.
Ros, E., Mota, S., Fernández, F. J., Toro, F. J., & Bernier, J. (2005). ECG characterization of paroxysmal atrial fibrillation: Parameter extraction and automatic diagnosis algorithm. *Computers in Biology and Medicine*, *34*, 679–696.
Satija, U., Ramkumar, B., & Manikandan, M. S. (2017). Real-time signal quality-aware ecg telemetry system for IoT-based health care monitoring. *IEEE Internet of Things Journal*, *4*(3), 815–823.
Schnabel, R., Yin, X., Gona, P., Larson, M., Beiser, A., Mcmanus, D., ... Levy, D. (2015). 50 year trends in atrial fibrillation prevalence, incidence, risk factors, and mortality in the framingham heart study: A cohort study. *Lancet*, *386*, 154–162.

Sehamby, R., & Singh, B. (2016). Noise cancellation using adaptive filtering in ECG signals: Application to biotelemetry. *International Journal of Bio-Science and Bio-Technology, 8*, 237–244.

Sološenko, A., Petrėnas, A., Marozas, V., & Sörnmo, L. (2016). Modeling of the photoplethysmogram during atrial fibrillation. *Computers in Biology and Medicine, 81*, 130–138.

Sörnmo, L., & Laguna, P. (2005). *ECG signal processing: Heart rate variability*. Elsevier Academic Press.

Stergiou, G., Alpert, B., Mieke, S., Asmar, R., Atkins, N., Eckert, S., ... O'Brien, E. (2018). A universal standard for the validation of blood pressure measuring devices: Association for the Advancement of Medical Instrumentation/European Society of Hypertension/International Organization for Standardization (AAMI/ESH/ISO) collaboration statement. *Hypertension, 71*, HYPERTENSIONAHA.117.10237.

Tamura, T., Maeda, Y., Sekine, M., & Yoshida, M. (2014). Wearable photoplethysmographic sensors—Past and present. *Electronics, 3*(2), 282–302.

Task Force of the European Society of Cardiology the North American Society of Pacing Electrophysiology. (1996). Heart rate variability. *Circulation, 93*(5), 1043–1065.

Tavel, M. (2006). Cardiac auscultation a glorious past—And it does have a future!. *Circulation, 113*, 1255–1259.

Thakor, N. V., & Zhu, Y. S. (1991). Applications of adaptive filtering to ecg analysis: Noise cancellation and arrhythmia detection. *IEEE Transactions on Biomedical Engineering, 38*(8), 785–794.

Turitto, G., Benson, D., Wong, B., & El-Sherif, N. (2013) Signal averaged ECG [Online], 2, 209–222.

Vos, C., Pisters, R., Nieuwlaat, R., Prins, M., Tieleman, R., Coelen, R., ... Crijns, H. (2010). Progression from paroxysmal to persistent atrial fibrillation. *Journal of the American College of Cardiology, 55*, 725–731.

Wann, L. S., Calkins, H., Chen, L. Y., & Cigarroa, J. E. (2019). 2019 AHA/ACC/HRS focused update of the 2014 AHA/ACC/HRS guideline for the management of patients with atrial fibrillation a report of the American College of Cardiology/ American Heart Association Task Force on Clinical Practice Guidelines and the Heart Rhythm Society. *Journal of the American College of Cardiology, 74*(1), 104–132.

Watanabe, E., Arakawa, T., Uchiyama, T., Tong, M., Yasui, K., Takeuchi, H., ... Hishida, H. (2007). Prognostic significance of circadian variability of RR and QT intervals and QT dynamicity in patients with chronic heart failure. *Heart Rhythm, 4*, 999–1005.

William, A., Kanbour, M., Callahan, T., Bhargava, M., Varma, N., Rickard, J., ... Tarakji, K. (2018). Assessing the accuracy of an automated atrial fibrillation detection algorithm using smartphone technology: The IREAD study. *Heart Rhythm, 15*, 1561–1565.

Wilson, F. N., Johnston, F. D., Macleod, A. G., & Barker, P. S. (1934). Electrocardiograms that represent the potential variations of a single electrode. *American Heart Journal, 9*(4), 447–458.

Zakrzewski, A. M., Huang, A. Y., Zubajlo, R., & Anthony, B. W. (2018). Real-time blood pressure estimation from force-measured ultrasound. *IEEE Transactions on Bio-Medical Engineering, 65*(11), 2405–2416.

Zaprutko, T., Zaprutko, J., Baszko, A., Sawicka, D., Szalek, A., Dymecka, M., ... Nowakowska, E. (2019). Feasibility of atrial fibrillation screening with mobile health technologies at pharmacies. *Journal of Cardiovascular Pharmacology and Therapeutics*, page ePublished ahead of print.

Zheng, Y., Poon, C. C. Y., Yan, B. P., & Lau, J. Y. W. (2016). Pulse arrival time based cuff-less and 24-h wearable blood pressure monitoring and its diagnostic value in hypertension. *Journal of Medical Systems*, *40*(9), 195.

Zorzi, A., Pelliccia, A., & Corrado, D. (2018). Inherited cardiomyopathies and sports participation. *Netherlands Heart Journal*, *26*, 154–165.

CHAPTER 3

Systems, sensors, and devices in personal healthcare applications

Jens Mühlsteff[1], Warner ten Kate[1], Alberto Bonomi[1], Illapha Cuba Gyllensten[1], Paulo de Carvalho[2], Alexandru Pielmus[3], and Reinhold Orglmeister[3]
[1]Philips Research, Eindhoven, The Netherlands
[2]Center for Informatics and Systems of the University of Coimbra, Department of Informatics Engineering, University of Coimbra, Coimbra, Portugal
[3]Electronics and Medical Signal Processing, Technische Universität Berlin, Berlin, Germany

3.1 Patient monitoring in personal healthcare settings

Any monitoring system has to reliably acquire vital signs from a patient and automatically notify or alarm a caregiver so that the caregiver can react with an appropriate action. This is the basic primary functionality of monitoring systems across various care settings, ranging from the hospital to the home.

Automated patient monitoring has been traditionally restricted to acute settings in hospitals (Fig. 3.1), such as in the operating room or intensive care units, where vital signs are obtained in relatively well-defined and controlled circumstances. Patients are mostly immobile and are supervised by trained medical staff. However, there is a trend toward ubiquitous monitoring across the complete continuum of care. This includes monitoring of patients in the intermediate units within the hospital with extension to the home after the patient is discharged.

Personal healthcare applications require highly robust and easy-to-use vital body sign sensors that can accommodate for patient mobility and

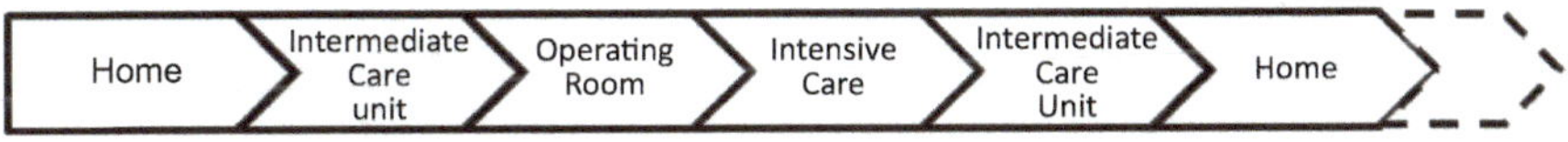
Home
Intermediate Care unit
Operating Room
Intensive Care
Intermediate Care Unit
Home

Figure 3.1 Patient monitoring has been well established and accepted in high-acuity areas such as the operating room and the intensive care unit. In personal healthcare applications, monitoring extends to intermediate care units of the hospital and to the home, where new requirements for sensors and measurements systems need to be taken into account.

Personalized Health Systems for Cardiovascular Disease
DOI: https://doi.org/10.1016/B978-0-12-818950-4.00014-8

require little or no interaction with care providers. Measurements are typically not supervised and are mostly done by the patients themselves. Also, to enable actionable and appropriate interventions, there must be a means for sending notifications or alarms to caregivers in remote locations, such as a hospital or a call center. Examples of commercialized personal healthcare (PHC) devices are wrist watches for activity and pulse measurements, patch devices for detection of arrhythmias, 24-hour blood pressure (BP) and electrocardiogram (ECG) Holter devices, and wearable external defibrillators for patients at high risk for cardiac arrest (Erath, Vamos, Sirat, & Hohnloser, 2017); the defibrillators automatically apply an electrical shock upon a detected event.

3.2 Application-driven sensor research and device development

3.2.1 The requirements that personal healthcare applications place on devices and systems

3.2.1.1 Trends

A major trend in healthcare systems is the transition from a fee-for-service system to a value-based care system (https://www.cognizant.com/whitepapers/how-providers-can-reshape-their-operations-to-master-value-based-reimbursements-codex3717.pdf) with an increasing emphasis on patient-centric quality metrics. The ability to adapt the care plan to the patient's personal situation will become a key factor in the care that is offered.

Ideally, to assess the patient's personal situation, two contributions need to be taken into account: in a direct sense, the individual health state of the care recipient and, in an indirect sense, the actual context in which the care recipient is embedded. Examples of the first concern metrics that inform about the state of the disease, disorder, or decline being treated, including parameters such as BP, heart rate, respiration rate, posture, and degree of mobility. Examples of the second cover information such as the level and type of activities in which the patient engages, the amount of walking the patient does, times of medication intake, eating and drinking behavior, and sleeping behavior. When the treatment is in a hospital, this context is usually implied, whereas when the patient is monitored at home, an additional sensing system to monitor the context might be effective in improving the care.

Another prominent trend is to reduce costs and to increase the efficiency of the healthcare systems. One objective is to minimize the length of stay in the hospital while preventing early readmissions. This may mean that the patient is monitored for a limited period after early discharge. This is enabled by telemonitoring solutions (Majumder, Mondal, & Jamal, 2017), in which vital sign data are measured and transmitted to the hospital for monitoring (White, n.d.). Concerning the reduction of admissions and readmissions, home-monitoring systems can be effective in predicting health worsening in the population segment at risk (Op den Buijs et al., 2018).

Similarly, rehabilitation can benefit from telemonitoring as well. After surgery, people need to perform exercises to regain their abilities. A telemonitoring system enables the patient to exercise without visiting the therapist. A smart system can provide feedback to the patient, for example, on the exercise quality without the therapist's consultation (Kraal et al., 2017). A summary report enables the therapist to determine possible adjustments of the care plan (Kraal et al., 2017).

There are different ways to structure application scenarios. An example is shown in Fig. 3.2. In the first layer, the main functions are determined, for instance, screening, post event, coaching, medication management, and chronic disease management. In the second layer, the specific health problem is defined. Obviously, functions can overlap, since a chronic disease program includes often coaching aspects as well as medication treatment and adaptations.

In summary, developments in PHC are driven by needs in terms of early discharge, remote rehabilitation, and telecare with systems grading from out-hospital into PHC. For managing chronic diseases or declining

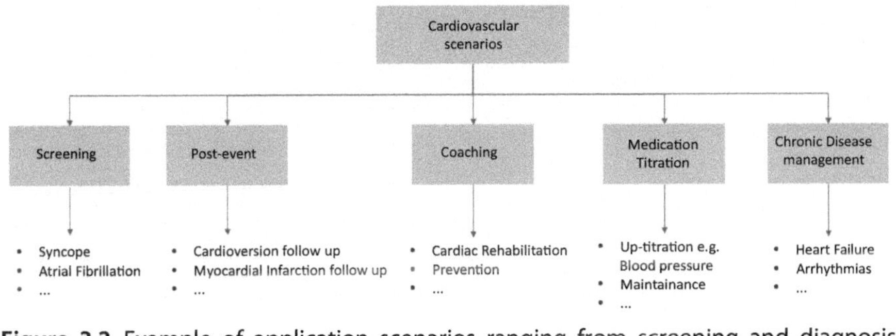

Figure 3.2 Example of application scenarios ranging from screening and diagnosis to chronic disease management.

abilities, a more sustaining remote monitoring system can be of help. In case of a skilled nursing home facility, the monitoring system is confined to the facility's premises; in case of independent living, there is a true telemonitoring system in place connecting the homes with a remote care or help center (The National Careline, Telecare Support).

3.2.1.2 Requirement drivers

A first essential aspect in the development of PHC sensors is that unsupervised measurements of mobile patients typically lead to ill-defined measurement conditions. Dedicated strategies are needed for proper handling and interpretation of uncertain and poorly reproducible out-of-hospital scenarios. While the clinical environment provides controlled conditions, for example, in assessing heart rate or BP, in the at-home setting, the daily life activities lead to a significantly larger dynamic range of subsequent measurements. In general, the home measurement will need some (automated) cleaning or filtering of the measurements to get meaningful information.

Next, the rate at which measurements are to be taken affects the sensing system. Static information does not change during the period of observation or is revised only after a longer time period. Such information includes age, gender, height, and medication prescription. These are typically acquired through questionnaires or at intake through a one-time measurement. Dynamic information may lead to continuous sampling and streaming of data but can also be processed in batches. Sampling rates of signals and parameters can vary a lot from the kilohertz level for an ECG signal to only once or a few times per day, for example, for weight.

A third aspect is the required precision and accuracy of the sensed vital parameter. On the one hand this concerns the health quantity itself that is being measured, on the other hand it might be influenced by the subsequent monitoring process that is using the data. For example, in cardiovascular applications the quality of ECG measurements can be affected by motion artifacts or suboptimal contact between skin and sensing electrodes. As another example, BP might be needed in reliable absolute values, while in some other applications only trend-information might be sufficient without knowing the precise absolute value for example, when detecting a BP regulation failure leading to loss of consciousness and fall. When monitoring general health it might be sufficient to track sleeping time, and bed leaves during the sleep (e.g., for toileting), while when treating posttraumatic stress disorder, the sleep stages need to be determined as well. The monitoring process may analyze the signals for emergency events such that alerts can be raised to a caregiver, but may also extract patterns from the data to detect anomalies or predict future care needs. For reliable and accurate detection, the sensor signals should be highly accurate and exhibit large signal-to-noise ratios (SNR). A major issue in these settings can be a high false alarm rate.

The fourth and perhaps most important requirement concerns the user experience (UX). It is key for a system to be accepted and finally be used as intended, which requires a seamless integration into a users' daily routines and life. Ease of use encompasses items such as comfort to wear and limited self-explaining interactions for operating a device such as initialization of a measurement, a simple power management (frequency to recharge) or a transparent handling of notifications or alarms.

Sensor embodiments differ widely. A sensor can be carried in the pocket or purse, such as with mobile phones, it can be carried as a pendant or wrist-worn device. Other options include the attachment on belts or bra, but might also be needed to be closely coupled to a body part or the skin like a plaster. Obviously, the level of comfort ranges with the attachment method, together with the form factor (shape) and weight of the device. Waterproofing and resistance is also important to ensure continuity in the measurements as showers and water activities can cause lowered coverage and adherence for wearable devices.

An alternative to provide patients with sensors to be carried around is to use external, and in particular wall-mounted sensors. They can offer a rich range of information about the user. Sensors like passive infrared, door open-close switches, and power sensors (Fibaro, n.d.) typically enable contextual and behavioral characterization of the user in indoors spaces but also can provide health related parameters (Robben, Englebienne, Pol, & Krose, 2012; Skubic, Alexander, Popescu, Rantz, & Keller, 2009). Other sensing modalities, such as radar- and camera-based sensors, enable the measurement of a range of vital signs, such as heart rate and respiration rate (Emerald, From Wearables to Invisibles). Wall-mounted sensors increase user comfort because of their unobtrusiveness. However, cameras might be experienced to compromise privacy. Another drawback of wall-mounted sensors is their limited range of observation, such as excluding out-of-house usage, and the potential need to install several sensors to cover wide spaces. In addition, it might be difficult to distinguish between multiple people or pets who are also present in the home.

A fifth driver concerns the group of enabling requirements, such as to contribute to environmental sustainability and to ensure a positive financial balance in manufacturing and operating the system. Costs arise from the components that are used, that is, the bill of material composed by the number and type of sensors; the packaging; the installation effort; the commissioning (which possibly can be automated); and maintenance, including replacement and refurbishment. Finally, infrastructure and personnel (emergency response call center, help desk) contribute significantly to the costs.

The combination of all of these drivers will lead to different solutions in terms of the sensing system. For example, when BP is to be measured on a daily basis with reliable accuracy, the use of a cuff would be preferred and acceptable to the user. However, if continuous measurement is required, for example, to find out how BP changes in response to the user's activities, a lightweight, comfortable wearable device would satisfy most of the technical requirements to extract BP change but could not provide the absolute BP level.

3.2.2 Core system components

Core technical components of a typical smart sensor system are shown in Fig. 3.3. The sensor system consists of the transducer, in which a vital sign is translated into electrical signals, the processing unit to operate the sensor and to do appropriate preprocessing of the signals already locally at the patient, means for power management and for data storage, and a user interface. Data are exchanged by wired or wireless means to the cloud, call center, or hospital. Various standardized radio options have been commercialized to communicate to a hub device (e.g., a smartphone) via Zigbee or Bluetooth.

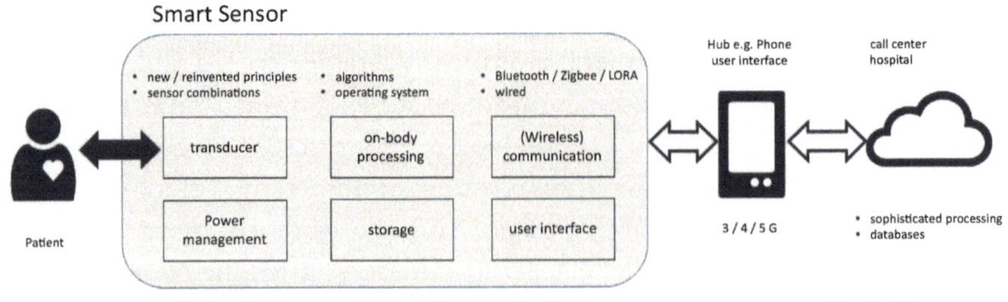

Figure 3.3 Technical components of a typical smart sensor system, including communication to the cloud or call center.

Relevant requirements for a system design are as follows:

1. Parameter to be measured
   a. Disease or application specific
   b. Context information
   c. Performance metrics
2. Technical
   a. Accuracy: resolution, SNR
   b. Sampling rate
   c. Processing power: local on-body processing versus processing in the cloud
   d. Wireless, bandwidth
   e. Battery power consumption
   f. Robustness
   g. Time stamping, syncing to other devices
   h. Connectivity
3. UX: ease of use, comfort
   a. Intrusiveness, stigmatizing
   b. Intuitive, simple operation
   c. On-body, wearable, or wall-mounted
   d. Form factor: size, weight
   e. Battery handling
4. Manufacturing
   a. Bill of materials
   b. Environmental sustainability
   c. Installation, commissioning (automated)
   d. Replacement, refurbishing
5. Business
   a. Payment schemes
   b. System deployment
   c. Education of staff
   d. Sales channel
   e. Maintenance
   f. Regulatory

3.2.3 Cardiovascular parameters for personal healthcare applications

Cardiovascular parameters to be acquired for a specific application have to be defined in close collaboration with the medical experts. Parameters of interest comprise the whole spectrum of the established ones used in hospitals. Basic parameters, also known as the vital signs, are heart/pulse rate, heart rate variability, respiration rate, oxygen saturation, BP, and core body temperature. More specific parameters for heart performance include detection of various arrhythmias, contractility, stroke volume, and cardiac

Table 3.1 Cardiovascular parameters relevant to personal healthcare applications.

Parameter	Normal values/comment
Heart rate	60–80 bpm
Respiration rate	12–14 min^{-1}
Blood pressure: systolic/diastolic	120/80 mmHg
Arterial oxygenation	98%–100%
Body weight	60–100 kg, dependent on body height
Core temperature	36.8°C
Motion, activities • At rest, posture • Quantified activity level	No clinically established metrics and values
Biomarkers • Glucose • B-type natriuretic peptide (BNP) • Lactate	80–120 mg/dL < 100 pg/m, 1,3 mmol/L
Arrhythmias • Atrial fibrillation • ST changes • Ventricular tachycardia	Detection established for diagnostic purposes
Cardiac output	4–8 L/min
Systemic vascular resistance	800–1400 dyn · s/cm^5
Pulmonary capillary wedge pressure	2–15 mmHg
Central venous pressure	3–8 mmHg
Systolic heart times • Pre-ejection period • Left ventricular contraction time • Diastolic time	70–100 ms 200–320 ms
Fluid accumulation • In the lung • In the periphery	For example, in patients with heart failure

output. Table 3.1 lists the most relevant parameters used in clinical practice to investigate the health status of a patient.

3.2.4 Devices for personal healthcare: An overview

Different classes of devices for PHC application have been established. Those can be classified as body worn, off-body, and spot-check measurement devices.

3.2.4.1 Body-worn devices

Body-worn devices include all devices that are attached to or worn continuously by the subject. Such devices are used mainly in situations in which continuous monitoring of vital signs is required, for example, for screening of arrhythmias or for monitoring of cardiac function in patients at risk of sudden cardiac arrest. Established measurement devices for diagnostic and screening purposes are ECG Holter and BP Holter monitors, for which the typical measurement period is about 24 hours.

Design criteria include robust and reliable data acquisition, ease of use, comfort, and biocompatibility. Components that are to be in direct contact with the skin, such as electrodes, should provide no or low skin irritation and form factors (housings) at body locations that will minimally interfere with the user's activities. Since patients are typically mobile, the system concept should include ways to deal with associated artifacts. Intuitive user interfaces are required, and the device often includes some means to transfer data from the patient location to a receiving station at the hospital or call center.

Examples are wrist watches, which are very popular for fitness applications; electronic plasters or patches, which are developed and commercialized mainly for diagnostic purposes; and sensors integrated into textiles for management of chronic conditions such as heart failure.

3.2.4.1.1 Off-body devices placed in a patient's vicinity

Less obtrusive are off-body devices, in which no sensors are attached to the subject's body. Here, vital signs are either monitored remotely by contactless methods or when a patient comes naturally into the vicinity of sensors. These measurement scenarios are often ill defined, since the availability of signals is limited to certain periods when the patient is within reach of the particular sensors. However, humans typically follow daily routines (sleeping in a bed, washing in a bathroom, sitting in a chair, going to the toilet, etc.), and sensor devices embedded in their environment have the potential to capture patient measurements at consistent times of the day. Examples of those sensors and devices include cameras, radar, or sensors integrated into objects that are important in their daily routine, such as the bed, toilet, chair, smart TV, or smart mirrors.

3.2.5 Devices for spot checks of vital parameters

Dedicated devices for spot check measurements have been used for many decades. Most prominent are thermometers for fever detection; others include BP monitors for self-measurements, weight scales for weight control, and devices to assess the blood for glucose levels. Weight scales have been augmented for assessment of body compositions. The patient consciously trigger a measurement. User interfaces have become more user friendly, for example, in guiding by voice control a measurement procedure to document measurements. Recently, measurement options have been integrated into smartphones via apps.

3.3 Personal healthcare sensing technologies

3.3.1 Overview of relevant sensing principles

Sensors are basic ingredients in personal health care applications, which ideally should gather medically relevant parameters with no impact on a consumer's quality of life (Abbas et al., 2009). Therefore the design guideline for these sensors is oriented on customer needs while at the same time ensuring accurate measurements which is essential for acceptance by the medical community. There is significant development effort in advanced sensing technologies in often ill-defined measurement conditions with sensors seamlessly embedded into a patient's daily routines.

It is impossible to capture all technologies being under development or being researched (Teichmann et al., 2012). Therefore this section can only provide a snapshot of technical approaches for a few examples. Various important technologies with relevance for PHC applications will be briefly introduced.

3.3.1.1 Capacitive or dry electrodes

In contrast to common adhesive gel electrodes, capacitive (electric field) sensors have the ability to measure electrophysiological signals (e.g., electrocardiogram, electroencephalogram) without a galvanic skin contact. In this technique, the sensor electrode is coupled capacitively to the skin of the user (Atallah et al., 2014). Measuring through clothes is relevant, since this eliminates many of the side effects caused by adhesive gel electrodes. Benefits include the avoidance of skin irritation (typical with adhesive electrodes), more freedom of movement, and the ability to measure with clothes on and without lengthy preparation. Drawbacks include a higher susceptibility to artifacts by many sources, such as motion or electric charges, which result in a lower SNR. The approach has been even tested for ECG in monitoring applications in cars (Walter, Eilebrecht, Wartzek, & Leonhardt, 2011).

3.3.1.2 Photoplethysmography

Heart rate measurements have usually been done with chest belts, by which electrodes in textiles or stiff bands sense the ECG at the thorax to deduce the heart rate. However, the attachment of the chest belt is cumbersome, and a longer period of attachment of the belt is considered uncomfortable, since the belts do not stay in place and may cause skin irritations. In particular, older adults with limited mobility have problems in attaching these systems. More recently, continuous strapless monitoring of pulse rate with a single wrist-worn device (smart watch) has been realized. The basic principle is based on reflective photoplethysmography (PPG) complemented by intelligent signal fusion with accelerometer data and consecutive robust parameter extraction. PPG sensors optically detect blood volume changes in a superficial area of the skin. Nowadays, these sensors allow monitoring even during challenging conditions such as while doing sports. The wrist is one of the most suitable places for wearable devices, as many people are used to wearing a watch. An active research area using smart watches is detection of arrhythmias, such as atrial fibrillation (Bonomi et al., 2017).

3.3.1.3 Heart sound analysis

Heart sounds have been used to assess multiple parameters related to the mechanical status of the heart, for example, the heart valve. One of the main applications has been in hemodynamics and contractility assessment. This is based on the fact that myocardial relaxation and contraction are governed by intracellular recycling of calcium ions. The timings of these basic cardiac events are directly related to the health of the cardiac cells (Oh & Tajik, 2003) and determine the ability of the myocardium to achieve blood delivery according to the metabolic requirements of the organs. Of major importance are the systolic time intervals (STIs) of the left ventricle, since it is this ventricle's function to ensure the blood flow in the systemic circulation. Because myocardial relaxation and contraction are controlled by intracellular recycling of calcium ions, the timings of these cardiac events relate directly to the health of myocardial cells (Gillebert, Leite-Moreira, & de Hert, 2000; Gillebert, Van de Veire, de Buyzere, & Sutter, 2004). Indeed, it is well known that the ratio between the main STIs, that is, the ratio between the preejection period and the left ventricle ejection time, is inversely correlated to ejection fraction and heart failure (Tavakolian, 2016). On the other hand, the amount of blood ejected in each heart stroke is directly related to the so-called preload, that is, the degree to which the ventricles are stretched before contracting, and the afterload, which relates to the pressure the left ventricle has to overcome to eject blood to the aorta. Preload and afterload influence the main STIs as well (Hassan & Turner, 1983); therefore STIs have been used to measure cardiac output (Couceiro et al., 2011). Carvalho et al. (2010) have shown that heart sounds are among the most reliable modalities to measure STIs compared to echocardiography, which is the current gold standard. The first (S1) and the second (S2) heart sounds encode information related to the movement of the aortic valve cusps. Hence using heart sounds as a reference for STI measurement is not a new idea. It was a common practice prior to the introduction of ultrasound. The procedure was based on the combination of the carotid pulse, the heart sounds recorded in the phonocardiogram, and the ECG. By neglecting the time delay caused by pulse propagation, the carotid pulse wave was analyzed to identify the aortic valve timings and enabled the estimation of the left ventricular ejection time (LVET). The preejection period was measured indirectly by subtracting LVET from QS2 (Newlin & Levenson, 1979; Tavel, 1974), where QS2 is the time interval from the ECG Q-peak to S2. Direct measurement of STIs have been proposed. Buxi, Redoute, and Yuce (2015) suggest using the closing instant of the atrioventricular valve (assessed by its peak in intensity of the S1 sound) as a marker of the aortic valve opening. However, it is well known that there is an average time difference of 30 ms between the atrioventricular valve closing and the onset of opening of the aortic valve (Tavel, 1974). More recently, Paiva et al. (2009) have introduced a method to identify the opening instant of the aortic valve using the S1 sound.

3.3.1.4 Ballistocardiography

Inside the human body there are a number of motion sources due to mechanical movements, including the heart (pump movement, heart valve movements), respiration, digestion, the voice, snoring, flows, and congestion. These vibrations propagate through the body, and can be detected at the body surface passively and noninvasively. For instance, it is possible to detect heart movement with ballistocardiography. This is a technique of measuring the movements of the body imparted by the ballistic forces (recoil and impact) associated with cardiac contraction and ejection of blood and with the deceleration of blood flow through the large blood vessels. These minute movements are translated by a pickup device (e.g., a piezoelectric sensor or highly sensitive accelerometer) and are then suitably amplified and recorded. This technique is very prone to motion artifacts. Applications of the technique have been for detection of respiration and pulse rate from the chest via a wearable device (Jin, Yin, Morren, Duric, & Aarts, 2009) or embodiments integrated into weight scales or beds (Brüser, Kerekes, Winter, & Leonhardt, 2012).

3.3.1.5 Blood pressure inference via surrogate measures

Arterial blood pressure (ABP) is the pressure exerted by the blood on the walls of vessels, which shows significant changes during a patient's day which can be normal variations (night dip, a morning rise) or critical such as sudden drops or overshoots, for example, due to circulatory regulation compromise. Many PHC applications need access to reliable, comfortable, and preferably continuously measured ABP, for example, for syncope (faint) detection, or cardiac rehabilitation or to characterize the impact of apnea events on the circulatory system during sleep.

However, state-of-the-art BP devices use the sphygmomanometric occlusive cuff that allows for noninvasive intermittent measurements only at a time scale of minutes. This technique is based on either the auscultatory or the oscillometric method, in which a cuff is placed on one arm above the elbow and the patient must sit quietly during the measurement. The cuff has to be inflated up to the point at which the brachial artery is completely occluded, which makes the device impractical for frequent and ambulatory measurements. Patients report pain due to the applied pressure, skin trauma, and difficulty applying the cuff. These type of BP measurements disturb the sleep (Heude, Bourgin, Feigel, & Escourrou, 1996) (Fig. 3.4).

Given these limitations, BP measurements without application of an external pressure are being researched. The most common approaches are pulse wave velocimetry and pulse shape analysis or a combination of the two, in which pulses detected at one or various sites of the arterial tree are analyzed for BP inference (Buxi et al., 2015; Mukkamala et al., 2015). An intensively investigated surrogate is the pulse arrival time (PAT), which is defined as the time interval between the peak of the R wave of the ECG and the onset of a peripheral plethysmographic pulse (Zhang et al., 2017). To infer the BP from the PAT requires an initiation procedure via a reference BP measurement to determine open parameters of an inference model. The validity or reinitialization of these model parameters is a major challenge and often not well understood. Another aspect is a missing consensus on an objective performance of such devices via an

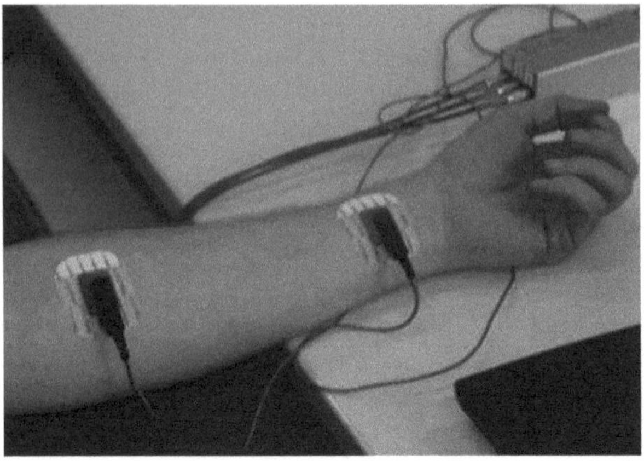

Figure 3.4 Pulse transit time is the time that it takes for a pressure wave to travel a certain distance along the cardiovascular tree. Here, two piezoelectric sensors detect the passing of a pressure pulse. It is common to replace the proximal (first) sensor by an electrocardiogram signal.

appropriate standard, which is currently being defined (http://www.iso.org/standard/71161.html).

3.3.1.6 Radar-based vital sign measurement

Radar is an interesting sensing principle to monitor basic vital signs comfortably without body contact and with low-cost radar sensors (Emerald, From Wearables to Invisibles; Thiel, Kreiseler, & Seifert, 2009). It uses electromagnetic waves as sensitive probes, which are reflected at the chest wall and undergo a Doppler frequency shift if the chest wall is moving due to the subject's respiration (Muehlsteff, Pinter, & Morren, 2009) (Fig. 3.5). The technique is sensitive enough to even detect heartbeat information. However, any motion by a subject causes artifacts, which limit the applicability. Artifact handling is a topic of current research. Radar has intrinsic advantages as well as disadvantages, which have to be considered for each particular monitoring scenario. Commercial devices exist for sleep monitoring (http://www.resmed.com/us/en/consumer/s-plus.html).

3.3.1.7 Camera-based sensing methods

There have been tremendous improvements in video-based vital sign monitoring, mainly driven by technical progress in camera technologies and video-processing algorithms accompanied by available processing

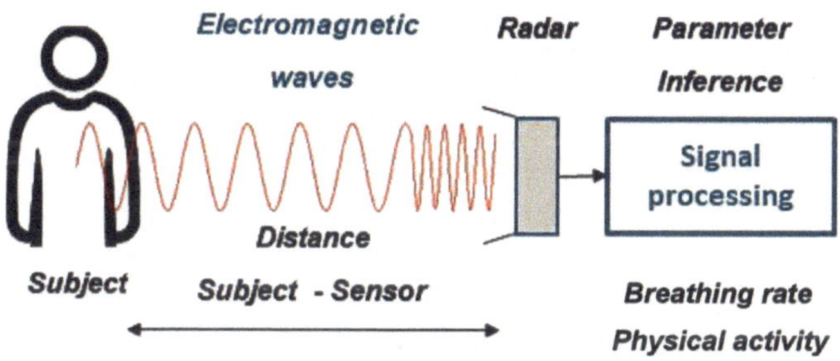

Figure 3.5 Basic principles of using electromagnetic wave as a sensitive probe for detecting a subject's vital signs.

power. Measurement concepts are based on single cameras, thermal infrared cameras, time-of-flight cameras, stereo techniques, or structured light (Abbas, Heiman, Orlikowsky, & Leonhardt, 2009; Tarassenko et al., 2014). The main driver here was the gaming industry, where Kinect is one of the most prominent examples (Han, Shao, Xu, & Shotton, 2013). Additionally, smartphones have been become ubiquitous with high-quality cameras as standard sensors. A camera offers a multitude of signals related to color changes and motion in a video sequence at the same time. Even with simple and low-cost cameras, respiration of a person can be measured by a barcode reader (Bartula, Tigges, & Muehlsteff, 2013).

Most of the research on vital sign measurements reported in literature refers to feasibility studies only, without focusing on a solid assessment of sensor system performance. The applicability of this method depends strongly on the use case, its susceptibility to varying lighting conditions, relative movements, and cumbersome and manual definition of the regions of interest in a video.

Cameras offer access to context information, such as subject identification via face recognition (for which many algorithms already exist) as well as measures of activities and motion in a scene.

3.3.1.8 Motion sensors

Patient mobility is considered the sixth vital sign, and physical activity is an important indicator of patient quality of life and disease progression. In monitoring human movement, one is interested in the time series of the subsequent positions at which the human limbs are located. This information in turn enables the extraction of further information, such as whether the user is sitting, lying, standing, or walking. The sensor signals can also be used to determine whether the user is tripping or slipping, is rising from a chair, or is falling, for example. Further information concerns the quality of these movements: how stable, how fast is the walking, how much energy is expended, and so on.

A first division of the sensing approaches to capture human movement is in on-body and off-body systems.

Off-body sensing systems can provide more user comfort. In some systems, however, the user is supposed to wear markers or tags that the sensing system uses to identify the particular body part (e.g., limb). Markers can be passive (reflecting) or active (radiating, such as blinking light emitters).

The main off-body motion-capturing systems are cameras and radar (Emerald, From Wearables to Invisibles). Their signals hold absolute location information. The information is already expressed in the global coordinate system aside from a fixed calibration for location and orientation (rotation) of the capturing camera. Since these sensors provide position information, velocity and acceleration can be determined by differentiation of the signals. A drawback of off-body sensors is their restricted viewing angle, possibly necessitating installation of a range of sensors, which subsequently need to be synchronized and to be aligned for proper cooperation. Besides a limited viewing angle, the usability of their signals may be impeded by occlusion, and additional measures may be needed to identify and distinguish between different people and/or pets.

On-body sensing systems can range from a single wearable device, hosting one or more sensing modalities, to a fully covering body sensor network (BSN) (Pflugradt et al., 2015). Wearing comfort relates to the number of attachment points, and the application of a BSN should be driven by the application's need for richer, more precise and accurate data. Also, the intrinsic costs will rise with the larger set of sensors and devices together with system complexity and power load for the needed communication.

The main on-body motion-capturing sensors are the accelerometer, gyroscope, magnetometer, and air pressure sensor. Sensitive on-body accelerometers can be successfully used to measure, besides human movement, vital signs such as heart rate and respiration rate and other forms of health information, such as pressure sensors (not to be confused with air pressure sensors) responding to the force between two objects. They can be used in gloves to measure grip strength or as insoles to measure weight distribution and step taking (Komi, Roberts, & Rothberg, 2008; Razak, Zayegh, Begg, & Wahab, 2012).

Obviously, the same parameters can often be acquired by different technologies. The decision on a concrete design will depend on the specific requirements.

3.4 Implementation examples

Example 1: Monitoring congestive heart failure patients using a wearable vest.

In this example we will detail a wearable sensor solution for the monitoring of heart failure. The clinical syndrome of heart failure occurs when the heart has lost its ability to deliver adequate blood flow to the body's organs at normal cardiac filling pressures. It can be either acute or chronic and is a common condition affecting an estimated 1%–2% of the European and U.S. population.

In heart failure the body tries to compensate for the lack of blood perfusion through a neurohormonal signaling process similar to the body's response to blood loss: increasing central blood volumes and pressures through fluid retention and peripheral vasoconstriction (reducing the blood vessels' diameter) to increase cardiac output and preserve perfusion of the central organs. Although corrective in the short run, over time (if the causative factor remains) this neurohormonal activation leads to maladaptive processes of cardiac remodeling, ventricular dilation, and worsening contractility of the heart, as well as deleterious effects in other organs and tissues. Unfortunately, this results in a negative feedback loop of progressively worsening cardiac function, with symptoms such as reduced exercise tolerance and fatigue and fluid buildup in the lungs, stomach, and legs, causing breathlessness, loss of appetite, and leg swelling. This is a dire situation, and once the diagnosis has been made, the prognosis is comparable to that of most common cancers. Medications are typically initiated to protect against these maladaptive processes, inhibit adverse remodeling of the heart, and stimulate excretion of excess fluids.

In the past decades, new drugs have improved the effectiveness of heart failure treatment, in particular in patients with reduced ejection fraction. However, despite these improvements, patients often experience periods of worsening symptoms requiring hospitalization, such as acute heart failure. These periods are associated with an increase in mortality and morbidity following discharge and are responsible for most of the costs related to heart failure care. With this background, strategies have been proposed to monitor heart failure more closely so that these situations can be averted. The hypothesis is that monitored signals could be integrated into the care of heart failure patients so that changes indicative of an upcoming episode of acute heart failure could be acted upon to improve management, avert the need for hospitalization, and possibly improve the patient's prognosis (Zsilinszka et al., 2017).

There are many different precipitating factors that can cause an episode of acute heart failure from stable heart failure, including arrhythmias, respiratory infection or other infections, nonadherence to medication, nonadherence to diet and fluids, ischemia and angina, heart failure disease progression, worsening renal function, valvular disease, hypertension, anemia, chronic obstructive pulmonary disease, or asthma; in many cases the cause is unknown. However, whatever the precipitating factor, signs of congestion are the most common presentation of acute heart failure. Outright cases of very low cardiac output, that is, cardiogenic shock, are much less common. Congestion and fluid buildup have therefore been seen as the common pathway to acute heart failure and a crucial monitoring target.

In particular, fluid buildup in the lungs is crucial to avoid. Increased pressures in the lung capillaries increase the fluid in the interstitial space of the lung, and if the lung interstitial buffer is overloaded with fluids, then fluids start leaking out into the air spaces of the lung, the alveoli, hindering the red blood cells from exchanging carbon dioxide for oxygen (Fig. 3.6). This situation can turn into a medical emergency, as it can lead to a deteriorating spiral with decreasing oxygenation starving the already weakened heart muscle and other organs. In turn, this leads to further neurohormonal activation with higher pressures and more fluids transuding to the air spaces, ultimately suffocating the patient unless rapid intervention is initiated.

Systems to monitor increasing congestion include implanted pressure sensors in the lung, and monitoring this together with adjustments has shown promise in reducing hospitalization and mortality in patients with unstable symptomatic heart failure (Abraham et al., 2011). Implantable sensors require surgical intervention and may not be suitable for all patients; therefore approaches to monitoring the fluid levels indirectly by using noninvasive sensors have been researched. Higher water content increases the conductivity of the chest, and this could be measured through various setups and technologies, such as radiofrequency technology (Amir et al., 2017), a gel electrode setup (Shochat et al., 2015), multiple gel

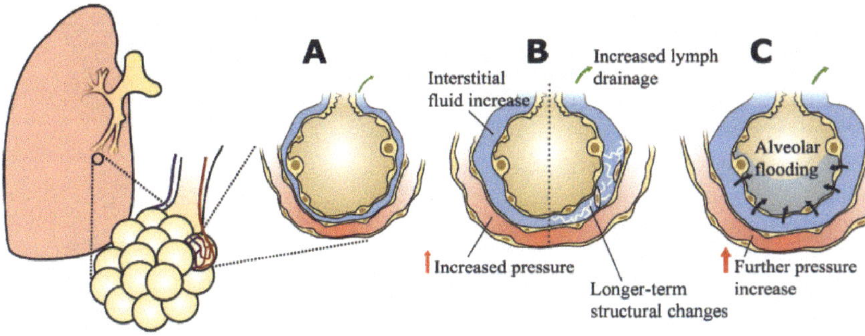

Figure 3.6 The spongelike lung tissue is made up of hundreds of millions of small bubble-shaped alveoli that connect to progressively larger air ducts. The thin walls of the alveoli and capillaries enable carbon dioxide to be exchanged for oxygen. Progression of increasing pulmonary congestion is shown from left to right. (A) Schematic representation of a normal alveolus. (B) Increasing pressure and interstitial edema with associated triggering of increased lymph drainage. (C) As fluids overload the drainage, the alveolus starts to flood and is no longer providing a site for blood to exchange carbon dioxide for oxygen. *Figure of alveolus adapted by author from source: Ware, L. B., & Matthay, M. A. Acute pulmonary edema.* New England Journal of Medicine 353*(2), 2788–2796.*

electrodes allowing impedance "imaging" (Anand et al., 2012), using the standard ECG setup of gel electrodes (Skrabal, Pichler, Gratze, & Holler, 2014), and a dry electrode wearable system (Gyllensten et al., 2016). Most of these are in a research stage. For continuous monitoring, the setup has to be patient-friendly and reliable. Furthermore, the sensor data need to be interpreted and used in a way that can lead to actionable changes in the care of the patient through either self-care or physician-directed medication changes.

Wearable monitoring of impedance presents many technical challenges. One issue is keeping electrode distances comparable and reproducible for longitudinal monitoring while allowing easy application. Another issue is ensuring even electrode coverage and reliable electrodes with limited noise to avoid impedance mismatch and other technical issues that can arise from measurements, such as parasitic capacitance and cross-talk (Ayllón, Gil-Pita, and Seoane, 2016). Nevertheless, by using algorithms to filter and detect issues together with a vest with integrated textile electrodes in a tetrapolar configuration, patients could produce reproducible measurements on their own (Fig. 3.7).

Fundamentally, measuring impedance from on-body electrodes will be affected by the chest morphology and body composition of the patient being measured. Therefore although conductivity increases and resistance

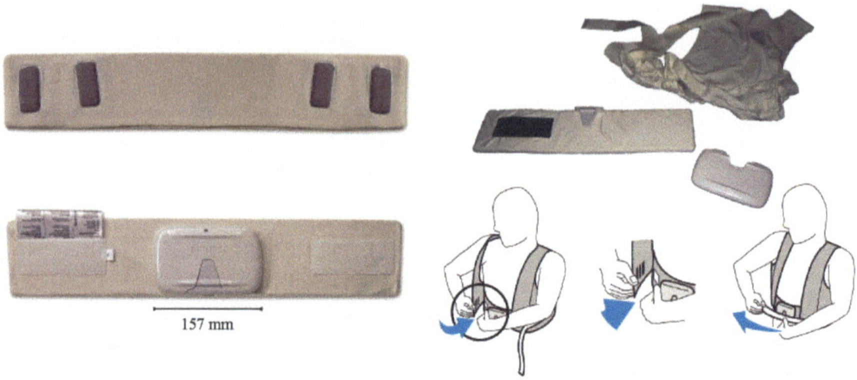

Figure 3.7 *Upper left*: The electrode belt with four textile electrodes that are placed in contact with the skin around the thorax. *Lower left*: The outside of the electrode belt connected to the measurement device box. *Upper right*: The disassembled system: electrode belt vest with strap, and measurement device box. *Lower right*: The assembly and fastening procedure for measuring thoracic bioimpedance.

of the tissue decreases with increased congestion (Fig. 3.8), absolute impedance values vary between patients (Fig. 3.9).

Tracking individual changes and detecting trends have been among the most common ways to treat longitudinal impedance measurements and avoid the baseline issue. Although this approach has shown some promise, the high false alert rate is a problem, and there is some evidence of difficulty in using trend alerts to guide care (Böhm et al., 2016; Radhakrishnan, Bowles, Hanlon, Topaz, & Chittams, 2013; Skrabal et al., 2014). When analyzing actions following calls to patients with an implanted device with impedance alerts ($N = 155$; average follow-up: 34 months), Smeets et al. found that the majority led to heart failure education compared to an intervention (411 vs 87), and among the interventions only half led to medication changes and half to further consultation (Smeets et al., 2017).

An underexplored avenue is to try to establish reference values by incorporating complementary measurements to the bioimpedance measurement. Mathematical models from baseline characteristics have seen some recent work (Cuba-Gyllensten et al., 2016; Rezaeieh, Zamani, Bialkowski, & Abbosh, 2017; Shochat et al., 2015). Yet heart failure patients are regularly seen in the hospital for follow-up, and much data are captured at admission, where available tests can be quite comprehensive, including chest X-rays, ultrasound B-lines, and clinical assessment. These can all be used to tailor reference values for impedance measurements and to connect the care circle closer to the home for the patient.

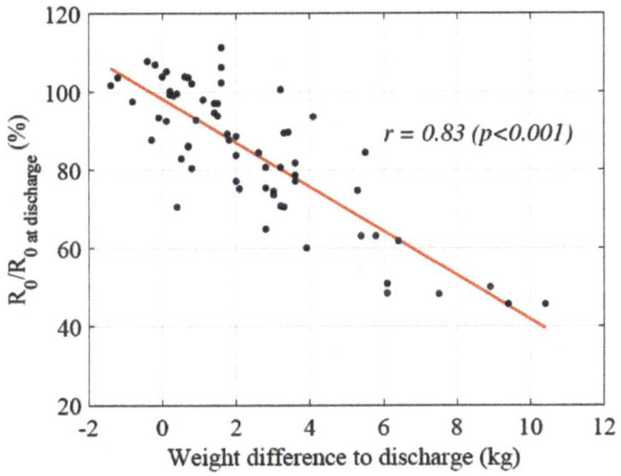

Figure 3.8 Weight (fluid) loss versus relative impedance change in hospitalized acute heart failure patients during treatment.

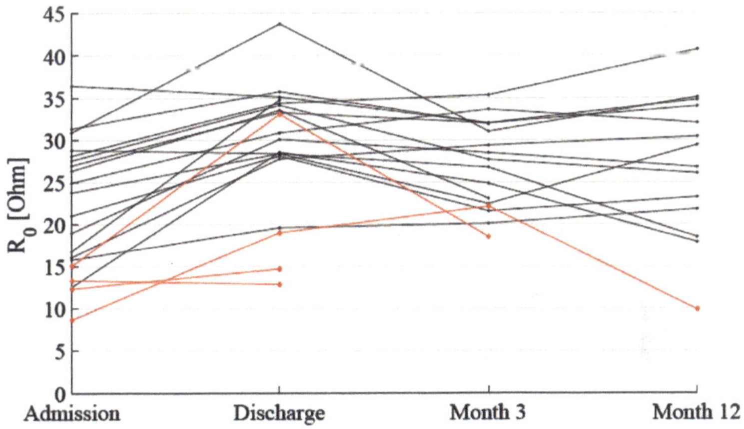

Figure 3.9 Absolute values of impedance from admission to 12-month follow-up.

Currently, there is plenty of evidence that impedance can track and provide insights into the patient's state and the risk of worsening heart failure better than common clinical tools such as weight gain. Furthermore, this measurement can be implemented in a smart textile solution and tracked by patients themselves (Darling et al., 2017). Yet its use for clinical guidance and improving patient care has not yet been realized. The stage is set for an integrated solution that could provide the next level of remote monitoring and the next step in heart failure care.

Example 2: Atrial fibrillation detection based on photoplethysmography with a smart watch.

Arrhythmia is a common cardiac condition characterized by an abnormal or irregular heartbeat pattern. In a healthy person the heart contraction is initiated by an electrical impulse generated in the right atrium that propagates as an action potential of the heart muscle cells to trigger synchronous contraction of the heart chambers and deliver blood, oxygen, and nutrients to the peripheral organs. In patients who are affected by arrhythmia, this process is disrupted by uncoordinated excitation of the heart muscle cells or by interruption in the propagation of the action potential from the atrium to the ventricle. The most common type of arrhythmia in the population is atrial fibrillation. Atrial fibrillation is a pathological condition in which the heart contraction is triggered by excitation of multiple locations of the atrium, as represented in Fig. 3.10. This causes quivering of the upper chambers and an irregular and fast contraction of the ventricles.

Atrial fibrillation results in a compromised pumping function of the heart. There is a high risk of blood clotting in the atrium, owing to stagnation of blood, and the patient may perceive symptoms such as palpitations, fatigue, and breathlessness. However, it is not uncommon for

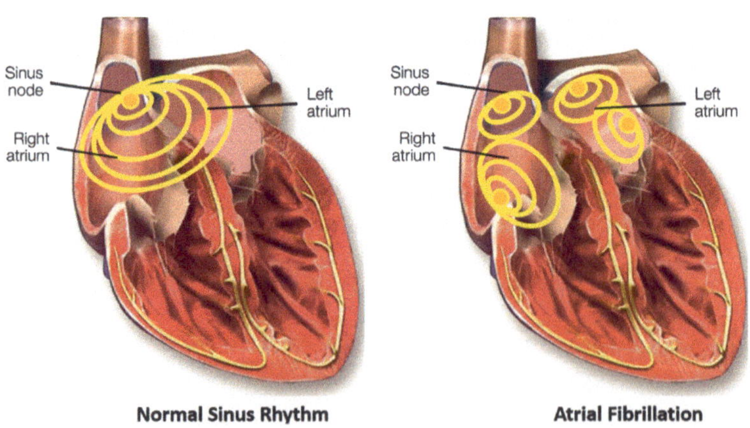

Figure 3.10 Visual representation of the atrial electrical activity in normal sinus rhythm condition (*left*) and during atrial fibrillation (*right*). As can be seen, during atrial fibrillation a common type of arrhythmia, atrial electrical activity is governed by electrical impulses generated outside the sinus node, causing asynchronous contraction of the upper atrial chambers and irregular propagation of the impulse to the ventricles via the AV node.

physicians to encounter patients who do not perceive any symptoms of atrial fibrillation. Atrial fibrillation is often first discovered in elderly individuals incidentally during routine pulse palpation or BP testing at the doctor's office. For this reason, atrial fibrillation is known to be a silent condition with serious health consequences for the patient.

It is estimated that about four million people in Europe suffer from atrial fibrillation. Atrial fibrillation is a growing problem in our aging society because of its large incidence in the elderly. Fig. 3.11 shows the number of patients with diagnosed AF in relation to their age in the United States. After the age of 60 the incidence of atrial fibrillation rises sharply. It has been projected that because of our aging society and the increased survival from cardiovascular diseases, the population of patients with atrial fibrillation will double within 5 years.

Identifying a single major root cause of atrial fibrillation is impossible. Several factors seem to be strongly linked with onset of atrial fibrillation. Some of these factors are age, high BP, and coronary and valve diseases. Obesity, diabetes, sleep apnea, alcohol, use and sedentary behavior, which are factors that worsen a person's heart health, are also potential risk factors for atrial fibrillation. The major health consequences of atrial fibrillation are that it sharply increases the risk for embolic stroke by five times,

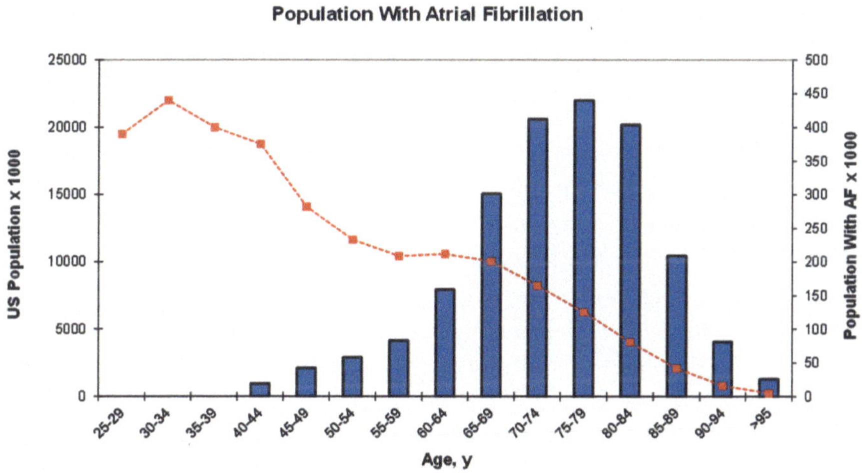

Figure 3.11 Data on the incidence and total size of the patient population having a diagnosis for atrial fibrillation in the United States. *The graph is based on data published by Feinberg, W. M., Blackshear, J. L., Laupacis, A., Kronmal, R., &Hart, R. G. (1995). Prevalence, age distribution, and gender of patients with atrial fibrillation.* Analysis and Implications Archives of Internal Medicine, 155*(5), 469–473.*

leads to increased hospitalization and readmission rates for cardiac patients, and contributes to worsening heart failure. For this reason, widespread screening of atrial fibrillation has been the target of several national initiatives to reduce stroke risk and mitigate the unsustainable societal and healthcare costs of the condition.

Several sensor-based solutions are available to screen and diagnose patients for atrial fibrillation. These differ in terms of cost, monitoring duration, and diagnostic quality. The most accurate and relatively cheap solution for diagnosis of atrial fibrillation is represented by multilead (typically 12 leads) ECG testing with the patient resting in the doctor's office. Portable ambulatory ECG monitoring devices have also been developed to allow for prolonged detection of atrial fibrillation in free-living conditions. Alternative solutions to enable the documentation of arrhythmias for several weeks up to years are represented by implantable ECG monitoring devices. However, they are typically expensive and therefore are not widely used in the patient population. All these ECG-based diagnostic systems aim to measure and document heart rhythm irregularities as well as the atrial electrical activity. Increased monitoring duration is a key requirement to capture sporadic and intermittent (paroxysmal) atrial fibrillation episodes. This need for long-term monitoring was stressed for the first time by the CRYSTAL AF trial, which showed a large difference in the capacity to diagnose AF in stroke survivors between implantable and periodic 24-hour Holter testing. Twelve times more patients were found to suffer from atrial fibrillation when using implantable devices to monitor heart rhythm than when clinical spot checks with Holter were done.

The asymptomatic and sporadic nature of atrial fibrillation poses the need for long-term and unobtrusive patient monitoring. New advances in personal health monitoring technologies coupled to smartphone systems are now allowing for frequent cardiac monitoring, providing options for more effective diagnosis of atrial fibrillation. A few examples include the use of smartphone camera and flashlight to measure the irregularity of cardiac pulse via finger PPG and detect atrial fibrillation or ECG monitoring systems connected to smartphones for real-time signal analysis and ECG transmission for expert review.

Smart wearable devices such as smart watches and health bands have recently been proposed as a viable means for long-term monitoring of atrial fibrillation. These systems have not yet been integrated into clinical pathways, and their clinical value is still under scrutiny by the scientific community. The quality of the measurements provided by these devices depends largely on two aspects: (1) the accuracy of atrial fibrillation detection algorithms and the propensity to offer low false positive rate and (2) the device's beat detection and noise rejection capabilities. Up to now, only one scientific report has tested the false-positive rate for atrial fibrillation detection using a wrist-wearable PPG sensor in free-living conditions (Bonomi et al., 2018). Concerns related to large false-positive behavior have been raised by the clinical community, which is directly affected by increased patient concerns due to suspicious atrial fibrillation alarms provided by the monitoring device. The signal quality depends on motion artifacts, which need to be removed before detecting heart beat irregularity and atrial fibrillation. This leads to decreased monitoring coverage in free-living conditions, owing to patient motion. Smart watches and health bands enabling long-term monitoring of arrhythmia often offer the possibility of collecting ECG documentation during cardiac events for allowing expert review of the patient data. Indeed, only ECG signals can be used for final diagnosis of atrial fibrillation. It is still unknown whether specific landmarks of disorganized atrial activity, typical of atrial fibrillation, can be extracted from the pulse waveform measured by a PPG sensor and allow clinicians to discriminate between arrhythmias for diagnostic purposes (Fig. 3.12).

Smart watches and health bands equipped with PPG sensors can also be used to accurately measure heart rate and identify episodes of heart rates that are too low (bradycardia) or too high (tachycardia) (Bonomi et al., 2017). This feature is helpful to support physicians in characterizing the patient's cardiac state during periods in which the patient is symptomatic. For example, falling or dizziness could be linked to bradycardic

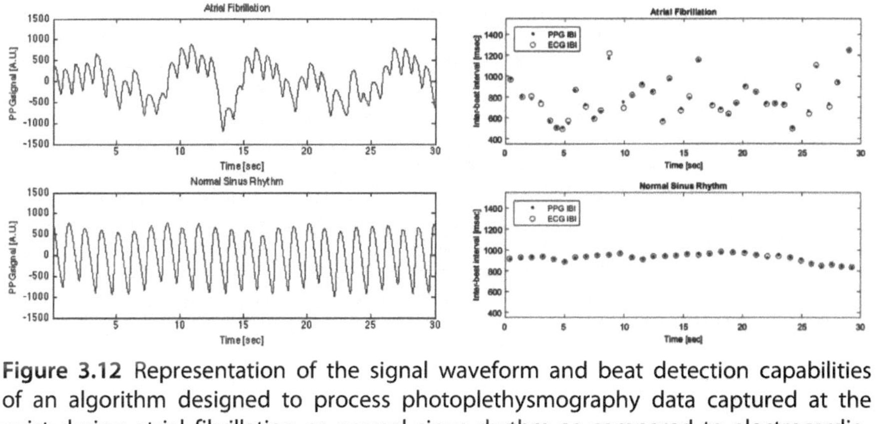

Figure 3.12 Representation of the signal waveform and beat detection capabilities of an algorithm designed to process photoplethysmography data captured at the wrist during atrial fibrillation or normal sinus rhythm as compared to electrocardiogram measurements.

events, while palpitation may be associated with tachycardia. Such correspondences between symptoms and heart rate may be used to improve medication titration.

Still underexplored is the feasibility of detecting ventricular arrhythmias with long-term monitoring devices equipped with PPG sensors. Ventricular arrhythmias such as ventricular tachycardia or ventricular fibrillation are potentially life-threatening conditions during which the patient often loses consciousness. In such situations, often leading up to cardiac arrest, prompt emergency care is necessary. The connectivity, geolocalization, and communication features offered by smart watches together with the PPG sensing modality offered by these platforms may represent a viable solution to detect life-threatening arrhythmias and prompt intervention to mitigate the risk for sudden deaths.

To conclude, the ability to screen and monitor atrial fibrillation in patients who are at risk for stroke and worsening of health due to cardiovascular disease is a clinical unmet need. Smart watches equipped with PPG technology and augmented with ECG spot-check functionalities offer an accurate solution for long-term and opportunistic atrial fibrillation detection. By combining advanced algorithms for arrhythmia detection in consumer-friendly technology, we can achieve a breakthrough in arrhythmia monitoring for improving patient management and health outcomes in individuals who are at risk for severe adverse health events related to arrhythmia.

Example 3: Body sensor network.

Advances in electronic miniaturization, power efficiency, and wireless communication allow for small, unobtrusive sensors to continuously monitor vital signs. A BSN or, alternatively, a body area network, consists of multiple, usually wireless sensors worn by the subject (Fig. 3.13). These may be attached by different means, such as with belts or adhesives, integrated into clothes, or even subcutaneously. The acquired signals are bundled together to characterize the measured subject. Use cases cover a very broad area and can range from wellness applications to operating room settings. The need for body-spanning BSNs arises because biosignals, be they distinct or homogeneous, need to be collected at different locations. Connecting these sites with cables is often not desirable, since the cables either impede daily activities or drastically interfere with medical procedures (Imhoff, 2004; Wallin & Wajntraub, 2004).

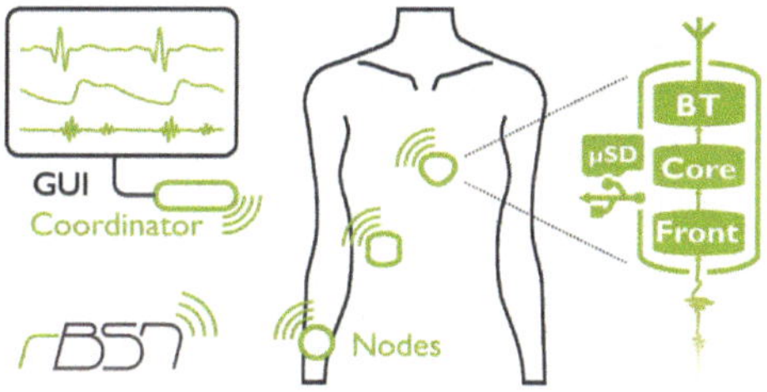

Figure 3.13 A body area network.

Because a BSN is designed to be wearable, its constituent nodes need to be compliant in application and use. Unobtrusive measurement locations and small sensors contribute to this aspect. Especially for wireless nodes, minimal power consumption is critical in long-term monitoring, such as during sleep diagnostics. Low-power devices can also be manufactured in smaller sizes, owing to their reduced battery requirements. The network architecture can theoretically take any shape, such as a fully distributed mesh or a star architecture with a master or coordinator node, depending on the use case. The hallmark of a BSN is scalability; the network enables the addition of different nodes to fulfill specific monitoring needs while maintaining synchronicity. Synchronous operation is necessary between all nodes, as the samples of different signals need to be unambiguously associated with each other (Rhee, Lee, Kim, Serpedin, & Wu, 2009; Wu, Chaudhari, & Serpedin, 2011). The jitter and drift of sampling times, prominently present in wireless networks, can be minimized and the latter even removed by using software or hardware synchronization schemes. The robustness of the system is reflected in its reliability in acquiring and storing biosignals without distortion or dropouts. Some complex or high-rate data may need processing before storage. The nodes should provide enough computing power to perform at least minimal online processing, such as downsampling and compression. The data must then be stored locally for later downloading and/or streamed over an uplink channel to a central repository. It should be kept in mind that wireless links are inherently error prone. Furthermore, streaming and communication over a wireless protocol is very power consuming; accordingly, the smaller the required bandwidth, the longer the system runtime.

There are virtually no restrictions on the node and sensor types employed in a BSN. The network can be a mix of wired or wireless, stand-alone or modular, and clustered or distributed nodes. The biosignal acquisition modalities can be either invasive or noninvasive, such as ECG, PPG, impedance plethysmography (IPG), actigraphy, and BP. With the advent of integrated analog front ends for most of the mentioned biosignals, the development and space requirements are drastically reduced. This enables small, power-efficient nodes even with multiple sensors, which return more consistent data owing to the standardized circuitry. Additionally, some or most of the digital signal processing is already taken care of on these front end chips (e.g., filtering, offset removal, fast Fourier transform), freeing the central controller for other tasks, such as compression, storage, and communication. Parameter extraction and processing usually happen after the data from all nodes have been centralized because nodes usually have no means of outputting it to the user. They may also lack the computational power to calculate them, or the processing necessitates data from multiple nodes, such as for pulse transit times.

The practical considerations in this paragraph are based on the robust Body Sensor Network developed at the Chair of Electronics and Medical Signal Processing at TU Berlin (Pflugradt et al., 2015). The network communicates and streams via the Bluetooth 5.0 protocol and is synchronized via ShockBurst technology to less than 1 μs jitter and zero long-term drift. Its star topology can flexibly accommodate up to 16 nodes, each built around a STM32L476 microcontroller for data handling and a NRF52840 SoC for Bluetooth. The power is delivered by rechargeable lithium-ion batteries, delivering an active system runtime, dependent on front end and battery capacity (1.1–7.98 Watt hours), of 12–48 hours. Sampling rates as high as 4 kHz and resolutions up to 32 bits can be reached, depending on the recorded signals. The data are always stored locally to an SD card and optionally streamed to a computer for live signal quality assessment. The measured signals include but are not limited to ECG, PPG, IPG, pressure, audio, and 9-axis actigraphy. Most of these signals are recorded by integrated analog front ends, such as the Texas Instruments AFE4490, ADS1292R, or Analog Devices AD5933, but some specialized hardware, for example, for the IPG current pumps, is designed and built in-house. The system allows these various biosignals to be measured wirelessly and robustly. Its synchronization accuracy enables long-term measurements as well as the precise calculation of signal runtimes to different anatomical locations. The possibility of using a flexible number of nodes and sensors in each setting, while retaining a consistent system behavior and data, highlights the advantages of BSNs in modern monitoring and diagnostics.

3.5 Conclusions

This chapter dealt with the typical steps for application-driven development of a monitoring solution for PHC use cases. PHC involves extending monitoring outside the classical hospital setting. It expands in-hospital care to the postdischarge phase of patients but also enables health monitoring while the patient is not in an acute phase of illness or otherwise needing intervention. In designing solutions for PHC monitoring, new and different requirements have to be met in comparison with the state-of-the-art monitoring solutions used in acute care in the hospital.

The chapter provided an overview of the different aspects that play a key role in defining the requirements and how they can be addressed. This concerns in particular a clear understanding of the disease and its treatment, complemented by the medical vital signs to be measured. Often, various sensing methods for these medical parameters are available, offering different implementations for a particular use case, such as using wearables or contactless approaches. It is important to have deep knowledge of the medical problem to be solved in order to arrive at an optimal and commercially successful solution. Also, the user experience plays an important role in acceptance of a solution, especially in monitoring situations outside of acute care. Accordingly, the wearing comfort of the device, the level of intrusiveness into daily life, and ease of handling must be taken into consideration. Cost plays another important role in all performance, usability, and technical design decisions.

In conclusion, designing PHC devices requires a comprehensive understanding of the user and system requirements. A thorough analysis of the application scenario has to be translated into options to realize the solution technically by appropriate sensing technologies and signal-processing methods. Then the selected approach has to be tailored and tested in the envisioned use case. This testing precedes the large effort that will be assigned to intensive verification and validation of the approach needed to get approval from regulatory bodies. Given the different backgrounds that need to come together in analyzing all these aspects, a multidisciplinary team is recommended for optimal solutions.

References

Abbas, A. K., Heiman, K., Orlikowsky, T., & Leonhardt, S. (2009). *Non-contact respiratory monitoring based on real-time IR-thermography*. World congress on medical physics and biomedical engineering (pp. 1306–1309). Berlin, Heidelberg: Springer, September 7–12, 2009, Munich, Germany.

Abraham, W. T., Adamson, P. B., Bourge, R. C., Aaron, M. F., Costanzo, M. R., Stevenson, L. W., & Weiner, S. (2011). Wireless pulmonary artery haemodynamic monitoring in chronic heart failure: A randomised controlled trial. *The Lancet, 377* (9766), 658–666.

Amir, O., Ben-Gal, T., Weinstein, J. M., Schliamser, J., Burkhoff, D., Abbo, A., & Abraham, W. T. (2017). Evaluation of remote dielectric sensing (ReDS) technology-guided therapy for decreasing heart failure re-hospitalizations. *International Journal of Cardiology, 240*, 279–284.

Anand, I. S., Tang, W. W., Greenberg, B. H., Chakravarthy, N., Libbus, I., & Katra, R. P. Music Investigators. (2012). Design and performance of a multisensor heart failure monitoring algorithm: Results from the multisensor monitoring in congestive heart failure (MUSIC) study. *Journal of Cardiac Failure, 18*(4), 289–295.

Atallah, L., Serteyn, A., Meftah, M., Schellekens, M., Vullings, R., Bergmans, J. W. M., ... Oetomo, S. B. (2014). Unobtrusive ECG monitoring in the NICU using a capacitive sensing array. *Physiological Measurement, 35*(5), 895.

Ayllón, D., Gil-Pita, R., & Seoane, F. (2016). Detection and classification of measurement errors in bioimpedance spectroscopy. *PLoS One, 11*(6), e0156522.

Bartula, M., Tigges, T., & Muehlsteff, J. (2013, July). Camera-based system for contactless monitoring of respiration. In *2013 35th Annual International Conference of the IEEE Engineering in Medicine and Biology Society (EMBC)* (pp. 2672–2675). IEEE.

Bonomi, A. G., Eerikäinen, L. M., Schipper, F., Aarts, R. M., de Morree, H. M., & Dekker, L. (2017). Detecting episodes of brady- and tachycardia using photoplethysmography at the wrist in free-living conditions. *Computing in Cardiology.*

Bonomi, A. G., Schipper, F., Eerikäinen, L. M., Margarito, J., van Dinther, R., Muesch, G., ... Dekker, L. R. C. (2018). Atrial fibrillation detection using a novel cardiac ambulatory monitor based on photo-plethysmography at the wrist. *Journal of the American Heart Association*, 7(15), e009351.

Brüser, C., Kerekes, A., Winter, S., & Leonhardt, S. (2012). *Multi-channel optical sensor-array for measuring ballistocardiograms and respiratory activity in bed. 2012 Annual International Conference of the IEEE Engineering in Medicine and Biology Society* (pp. 5042–5045). IEEE.

Buxi, D., Redoute, J. M., & Yuce, M. R. (2015). A survey on signals and systems in ambulatory blood pressure monitoring using pulse transit time. *Physiological Measurement, 36*(3), R1.

Böhm, M., Drexler, H., Oswald, H., Rybak, K., Bosch, R., Butter, C., ... Bimmel, D. (2016). Fluid status telemedicine alerts for heart failure: A randomized controlled trial. *European Heart Journal, 37*(41), 3154–3163.

Carvalho, P., Paiva, R. P., Couceiro, R., Henriques, J., Antunes, M., Quintal, I., ... Aubert, X. (2010). Comparison of systolic time interval measurement modalities for portable devices. In *Conference of IEEE-EMBC.*

Couceiro, R., Carvalho, P., Paiva, R. P., Henriques, J., Antunes, M., Quintal, I., & Muehlsteff, J. (2011). Beat-to-beat cardiac output inference using heart sounds. *IEEE-EMBC.*

Cuba-Gyllensten, I., Gastelurrutia, P., Bonomi, A. G., Riistama, J., Bayes-Genis, A., & Aarts, R. M. (2016). A method to adapt thoracic impedance based on chest geometry and composition to assess congestion in heart failure patients. *Medical Engineering & Physics, 38*(6), 538–546.

Darling, C. E., Dovancescu, S., Saczynski, J. S., Riistama, J., Kuniyoshi, F. S., Rock, J., ... McManus, D. D. (2017). Bioimpedance-based heart failure deterioration prediction using a prototype fluid accumulation vest-mobile phone dyad: An observational study. *JMIR Cardio, 1*(1), e1.

Emerald, From Wearables to Invisibles. https://www.emeraldinno.com/.

Erath, J. W., Vamos, M., Sirat, A. S., & Hohnloser, S. H. (2017). The wearable cardioverter-defibrillator in a real-world clinical setting: Experience in 102 consecutive patients. *Clinical Research in Cardiology*, *106*(4), 300–306.

Feinberg, W. M., Blackshear, J. L., Laupacis, A., Kronmal, R., & Hart, R. G. (1995). Prevalence, age distribution, and gender of patients with atrial fibrillation. *Analysis and Implications Archives of Internal Medicine*, *155*(5), 469–473.

Fibaro. Motion Sensor FGMS-001, Door/Window Sensor FGDW-002, Walli Outlet FGWOE/F-011. http://www.fibaro.com.

Gillebert, T., Leite-Moreira, A., & de Hert, A. (2000). Load dependent diastolic left ventricular function in heart failure. *Heart Failure Reviews*, *5*, 345–356.

Gillebert, T., Van de Veire, N., de Buyzere, M., & Sutter, J. (2004). Time intervals, global function. *Use, limitations, European Heart Journal*, *25*, 2185–2186.

Gyllensten, I. C., Bonomi, A. G., Goode, K. M., Reiter, H., Habetha, J., Amft, O., & Cleland, J. G. (2016). Early indication of decompensated heart failure in patients on home-telemonitoring: A comparison of prediction algorithms based on daily weight and noninvasive transthoracic bio-impedance. *JMIR Medical Informatics*, *4*(1), e3.

Han, J., Shao, L., Xu, D., & Shotton, J. (2013). Enhanced computer vision with microsoft kinect sensor: A review. *IEEE Transactions on Cybernetics*, *43*(5), 1318–1334.

Hassan, S., & Turner, P. (1983). Systolic time intervals: A review of the method in the non-invasive investigation of cardiac function in health, disease, clinical pharmacology. *Postgraduate Medical Journal*, *59*, 423–434.

Heude, E., Bourgin, P., Feigel, P., & Escourrou, P. (1996). Ambulatory monitoring of blood pressure disturbs sleep and raises systolic pressure at night in patients suspected of suffering from sleep-disordered breathing. *Clinical Science*, *91*(1), 45–50.

https://www.cognizant.com/whitepapers/how-providers-can-reshape-their-operations-to-master-value-based-reimbursements-codex3717.pdf.

Imhoff, M. (2004). The spaghetti syndrome revisited. *Anesthesia & Analgesia*, *98*, 566–567.

Jin, A., Yin, B., Morren, G., Duric, H., & Aarts, R. M. (2009). *Performance evaluation of a tri-axial accelerometry-based respiration monitoring for ambient assisted living. 2009 Annual International Conference of the IEEE Engineering in Medicine and Biology Society* (pp. 5677–5680). IEEE.

Komi, E. R., Roberts, J. R., & Rothberg, S. J. (2008). Measurement and analysis of grip force during a golf shot. In *Proceeding of IMechE Part P: Journal Sports Engineering and Technology* Vol. 222, (pp. 23–35).

Kraal, J. J., Van den Akker-Van Marle, M. E., Abu-Hanna, A., Stut, W., Peek, N., & Kemps, H. M. C. (2017). Clinical and cost-effectiveness of home-based cardiac rehabilitation compared to conventional, centre-based cardiac rehabilitation: Results of the FIT@Home study. *European Journal of Preventive Cardiology*, PMID: 28534417.

Majumder, S., Mondal, T., & Jamal, M. (2017). Deen, wearable sensors for remote health monitoring. *Sensors*, *17*, 130. Available from https://doi.org/10.3390/s17010130.

Muehlsteff, J., Pinter, R., & Morren, G. (2009). *Comparison of respiration rate monitoring with a low-cost doppler-radar sensor and inductive thorax-plethysmography. World Congress on Medical Physics and Biomedical Engineering* (pp. 768–771). Berlin, Heidelberg: Springer, 2009, September 7–12, Munich, Germany.

Mukkamala, R., Hahn, J. O., Inan, O. T., Mestha, L. K., Kim, C. S., Töreyin, H., & Kyal, S. (2015). Toward ubiquitous blood pressure monitoring via pulse transit time: Theory and practice. *IEEE Transactions on Biomedical Engineering*, *62*(8), 1879–1901.

Newlin, D. B., & Levenson, R. (1979). Pre-ejection period: Measuring beta-adrenergic influences upon the heart. *Psychophysiology*, *16*, 546–553.

Oh, J., & Tajik, J. (2003). The return of cardiac time intervals. The Phonix is rising. *Journal of the American College of Cardiology*, *42*(8), 1471–1474.

Op den Buijs, J., Simons, M., Golas, S., Fischer, N., Felsted, J., Schertzer, L., ... Jethwani, K. (2018). Predictive modeling of 30-day emergency hospital transport of patients using a personal emergency response system: Prognostic retrospective study. *JMIR Medical Informatics*, *6*(4), e49.

Paiva, R., Carvalho, P., Henriques, J., Antunes, M., Muehlsteff, J., & Aubert, X. (2009). Assessing PEP, LVET from heart sounds: Algorithms, evaluation. In *International Conference of the IEEE Engineering in Medicine, Biology Society*.

Pflugradt, M., Mann, S., Tigges, T., et al. (2015). Multi-modal signal acquisition using a synchronized wireless body sensor network in geriatric patients. *Biomedical Engineering /Biomedizinische Technik*, *61*(1), 57–68, Retrieved September 9, 2019, from doi: 10.1515/bmt-2014-0178.

Radhakrishnan, K., Bowles, K., Hanlon, A., Topaz, M., & Chittams, J. (2013). A retrospective study on patient characteristics and telehealth alerts indicative of key medical events for heart failure patients at a home health agency. *Telemedicine and e-Health*, *19* (9), 664–670.

Razak, A. H. A., Zayegh, A., Begg, R. K., & Wahab, Y. (2012). Foot plantar pressure measurement system: A review. *Sensors*, *12*, 9884–9912.

Rezaeieh, S. A., Zamani, A., Bialkowski, K. S., & Abbosh, A. M. (2017). Novel microwave torso scanner for thoracic fluid accumulation diagnosis and monitoring. *Scientific Reports*, 7(1), 304.

Rhee, I. K., Lee, J., Kim, J., Serpedin, E., & Wu, Y. C. (2009). Clock synchronization in wireless sensor networks: An overview. *Sensors (Basel, Switzerland)*, *9*(1), 56–85.

Robben, S., Englebienne, G., Pol, M., & Krose, B. (2012). How is grandma doing? Predicting functional health status from binary ambient sensor data. *AAAI Technical Report FS – 12-01*.

Shochat, M., Shotan, A., Blondheim, D. S., Kazatsker, M., Dahan, I., Asif, A., ... Meisel, S. R. (2015). Derivation of baseline lung impedance in chronic heart failure patients: Use for monitoring pulmonary congestion and predicting admissions for decompensation. *Journal of Clinical Monitoring and Computing*, *29*(3), 341–349.

Skrabal, F., Pichler, G. P., Gratze, G., & Holler, A. (2014). Adding "hemodynamic and fluid leads" to the ECG. Part I: The electrical estimation of BNP, chronic heart failure (CHF) and extracellular fluid (ECF) accumulation. *Medical Engineering & Physics*, *36*(7), 896–904.

Skubic, M., Alexander, G., Popescu, M., Rantz, M., & Keller, J. (2009). A smart home application to eldercare: Current status and lessons learned. *Technology and Health Care*, *17*, 183–201.

Smeets, C. J., Vranken, J., Van der Auwera, J., Verbrugge, F. H., Mullens, W., Dupont, M., ... Storms, V. (2017). Bioimpedance alerts from cardiovascular implantable electronic devices: Observational study of diagnostic relevance and clinical outcomes. *Journal of Medical Internet Research*, *19*(11), e393.

Tarassenko, L., Villarroel, M., Guazzi, A., Jorge, J., Clifton, D. A., & Pugh, C. (2014). Non-contact video-based vital sign monitoring using ambient light and autoregressive models. *Physiological Measurement*, *35*(5), 807.

Tavakolian, K. (2016). Systolic time intervals and new measurement. *methods. Cardiovascular Engineering and Technology*, 7(2), 118.

Tavel, M. (1974). *Clinical phonocardiography, external pulse recording*. Year Book Medical Publishers, Inc.

Teichmann, D., Brüser, C., Eilebrecht, B., Abbas, A., Blanik, N., & Leonhardt, S. (2012, August). Non-contact monitoring techniques-Principles and applications. In *2012 Annual International Conference of the IEEE Engineering in Medicine and Biology Society* (pp. 1302–1305). IEEE.

The National Careline, Telecare Support. http://www.thenationalcareline.org/telecare/.

Thiel, F., Kreiseler, D., & Seifert, F. (2009). Non-contact detection of myocardium's mechanical activity by ultrawideband RF-radar and interpretation applying electrocardiography. *Review of Scientific Instruments*, *80*(11), 114302.

Wallin, M. K. E. B., & Wajntraub, S. (2004). Evaluation of bluetooth as a replacement for cables in intensive care and surgery. *Anesthesia & Analgesia*, *98*, 763–767.

Walter, M., Eilebrecht, B., Wartzek, T., & Leonhardt, S. (2011). The smart car seat: Personalized monitoring of vital signs in automotive applications. *Personal and Ubiquitous Computing*, *15*(7), 707–715.

White, D. *New approaches to patient monitoring aim to deliver better care at lower costs*. https://www.usa.philips.com/healthcare/innovation/research-and-exploration/connected-sensing/connectedsensing-monitoring.

Wu, Y., Chaudhari, Q., & Serpedin, E. (2011). Clock synchronization of wireless sensor networks. *IEEE Signal Processing Magazine*, *28*(1), 124–138.

www.iso.org/standard/71161.html.

www.resmed.com/us/en/consumer/s-plus.html.

Zhang, Q., Chen, X., Fang, Z., Xue, Y., Zhan, Q., Yang, T., & Xia, S. (2017). Cuff-less blood pressure measurement using pulse arrival time and a Kalman filter. *Journal of Micromechanics and Microengineering*, *27*(2), 024002.

Zsilinszka, R., Mentz, R. J., DeVore, A. D., Eapen, Z. J., Pang, P. S., & Hernandez, A. F. (2017). Acute heart failure: Alternatives to hospitalization. *JACC. Heart Failure*, *5*(5), 329–336.

CHAPTER 4

Signal processing for cardiovascular applications in p-health

Anna Maria Bianchi, Stefania Coelli, Riccardo Lolatto, Pierluigi Reali, and Giuseppe Baselli
Department of Electronics, Information, and Bioengineering, Politecnico di Milano, Milan, Italy

4.1 Introduction

The availability of many different sensors, both wearable and integrated into the environment, allow the generation of large amounts of data, which need to be properly processed and analyzed in order to be correctly interpreted. In clinical settings, vital sign analysis is usually performed through visual inspection for limited periods of time, while for monitoring purposes, simple processing procedures are mainly utilized for alarm generation. More complex and sophisticated procedures are also applied, but this is generally done by experts, who use proper processing toolboxes in an interactive way.

In p-health applications, signal processing implies a most intensive use of automatic analyses, resulting in synthesized information for the user and, when possible, in suggestions and advice about the correct actions to take. Specific processing strategies are required, which depend on the applications and aims of the analysis and sometimes are tailored to the user's characteristics (Banaee, Ahmed, & Loutfi, 2013; Fernandez-Llatas et al., 2016). Fig. 4.1 presents the general schema for a p-health application with a typical double-loop configuration in which data are generated by means of sensors provided to the patient (Cerutti, Bianchi, Coelli, & Tacchino, 2016).

In this double-loop configuration the processing step implies completely automatic procedures for analysis and interpretation, including proper synthesis of data for feedback and visualization, and expert professionals are not constantly included in the loop. Proper data processing and classification are key elements in the schema, providing users (patients

Personalized Health Systems for Cardiovascular Disease
DOI: https://doi.org/10.1016/B978-0-12-818950-4.00007-0

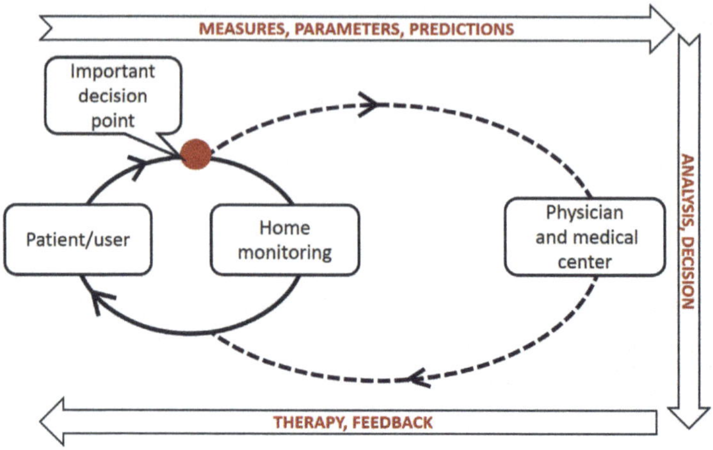

Figure 4.1 Double-loop schema for p-health applications. In the large loop (*dashed line*), raw data and extracted features are sent directly to the physician or to the clinical center to be evaluated in order to take action when necessary. In the small loop (*solid line*), the collected data are processed, and feedback is provided directly to the user. In a double-loop schema (*large arrows*), the data are collected and locally processed and classified, and feedback is then sent to the user. Only in case of need, selected data and alarms are sent to the experts. *Adapted from Cerutti, S., Bianchi, A., Coelli, S., & Tacchino, G. (2016). L'elaborazione dei segnali biomedici per ottenere parametri vitali significativi per il benessere e l'invecchiamento attivo. In Patron (Ed.),* Gruppo Nazionale di Biuoingegneria.

and/or clinicians) appropriate feedback and condensed information in presentations that can be used to suggest behaviors and therapies.

The loop between the user and the home monitoring system is chiefly about monitoring, and alarms can be added to draw the attention on selected situations. Also the loop between patient and medical centers, as well as the combination of the two loops need to incorporate an onboard "intelligence" that can automatically execute the following important functions:

- Pre-processing and noise reduction
- Extraction of relevant features from the signals
- Identification of worsening or hazard conditions
- Selection of informative time windows from the signals and, if required, transmission of data to a remote station for further interpretation
- Synthesis of the data
- Generation of alarms

- Provision of proper feedback to the user, particularly when a human expert is not involved (small loop)

Each of these items is strictly linked to specific applications, which require ad hoc implementations according to the addressed pathology, the patients' characteristics, and the available technologies. In the following paragraphs, the main strategies for signal processing in p-health applications are described. First, a general view of preprocessing and feature extraction is presented. In the following paragraphs the focus is mainly on electrocardiogram (ECG) and heart rate variability (HRV) signals, which are incorporated into a wide variety of applications in p-health systems addressed to cardiovascular patients.

4.2 Preprocessing

Signal preprocessing is intended to improve the signal-to-noise ratio (SNR) and to make the signal suitable for the following processing and feature extraction steps. Signal preprocessing takes a fundamental role in p-health applications when automatic signal evaluation is needed, as it aims to guarantee data quality, reliability of the extracted features, and high performance in the classification process.

4.2.1 Baseline and noise reduction

In the field of wearable sensors and mainly in the case of electrical signals, movements and sweating generate variations in the electrode-skin coupling, which produces motion artifacts and baseline drifts (An & Stylios, 2020). These can affect the processing procedures, such as zero-crossing and waveform detection, as well as the features that are extracted in the frequency and information domains (Banaee et al., 2013; Cohen, 1986; Pan & Tompkins, 1985a). In most of the applications a digital high-pass filter is used to remove the baseline offset. Attention must be paid to the linearity of the filter to preserve the signal waveform. On the other hand, when the information content of the very low frequencies of the signal is relevant (e.g., the mean value of a signal), more complex procedures could be required. A typical example is the ECG signal, in which the frequencies between 0.05 and 1 Hz are relevant to detect the ST interval displacement, which is associated with ischemic events. A high-pass filter applied for removal of baseline wandering could also affect the frequency range of interest; therefore baseline reduction is usually performed together with feature extraction. The baseline is estimated by interpolation (i.e., through cubic splines) of specific fiduciary points located on isoelectric values. This procedure is applied to the ongoing signal in real time or to the whole recorded signal before any other processing step. On the other hand, after selecting specific time frames for feature extraction, a second baseline elimination procedure (i.e., mean value subtraction) is recommended to guarantee the signal stationarity required for estimation of features in the time, frequency, or information domain. Fig. 4.2 shows an example of baseline wandering in an ECG signal (Sörnmo & Laguna, 2006).

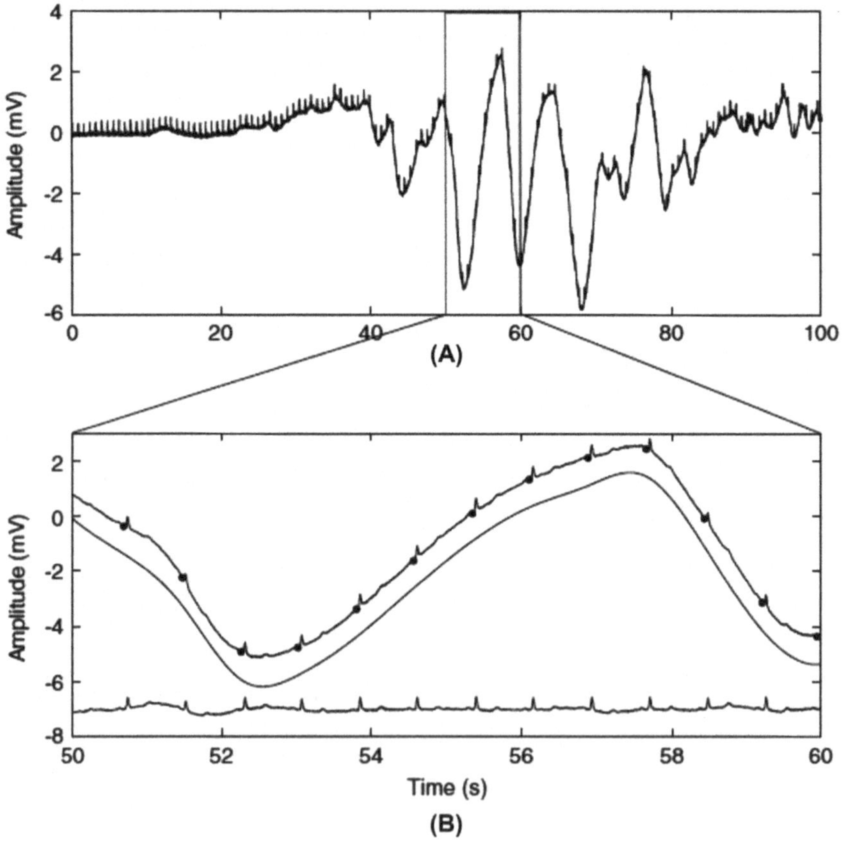

Figure 4.2 (A) The electrocardiographic (ECG) baseline wanders with large amplitude because of body movements. (B) A portion of the ECG and the estimated baseline obtained with cubic spline fitted to the series of knots (*black dots*). On the bottom, the final corrected ECG signal is shown. *From Sörnmo, L., & Laguna, P. (2006). Electrocardiogram (ECG) signal processing. In* Wiley Encyclopedia of Biomedical Engineering.

A low-pass filter is usually applied to reduce high-frequency artifacts or noise components, while notch digital filters are useful to eliminate residuals of the power line interference. In some cases, the frequency ranges of signal and noise overlap; therefore traditional filtering cannot be effectively applied. Optimal filters, including Kalman, Wiener, and Widrow filters, are useful in these situations, given that specific hypotheses on the signal and noise statistical properties and on their reciprocal interactions are fulfilled (Anderson, Moore, & Eslami, 1982). In other cases, ad hoc designs tailored to the device and the application are required.

4.2.2 Discarding corrupted frames

A signal that is extremely corrupted by noise, is absent, or is saturated could be a frequent situation in wearable or mobile devices. For this reason, it is fundamental to include procedures for the identification of artifact-contaminated signal segments that can be performed by analyzing specific waveform morphology features of the raw signals (Sukor, Redmond, & Lovell, 2011) or by comparing the extracted features with the expected variability ranges and distributions. When corrupted or missing signals are limited in time, proper interpolation allows reconstructing the missing data. It is worth noting that this is not done to recover the missing piece of information but rather is intended to make the signal more suitable for the following processing so that the results are not dependent on noise. In fact, the presence of even a few impulsive outliers in a time series or a few missing value, can strongly affect the estimation of time-domain and/or frequency-domain parameters. Median filters, as well as linear or higher-order interpolations, are used to replace the missing values. On the other hand, when the amount of corrupted signal overcomes a certain threshold, in the range of a unit percentage of the considered time frame, the best solution is to discard the frame.

4.3 Feature extraction

Many parameters (or features) can be extracted from any physiological signal. They constitute the quantitative information content and are the bases for describing, modeling, and classifying the patient's status and health condition as well as for detecting events of interest (Banaee et al., 2013). Clinical guidelines provide signal acquisition requirements (e.g., frequency bands and sampling rate) and the reference values that are usually employed in clinical settings. On the other hand, in p-health or mHealth applications the instrumentation is often unable to completely fulfill the clinical requirements, and the signals of interest are obtained in suboptimal configurations (e.g., limited frequency band in ECG or a limited number of leads in EEG). Moreover, sometimes the signals that are the gold standard in clinical application, cannot be reliably recorded at home; for example, an EEG recording is not reliable for sleep quality analysis at home, or a standard ECG lead are not aleìways possible for heart rate (Dias & Cunha, 2018). Thus it is very important to know the actual information that is possible to achieve from the available sensors and whether there are other different signals or features that correlate with the condition of interest. In that case, it is possible to use models that allow robust estimations from other available data. It is worth remembering that in p-health applications, the interest is usually more in detecting deviations from a baseline condition (physiological or pathological) than in diagnosis, which must be always performed according to clinical standards and in a clinical environment.

4.3.1 Time domain

In the case of stochastic signals, the typical features that are evaluated in the time domain are the first- or second-order statistics: mean value, variance, standard deviation, variation coefficient, autocorrelation, and cross-correlation functions (Cohen, 1986). These are reliable when the signals are properly calibrated and random variations in the offset have been properly removed. Otherwise, normalized measures are considered, and time-domain parameters are useful for evaluating variations with respect to a reference period (e.g., a baseline recorded in controlled conditions). The estimation of the above parameters requires stationarity (or pseudo-stationarity) of the signals in the considered time window, which implies that the correct choice of length of the observation window is a critical step. Often, the features are estimated on consecutive or overlapping time windows, and their time evolution is considered.

When the signals present deterministic content, common features are measured directly from signal waveforms: peak-to-peak amplitudes, peak values, time distance between peaks, areas under the curve, and so on.

A template waveform can be used for wave detection and recognition. The template is compared with the signal through different metrics that evaluate the distance (or the cross-correlation). The wave of interest is detected when the distance presents a minimum (or the cross-correlation presents a maximum). A matched filter can be used, with the impulse response obtained from the template; this is equivalent to the cross-correlation procedure. During long-lasting recordings, the waveform of interest may change in amplitude, or the baseline wandering may lead to erroneous results; therefore a signal equalization or normalization is required. Further, the waveform of interest may change with time; therefore the template should be made adaptive (e.g., the template can be a running average of the *N* last-detected waves) (Cohen, 1986; Tompkins, 2000).

The high selectivity of template-based methodologies allows detecting specific waves. They are not suitable in wearable applications where the morphology may not be a priori known (e.g., in a wearable ECG in which nonstandard leads are used or movements may alter electrode positions), and noise is often relevant. Different strategies are required that are based on other more stable characteristics of the waves. A typical example is the Pan-Tompkins algorithm for the detection of the QRS complex in the ECG (Pan & Tompkins, 1985a, 1985b), which is summarized in Fig. 4.3. The following steps are included: (1) bandpass filtering centered on the frequency content of the QRS complex; (2) the first derivative of

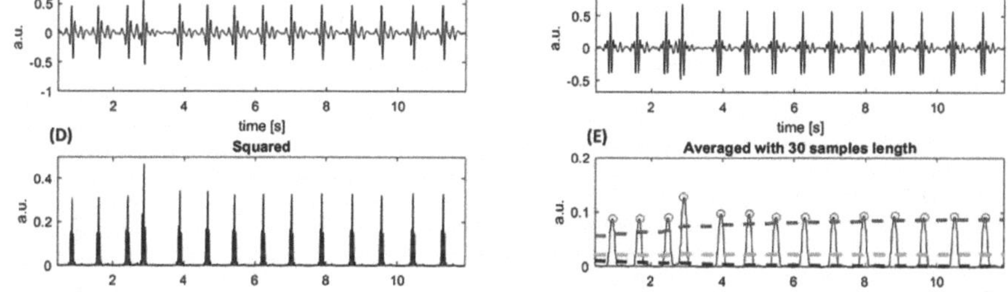

Figure 4.3 The steps of the Pan-Tompkins algorithm. The raw ECG signal (A) is band-pass filtered (B), and the derivative is calculated (C). The signal is then rectified by squaring (D) and averaging (E). The dashed lines in (D) represent the noise level (*black*), the adaptive threshold (*green*), and the signal level (*red*). *The figure was obtained using Sedghamiz, H. (2014). Complete pan tompkins implementation ECG QRS detector.*

the signal to put into evidence the high slope of the QRS; (3) making the signal all positive (absolute value or squared values are calculated); (4) low-pass filtering for obtaining a unique square wave; and (5) thresholding. The fiducial points are then obtained: R peaks as the max values on the original ECG contained in the time windows over the threshold, beginning and ending of the QRS derive from the length of the squared wave, and so on. The algorithm is also suitable for real-time implementation (Pan & Tompkins, 1985a).

Detection and time localization of specific waves correspond to the occurrence of physiological events (e.g. the cardiac beat); thus it is possible to obtain signals related to these events. The typical example is the HRV signal, or the series of the cardiac cycle duration (R-R intervals, RRI). HRV and RRI are reciprocal to one another and carry the same information. The term "HRV" is used also when the analyzed signal is RRI as defined by the Task Force of the European Society of Cardiology and the North American Society of Pacing and Electrophysiology (Task Force of the European Society, 1996). Similarly, other time series can be obtained from other signals, such as the sequence of the systolic and diastolic values from the blood pressure. Events that are detected on some specific signals are used for estimation of other data that cannot be recorded through wearable devices; an example is the time interval between the R peak on the ECG and the maximum value on the photoplethysmogram (PPG) at the periphery (e.g., at the wrist). This is the pulse transit time (PTT), which is the basis for noninvasive estimation of the blood pressure (Peter, Noury, & Cerny, 2014).

4.3.2 Frequency domain

In the analysis of processes characterized by a prevalent stochastic content, the frequency analysis provides information on how different rhythms contribute to the total variance of the signal and put into evidence and quantify the presence of specific oscillations. Two main approaches are commonly used: the nonparametric approach, which is based on the Fourier transform, and the parametric approach, which is based on the identification of a parametric model that generates the data sequence (Kay & Marple, 1981).

Nonparametric methods. The periodogram allows estimation of the power spectral density (PSD) through the direct application of the discrete

Fourier transform to the signal $s(n)$ composed of N samples (using the FFT algorithm) followed by a squaring of the resulting frequency representation $S(f)$ as in Eq. (4.1).

$$\mathrm{PSD}(f) = \frac{1}{N}|S(f)|^2 \tag{4.1}$$

where $S(f)$ is the Fourier Transform of the signal and PSD(f) is its power spectral density or spectrum. To reduce estimation variance and to obtain smoother spectra, an average of the PSDs calculated on multiple windows, consecutive or partially overlapping, is generally performed. The final result strongly depends on the number and length of the time windows in the average, on the percentage of their overlap, and on the windowing procedure (Kay & Marple, 1981).

Parametric methods. The signal is modeled as a stochastic process originated by filtering a white noise $w(0, s^2)$. In the frequency domain,

$$\mathrm{PSD}(f) = |H(f)|^2\sigma^2 \tag{4.2}$$

where σ^2 is the power (variance) of the input white noise and $H(f)$ is the frequency response of the filter. Usually, an autoregressive model in the form of Eq. (4.3),

$$H(z) = \frac{1}{\sum_{i=1}^{p} a_i z^{-i}} \tag{4.3}$$

can model a large variety of signals as a function of the model parameters a_i given that model order (p) is properly chosen (for details, see Stoica & Selen (2004)). One of the advantages of the parametric approach is that smoother PSDs are obtained and so averaging procedure is not required and shorter time frames in the signal can be analyzed, reducing the stationarity requirements. Also, a spectral decomposition is possible for an automatic calculation of the spectral power in the different frequency bands. Fig. 4.4 shows the parametric spectral estimation of the HRV signal. The correct choice of the transfer function $H(z)$ and the identification of its parameters could imply complex calculations and require a posteriori validation (Kay & Marple, 1981).

The sequence of single PSDs (parametric or nonparametric) as function of time on consecutive or overlapping frames constitutes the spectrogram and allows putting into evidence variations of the frequency content with time.

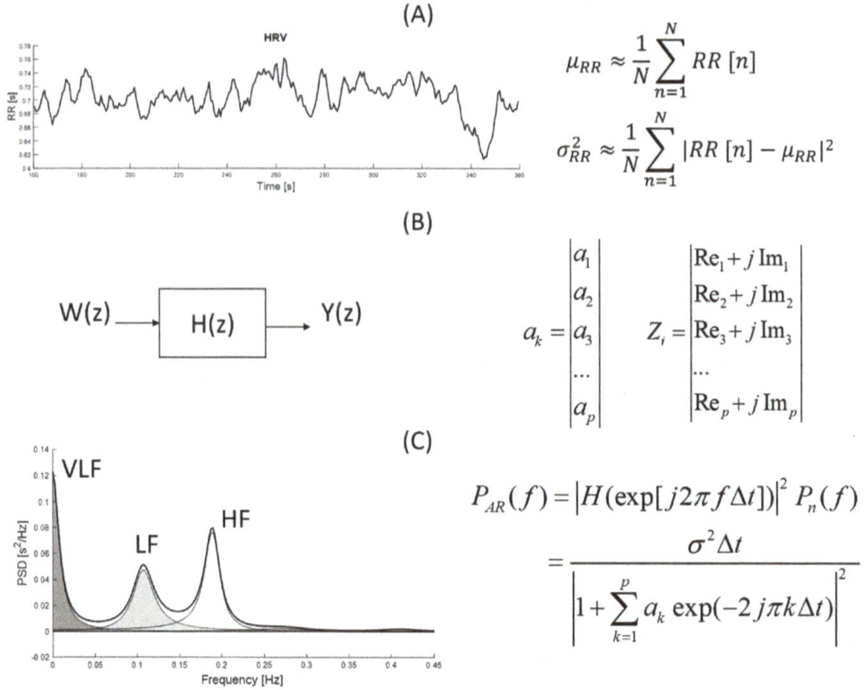

Figure 4.4 (A) The RR signal is represented as a function of the time. In the time domain it is possible to extract descriptive statistics, such as the mean (μRR) and the standard deviation $(\sigma^2{}_{RR})$ of the time series of N samples. (B) The RR can be modeled as the output of an AR model whose transfer function *H*(*z*) is described as a function of its coefficients a_k or as a function of its poles z_i. (C) The corresponding power spectral density $P_{AR}(f)$ can be then obtained, and by using the spectral decomposition method (Baselli et al., 1986) the HRV frequency components [very low frequency (VLF), low frequency (LF), and high frequency (HF)] can be extracted.

4.3.3 Information domain

Nonlinear and complexity features are often estimated for complementing the analysis of a signal. Some of them are now extensively used in biomedical applications. In particular, nonlinear and complexity measures have been shown to be useful in predicting cardiovascular events when they are applied to HRV (Henriques et al., 2020; Sassi et al., 2015).

Entropy: In information theory the complexity of a sequence can be measured with a quantity known as entropy, which represents the average information content in the sequence (Shannon, 1948). The entropy is used to measure the sequence predictability: if the entropy is low, the sequence is regular and can be predicted; if the entropy is high, the sequence is complex and cannot be predicted (Kolmogorov, 1965). The computation of the entropy needs long sequences, which are rarely available in physiological signals. Therefore metrics such as approximate entropy (ApEn) and sample entropy (SampEn) have been proposed to deal with short or midlength sequences (Sassi et al., 2015).

ApEn: Approximate entropy was introduced by Pincus (1991) as a measure of regularity and repeatability in short sequences. It was formulated as a simplified version of the Kolmogorov-Sinai entropy for nonlinear dynamic systems. Briefly, ApEn(m,r,N) of a sequence of N points is defined as the negative natural logarithm of the conditional probability that two sequences contain similar patterns of m points, with a tolerance r, for $m + 1$ points.

SampEn: The sample entropy was introduced (Richman & Moorman, 2000) as a new entropy measure SampEn(m,r,N). Again, it measures, with a tolerance r, the occurrence of patterns in a sequence, comparing them to a given one of length m. In this case it is computed as the ApEn, but the self-matches are excluded in computing the probabilities (Richman & Moorman, 2000).

In both cases, there is not a perfect rule for the selection of the parameters m and r. For HRV, r is usually considered to be in the range 10%–25% of the standard deviation of the signal, while the template length $m = 2$ is mostly used (Sassi et al., 2015)

Multiscale Entropy (MSE) was proposed to capture HRV fluctuations at different resolutions, that is, in a multiscale manner (Costa, Goldberger, & Peng, 2002). The first step in computing MSE is the construction of the coarse-grained time series. Given a time series of N points $\{xi\}$, the coarse-grained time series $\{yj(\tau)\}$, determined by the scale factor τ, is constructed as in Eq. (4.4)

$$y_j(\tau) = 1/\tau \sum\nolimits_{i=(j-1)\tau+1}^{j\tau} x_i, \text{for} 1 \le j \le N/\tau \tag{4.4}$$

For each of these new time series, an entropy measure is calculated (e.g., ApEn, SampEn), and the obtained value is plotted as a function of the coarse-graining scale factor, τ.

Lempel-Ziv Complexity (LZC): The measure of complexity introduced by Lempel and Ziv (Lempel & Ziv, 1976) assesses the so-called algorithmic complexity, which is defined as the minimum quantity of information needed to define a binary sequence. In the case of random strings, the algorithmic complexity is the length of the sequence itself (Ferrario,

Signorini, Magenes, & Cerutti, 2006; Migliorini, Mendez, & Bianchi, 2012). In fact, any compression effort will produce an information loss. The LZC quantifies the rate of new patterns arising with the temporal evolution of a sequence. To estimate the LZC for biological signals, the signal must be transformed into a symbolic sequence. This can be deconstructed to find distinct words, which are then encoded. If LZC(n) is the length of the encoded sequence, where n is the length of the sequence, the LZC can be computed as LZC(n) with $n < N$, with N the length of the series. For a totally random series a value for LZC(N) close to N is expected. The LZC in fact reflects the increase of new patterns along the sequence.

4.3.3.1 Fractal analysis

$1/f^{\alpha}$ slope or power law exponent α: Some time series are characterized by a power law spectral density (also referred to as "one-over-f") that can be expressed as $P(f) \propto 1/f\alpha$ (Cerutti, Esposti, Ferrario, Sassi, & Signorini, 2007). The computation of the exponent α of the spectrum is representative of its fractal-like behavior in the context of long-range correlation (Sassi et al., 2015). Two computational strategies have been proposed for the computation of its value (Task Force of the European Society, 1996). Both of them require the following steps:

- Compute the PSD of the time series (i.e. normal-to-normal RR intervals (NN intervals))
- Apply a robust regression in the log(power) versus log(frequency) axis in the range 10^{-4} to 10^{-2}

The exponent is the slope of this regression line. The second method (Bigger et al., 1996) also introduces the resampling of the NN interval series to regularly spaced time series and the integration of the PSD (logarithmic smoothing) over frequency with a fixed number of bins per decade. The two methods have been demonstrated to be technically equivalent.

This index is strongly correlated to the Detrended fluctuation analysis indices when a scaling law is present, but it does not permit separate analysis of the short- and long-term components, as for the DFA, which is also a method that is useful for the representation of the fractal behavior of the HRV, as is illustrated hereinafter.

Detrended fluctuation analysis (DFA): As the power law exponent, the DFA derives from the fractal analysis and is particularly suited for the analysis of scale-invariant signals (Henriques et al., 2020; Sassi et al., 2015).

Concerning application to HRV, it is often used to quantify self-similarity properties on a short scale. The DFA was introduced by Peng and coworkers in 1995 (Peng, Hausdorff, & Goldberger, 2000; Peng, Havlin, Stanley, & Goldberger, 1995) as a modified root mean square analysis of a random walk. In fact, in highly nonstationary physiological time series, the DFA permits the estimation of intrinsic self-similarity, avoiding spurious detections due to extrinsic trends. The computation algorithm starts with the integration of the time series. Next, it is divided into bins of equal length, n. In each bin, a least squares line fitting the data is estimated. Then the integrated time series is detrended by subtracting the estimated local trend in each bin. On this integrated and detrended time series, the root-mean-square fluctuation $F(n)$ is calculated. To determine the relationship between $F(n)$, the average fluctuation, and the bin size n, this computation is repeated over all time scales (bin sizes). Finally, the presence of a linear relationship on a log-log plot indicates self-similarity and a power law (fractal) scaling. The slope of the line relating $\log(F(n))$ to $\log(n)$ determines the scaling exponent.

Poincaré plot analysis: The Poincaré plot (or recurrence map) , in HRV analysis, is obtained as a scatterplot of the current R-R interval (NNn) against the preceding R-R interval (NNn-1) (Brennan, Palaniswami, & Kamen, 2002; Sassi et al., 2015). This visual quantitative tool provides information on the behavior of the heart in the function of the dispersion of points around the line of identity (Woo, Stevenson, Moser, Trelease, & Harper, 1992). The short-term variability is identified by the dispersion of the points perpendicular to the line of identity (width or SD1), which is equivalent to the standard deviation of successive differences of the RR series. The standard deviation of the RR intervals is represented by the "length," that is, the dispersion of the point along the line of identity, and it is a measure of long-term HRV (SD2). The ratio SD1/SD2 is also commonly used and is called SD12.

Information theory measures and fractal dimension analysis are highly dependent on the time series length N on which they are applied. Hence their application for p-health scenario can be challenging.

ApEN, SampEN, and MSE may be prone to inconsistency (Aktaruzzaman & Sassi, 2014), owing to the number of samples that are used to converge to the final value [e.g., 10^m or 30^m (Pincus & Goldberger, 1994)], since their results are very sensitive to the data length, particularly when $N < 200$. This issue has been faced by proposing parametric estimation of the entropy indexes (i.e., employing linear AR process), which have been shown to be useful when the series is short and free of artifacts. Anyway, the estimation reliability is dependent on the stationarity of the sequence.

Rivolta, Migliorini, Aktaruzzaman, Sassi, and Bianchi (2014) also showed the dependency of the Lempel-Ziv complexity index on the data length, suggesting the use of at least 1000 samples for a satisfactory estimation (5% of tolerance).

Also the power law exponent and the DFA reliability in HRV have been demonstrated to depend on the number of beats used for the estimation. In fact they describe the long-range correlation and long-term irregularity of a process; thus these methods are suited for the analysis of Holter signals (Cerutti et al., 2007). Of note, a short-range version of the DFA has been proposed by adjusting the range of scales (Peng et al., 1995).

4.4 Heart rate variability, a time series rich in information

Heart rate variability is a physiological time series that has much potential in p-health applications because of the noninvasivity of the measurement, the possibility of long-time monitoring through nonobtrusive devices, and its high sensitivity to the patient's status. In a complete review of the clinical use of HRV, many applications are listed as well as the features that are extensively employed in clinics and in research (Task Force of the European Society, 1996). Table 4.1 reports a list of the main HRV features with their physiological interpretation.

Fig. 4.4 shows an example of RR intervals (A) with the estimation of the mean value and variance. The AR model shown in (B) leads to the estimation of the power spectral density represented in (C). The parametric approach permits the decomposition and power estimation of the VLF (very low frequency), LF (low frequency) and HF (high frequency) components. These are associated with autonomic control exerted on the heart. HF, at the respiratory frequency, is an expression of the respiratory arrhythmia of the heart, which is mediated by the parasympathetic system through the vagal nerve; LF, centered on 0.1 Hz, is strictly linked with vascular oscillations and increases in correspondence of sympathetic activations. Thus the power associated with LF and HF components, in absolute and normalized units, as well as their ratio are good markers of the sympathovagal balance in the cardiovascular system. VLF accounts for

Table 4.1 List of commonly used features in heart rate variability analysis.

Variable	Unit	Description
Time domain: statistical measures		
SDNN	ms	Standard deviation of all NN intervals
SDANN	ms	Standard deviation of the averages of NN intervals in all 5-min segments of the entire recording
RMSSD	ms	The square root of the mean of the sum of the squares of differences between adjacent NN intervals
SDNN index	ms	Mean of the standard deviations of all NN intervals for all 5-min segments of the entire recording
SDSD	ms	Standard deviation of differences between adjacent NN intervals
NN50 count		Number of pairs of adjacent NN intervals differing by more than 50 ms in the entire recording
pNN50	%	NN50 count divided by the total number of all NN intervals
Time domain: geometric measures		
HRV triangular index		Total number of all NN intervals divided by the height of the histogram of all NN intervals measured on a discrete scale with bins of 1/128 s.
TINN	ms	Baseline width of the minimum square difference triangular interpolation of the highest peak of the histogram of all NN intervals
Differential index	ms	Difference between the widths of the histogram of differences between adjacent NN intervals measured at selected heights.
Logarithmic index	ms^{-1}	Coefficient φ of the negative exponential curve $ke - \varphi t$, which is the best approximation of the histogram of absolute differences between adjacent NN intervals
Frequency domain: short-term recordings (5 min)		
Total power	ms^2	The variance of NN intervals over the temporal segment ($f \approx \leq 0.4$ Hz)

(*Continued*)

Table 4.1 (Continued)

Variable	Unit	Description
VLF	ms^2	Power in very low frequency range ($f \leq 0.04$ Hz)
LF	ms^2	Power in low frequency range ($0.04 \leq f \leq 0.15$ Hz)
LF norm	—	LF power in normalized units: LF/(total power-VLF) × 100
HF	ms^2	Power in high frequency range ($0.15 \leq f \leq 0.4$ Hz)
HF norm	—	HF power in normalized units: HF/(total power-VLF) × 100
LF/HF		Ratio LF/HF
Frequency domain: long-term recordings (24 h)		
Total power	ms^2	Variance of all NN intervals ($f \approx \leq 0.4$ Hz)
ULF	ms^2	Power in the ultra low frequency range ($f \leq 0.003$ Hz)
VLF	ms^2	Power in the very low frequency range ($0.003 \leq f \leq 0.04$ Hz)
LF	ms^2	Power in the low frequency range ($0.04 \leq f \leq 0.15$ Hz)
HF	ms^2	Power in the high frequency range ($0.15 \leq f \leq 0.4$ Hz)
α		Slope of the linear interpolation of the spectrum in a log-log scale ($f \approx \leq 0.04$ Hz)
Information domain: nonlinear and nonstandard parameters		
DFA α2		DFA long-term scaling exponent, quantifies long-range dependence in a time series
DFA α1		DFA short-term scaling exponent, used to quantify short term complexity
Hurst exponent		Estimator for the evaluation of the self-similarity and the long-range correlation properties in a time series (1)
Poincaré plot (SD1, SD2, or SD12)	ms	Used as a graphical tool to summarize statistics, its parameters are directly related to standard temporal indices SDNN and SDSD
HRT	%	Heart rate turbulence quantify short-term fluctuation in sinus cycle length following ventricular premature complexes (2). It is quantified as % of occurrences of abnormal HRT.

(Continued)

Table 4.1 (Continued)

Variable	Unit	Description
DC/AC		Deceleration and acceleration capacity quantified using the phase-rectified signal averaging (PRSA) method
ApEn		Approximate entropy
SampEn		Sample entropy
MSE		Multiscale entropy

(1) (Hurst, 1951); (2) (Bauer et al., 2008).
Source: Adapted from Task Force of the European Society. (1996). Heart rate variability. Standards of measurement, physiological interpretation, and clinical use. *Task Force of the European Society of Cardiology and the North American Society of Pacing and Electrophysiology. European Heart Journal, 17*, 354–381. https://doi.org/10.1161/01.CIR.93.5.1043.

long-term oscillations, which include thermoregulation and long-term correlation phenomena.

An example of the application of fractal analysis to extract information from the HRV signal is shown in Fig. 4.5 (Sassi et al., 2015). It is shown that in the normal subject the spectral decay is slower than in pathological conditions. For example, the myocardial infarction (MI) is characterized by a steeper slope, meaning that the spectral exponent of a normal subject should be smaller than that of a post-MI subject. The DFA long-term exponent also shows differences in the two cases.

In HRV applications the Poincaré plots are mainly used as a graphical tool for the representation of statistical properties and to easily identify abnormalities in the RR signals (Woo et al., 1992). In Fig. 4.6 (Sassi et al., 2015) the Poincaré plot of a normal RR is compared with the one obtained from an RR characterized by the presence of ectopic beats.

4.4.1 How sampling frequency affects extracted features

In p-health applications, some aspects must be taken into consideration to provide reliable and trustable features. The first important consideration is about the signal from which the HRV is extracted. In Holter recordings and any case in which an actual ECG is available (e.g., a T-shirt with electrodes), the HRV is obtained as the series of RR time intervals. A critical aspect is related to the low sampling frequency, f_s, (or high sampling interval Δt) of the ECG, which introduces errors in the R peak detection and the following measurements (Merri, Farden, Mottley, & Titlebaum, 1990). The R peak is usually identified as the sample of the maximum value in the QRS complex (see Fig. 4.7), and an error $e(n)$

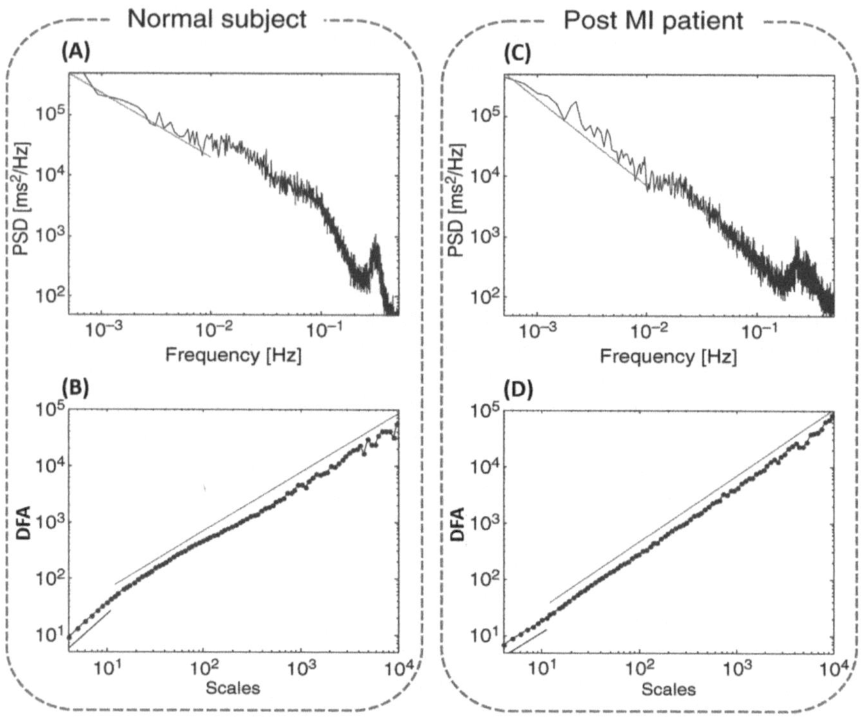

Figure 4.5 Power-law power spectral density at very low frequency (A and B) and DFA for long scales (C and D). As the frequency increases (or the scale decreases), the scaling breaks down when the higher heart rate variability spectral components become dominant. In a healthy subject (A and C), α is 1.07 and the DFA long-term exponent α_2 is equal to 1.04, while for myocardial infarction patient in (B) and (D) an $\alpha = 1.44$ and $\alpha_2 = 1.18$ are obtained. *From Sassi, R., Cerutti, S., Lombardi, F., Malik, M., Huikuri, H. V., Peng, C. -K., . . . Macfadyen, R. (2015). Advances in heart rate variability signal analysis: Joint position statement by the e-Cardiology ESC Working Group and the European Heart Rhythm Association co-endorsed by the Asia Pacific Heart Rhythm Society.* Europace: European Pacing, Arrhythmias, and Cardiac Electrophysiology: Journal of the Working Groups on Cardiac Pacing, Arrhythmias, and Cardiac Cellular Electrophysiology of the European Society of Cardiology, 17, *1341–1353.*

may occur with respect to the actual R peak. It results in a global error $d(n)$ added to the HRV signal, with zero mean and variance $\Delta t^2/6$, which affects the extracted features in the time and frequency domains.

In particular, in the frequency domain the PSD of the HRV series can be described as in Eqs. (4.5) and (4.6):

$$P_{\mathrm{mm}}(f) = P_{tt}(f) + P_{\mathrm{dd}}(f) \tag{4.5}$$

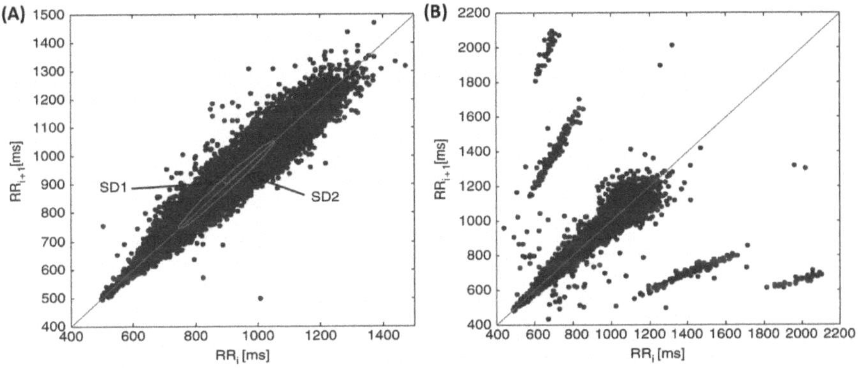

Figure 4.6 Traditional parameters SD1 and SD2 obtained from a Poincaré plot from a heart rate variability series of an healthy subject (A) and in presence of ectopic beats or other rhythm abnormalities (B). *From Sassi, R., Cerutti, S., Lombardi, F., Malik, M., Huikuri, H. V., Peng, C. -K., ... Macfadyen, R. (2015). Advances in heart rate variability signal analysis: Joint position statement by the e-Cardiology ESC Working Group and the European Heart Rhythm Association co-endorsed by the Asia Pacific Heart Rhythm Society.* Europace: European Pacing, Arrhythmias, and Cardiac Electrophysiology: Journal of the Working Groups on Cardiac Pacing, Arrhythmias, and Cardiac Cellular Electrophysiology of the European Society of Cardiology, 17, *1341–1353.*

where

$$P_{\mathrm{dd}}(f) = \frac{\Delta t^2}{6}\left[1 - \cos(2\pi f)\right] \tag{4.6}$$

This implies that the error depends on the sampling interval and on the frequency in the spectrum; thus it has more impact at higher frequencies (Merri et al., 1990). To reduce the error, interpolation procedures are recommended when it is not possible to have high sampling rates (Bianchi et al., 1993).

Wearable devices are likely to provide signals that are different from those of an ECG, such as signals from a photoplethysmogram (PPG), ballistocardiogram (BCG), or seismocardiogram (SCG). It is important to point out that their frequency content is much lower than that of an ECG, and sampling frequencies are also lower. Therefore Δt is larger with an intrinsic error in HRV parameters as described earlier. To partially solve this problem, interpolation procedures are strongly recommended in order to improve the detection of the fiducial points that are usually based on maxima and minima on the raw signals.

To date, the most commonly used method to deal with such a problem is the cubic spline interpolation of the PPG signal. This method was

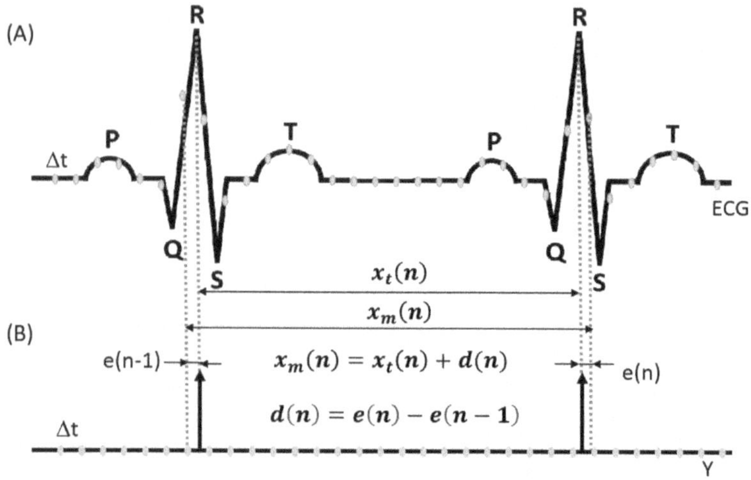

Figure 4.7 (A) simplified representation of two cardiac cycle of an ECG sampled with a sampling frequency of $1/\Delta t$. P, Q, R, S, and T indicate the conventional nomenclature of the ECG waves; $x_m(n)$ is the nth measured RR interval; $x_t(n)$ represents the true RR interval; and $e(n)$ are the measurement errors due to the finite sampling frequency. (B) Simulated ECG. The signal $Y(t)$ is obtained as a train of delta function synchronized with the occurrence of the R waves. The R peak detection is simulated by taking the samples of $Y(t)$ that are the closest to each delta function. *Adapted from Merri, M., Farden, D. C., Mottley, J. G., & Titlebaum, E. L. (1990). Sampling frequency of the electrocardiogram for spectral analysis of the heart rate variability.* IEEE Transactions on Bio-Medical Engineering 37, *99–106.*

found to adequately compensate for the loss of temporal resolution up to a sampling frequency of 20 Hz, guaranteeing accuracy similar to that of a PPG acquired at 200 Hz (Sun, Hu, Azorin-Peris, Kalawsky, & Greenwald, 2012). Alternatives to cubic spline interpolation include the approximation of signal peaks (or valleys) through regression with specific functions, for example, with a parabola approximation that can provide accuracy comparable to that of the cubic spline interpolation (Baek, Shin, Jin, & Cho, 2017). Another approach relies on fitting two distinct curves for the ascending and descending segments of the signal valleys and taking the intersection as a fiducial point. Fig. 4.8 shows an example of this method on a PPG signal sampled at 32 Hz, where the descending and ascending segments of each valley were fitted with an exponential curve and a linear curve, respectively. Table 4.2 shows the comparison among the interbeat intervals (IBI) computed on the original signal (original IBI), the IBI calculated through curve fitting (regression IBI), and RRI derived from a simultaneously acquired ECG sampled at 256 Hz. The average

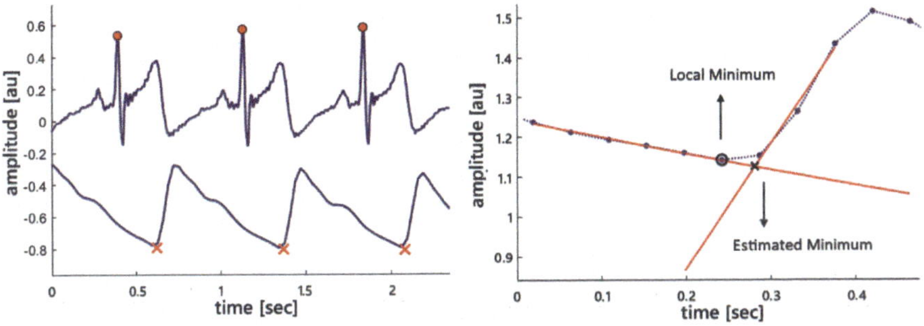

Figure 4.8 More accurate localization of photoplethysmogram (PPG) local minima through the interception of two distinct regression curves for the descending and ascending portions of the signal valleys. *Left*: Simultaneously acquired PPG and ECG signals, with highlighted R peaks (*red points*) and estimated minima (*red crosses*). *Right*: Detailed representation of a PPG valley: signal samples (*blue dots*), regression curves (*red*), local minimum directly identified on the signal (*black dot*), estimated minimum (*black cross*).

Table 4.2 Mean, standard deviation, variance, percentage difference of variance and 95% limits of agreement (LOA) of R-R intervals (RRI), regression interbeat intervals (IBI), and original IBI during rest and standing conditions.

		RRI	Regression IBI	Original IBI
Rest	Mean ± SD (ms)	740.4 ± 73.5	740.5 ± 74.6	740.5 ± 75.5
	Variance (ms^2)	5405.2	5566.4	5696.9
	95% LOA (ms)	—	± 12.3	± 27.0
Stand	Mean ± SD (ms)	600.8 ± 39.6	600.8 ± 40.4	600.9 ± 42.2
	Variance (ms^2)	1566.0	1630.5	1779.7
	95% LOA (ms)	—	± 10.6	± 26.9

SD, Standard deviation; *RRI*, R-R intervals; *IBI*, interbeat intervals; *LOA*, limits of agreement. The percentage difference of variance and the 95% LOA were computed by assuming RRI as the reference measure.

values, standard deviation, and variance, as well as the Bland-Altman 95% limits of agreement (LOA), indicate the error reduction obtained through interpolation in both resting and standing positions

Other, more robust fiducial points can be chosen, such as PPG maximum slope or PPG foot, as shown in Fig. 4.9 which are also used for the estimation of PTT.

Other signals that are often considered for HRV estimation and available on mobile systems are the ballistocardiogram (BCG) and the seismocardiogram (SCG), which are represented in Fig. 4.10A. These signals present multiphasic waveforms associated with each cardiac beat, and

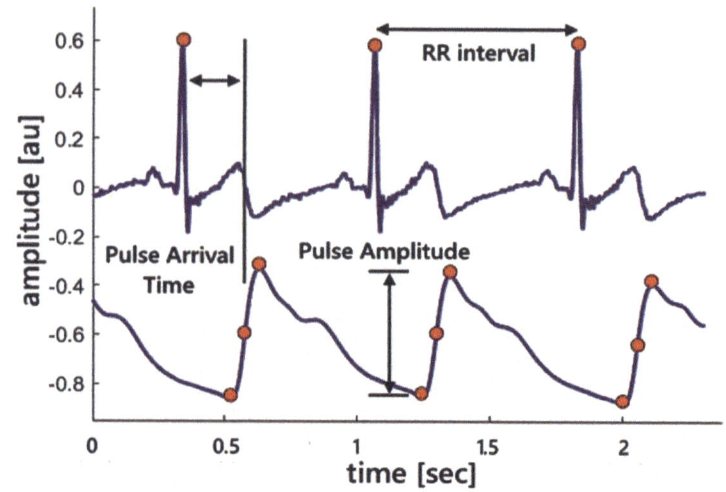

Figure 4.9 Fiducial points typically used for interbeat intervals and pulse transit time computation. photoplethysmogram (PPG) peaks and valleys can be detected directly on the signal, with algorithms that identify local maxima and minima. Instead, the maximum slope point can be detected by searching local maxima on the first derivative of the PPG signal (Chua, McDarby, & Heneghan, 2008).

maxima and minima have been associated with well-defined events in the cardiac cycle. On the other hand, the oscillating behavior makes more difficult to identify a fiducial point for the calculation of the HRV signal. For this reason, a recent paper proposed a different approach based on the estimation of the cepstrum, which is exemplified in Fig. 4.10B–D.

The cepstrum is defined as the inverse Fourier transform of the natural logarithmic of the spectrum $S_x = \{x\}$ of the signal x:

$$\text{CSP} = \text{real}(F^{-1} ln(|\text{Sx}|)) \tag{4.7}$$

Given the formulation reported by Kortelainen, Mendez, Bianchi, Matteucci, and Cerutti (2010), a peak value in the cepstrum represents a periodicity of the spectrum. Thus it provides the period of a signal, corresponding in this case to the peak located at the IBI lag time value.

It is recommended that the IBI be estimated by using a sliding window cepstrum analysis, and it was shown that if two events (heartbeats) are included in the analysis window, the interevent interval can be effectively obtained (Kortelainen et al., 2010; Migliorini et al., 2014).

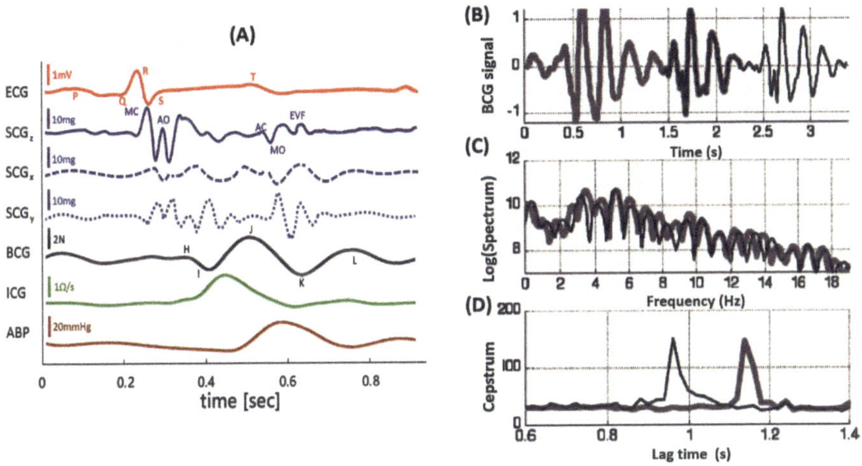

Figure 4.10 (A) Signals simultaneously acquired from one subject: ECG signal; seismocardiogram (SCG), which is provided with the dorsoventral axis (*z*), the right-to-left lateral axis (*x*), and the head-to-foot axis (*y*); ballistocardiogram (BCG); impedance cardiogram; and arterial blood pressure (ABP) measured at the finger. (B, C, and D) An example of application of the cepstrum to a BCG signal: (B) two heartbeats (*gray* and *black*) from a BCG signal are considered, (C) the corresponding spectra, and (D) the related cepstra. *(A) Adapted from Inan, O. T., Migeotte, P. -F., Park, K. —S., Etemadi, M., Tavakolian, K., Casanella, R., … Di Rienzo, M. (2015). Ballistocardiography and seismocardiography: A review of recent advances.* IEEE Journal of Biomedical and Health Informatics, 19, *1414—1427. https://doi.org/10.1109/JBHI.2014.2361732; (B—D) From Kortelainen, J. M., Mendez, M. O., Bianchi, A. M., Matteucci, M., & Cerutti, S. (2010). Sleep staging based on signals acquired through bed sensor.* IEEE Transactions on Information Technology in Biomedicine: A Publication of the IEEE Engineering in Medicine and Biology Society, 14, *776—785.*

To reduce the number of sensors that are positioned on the body and to make data collection more efficient and comfortable, an essential aspect that comes with wearable devices is the possibility of extracting as much information as possible from a single recorded signal. For example, deriving respiration activity from PPG or BCG is of great interest, both for the low cost of the devices and for their ease of use and comfort. To date, numerous techniques have been proposed to obtain the respiratory signal from PPG (e.g., see Fig. 4.11). Among these are the analysis of time-domain parameters (Lázaro, Gil, Bailón, Mincholé, & Laguna, 2013), the application of digital filters, wavelet decomposition or autoregressive models, the analysis of independent components, and the use of machine learning techniques.

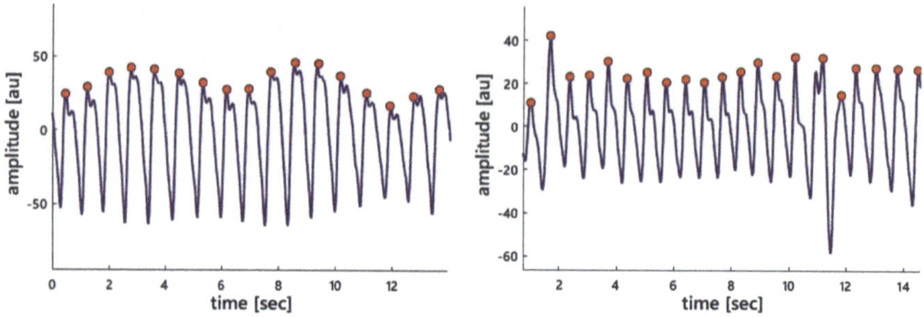

Figure 4.11 Identification of photoplethysmogram maxima in order to derive the respiratory signal. *Left*; A signal without noise. *Right*: A signal with artifacts.

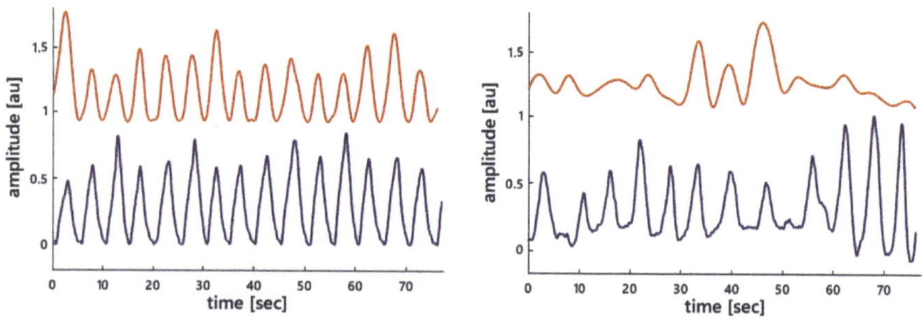

Figure 4.12 Derivation of the respiratory signal from photoplethysmogram (*orange*) and the breath signal (*blue*) acquired simultaneously by using a thoracic belt. *Left*: An example of a signal without noise. *Right*: A signal with artifacts.

Each of these methodologies shows a statistically irrelevant bias compared to the reference respiratory signal, but this happens when static conditions are considered. Indeed, the quality of the recorded PPG signal is fundamental for accurate breathing activity estimation, since high-frequency noise components would compromise its success, as shown in Figs. 4.11 and 4.12. The accuracy of such estimates was investigated in relation to the position of the PPG sensor, which can be applied on different regions of the body (Hartmann et al., 2019). These studies concluded that the best body regions are the forehead and the fingers. Interestingly, acquiring the PPG from the wrist, as is usually done by smart watches, may not always allow for a reliable estimate of the respiratory signal, owing to arm movements, which can considerably decrease the SNR of the recorded PPG signal.

4.4.1.1 *Some considerations in the use of photoplethysmogram*

In the absence of artifacts, PPG is an excellent candidate for the evaluation of cardiovascular parameters and the extraction of related signals, such as HR, HRV, and respiratory activity. However, many factors can affect the SNR and may lead to erroneous interpretation of the PPG signals, thus degrading the accuracy of the estimated parameters. For instance, the intensity of the ambient light and the subject's motion are two of the most common sources of artifacts (Allen, 2007), especially when wearable devices, such as wrist bands, are used. In recent years, many research groups have been proposing, with mixed luck, algorithms for the identification and removal of artifacts. Particular effort has been put into the improvement of wearable devices' performance, perhaps fostered by the broad diffusion of PPG wrist bands in many different applications, such as fitness, sleep, and continuous monitoring (Patel, Asch, & Volpp, 2015). However, the results achieved so far, even if promising, are still not enough to guarantee accurate estimation of HRV and cardiovascular parameters in the presence of motion, making the absence of large movements a major requirement for accurate interpretation of the obtained measures (Bent, Goldstein, Kibbe, & Dunn, 2002);(Reali, Tacchino, Rocco, Cerutti, & Bianchi, 2019) . This aspect becomes particularly important when the use of PPG wearable devices is considered for the daily life monitoring of cardiovascular patients.

4.4.2 Nonstationarity of the signals

The hypothesis of stationarity is the basis for the estimation of the features from a time series. On the other hand, stationarity in HRV, and in general in physiological signals, is not a usual condition, especially in ambulatory subjects during their daily activities. Commonly, the ongoing signals are divided into windows in which they can be considered stationary, and the features of interest are evaluated for each window. The window length should balance the need for stationarity with the need for a sufficient number of samples for the reliable estimation of the features. In literature there are several statistical tests (see Dwivedi & Subba Rao, 2011; Paparoditis, 2010; Priestley & Rao, 1969; von Sachs & Neumann, 2000) that allow the selection of approximately second-order stationary segments of signal. One of the most recent, for example, exploits wavelet analysis by examining the constancy of the computed Haar coefficients over a set of wavelet scales (Nason, 2013). It is designed to work with non-Gaussian data and is capable of identifying the location of the nonstationarities. Other tests are described by Constantine and Percival (2017). Other measures, based on time-frequency representation, such as the Kullback-Leibler divergence or the Shannon entropy, can be used to quantify the degree of nonstationarity in a time series and have been successfully applied to the EEG signal in several contexts (Núñez et al., 2017; Tong, Li, Zhu, & Thakor, 2007).

The analysis of nonstationarities is of high interest, as it provides the possibility of analyzing short and transient events. These events could be relevant, from a physiological or clinical point of view, or can describe the transition mechanisms from one stationary condition to another. For this purpose, is possible to find in the literature extensive use of linear decomposition (e.g., short-time Fourier transform and wavelet analysis) (Varanini, 2011) and quadratic (or energy) distributions belonging to the Cohen class (Mainardi, 2011), which find wide applications in HRV analysis. In addition, it is worth mentioning adaptive or time-variant autoregressive (TVAR) models, which exploit the adaptation of a recursive estimation to track varying signal characteristics. The advantage of this methodology is its suitability for real-time implementation, as the model parameters are updated each time a new sample is available.

4.4.2.1 Time-variant autoregressive model

The identification of the autoregressive (AR) parameters $\boldsymbol{a}(t)$, $t = 1, 2, \ldots, p$, of an AR model of order p, is usually performed by solving a linear prediction problem (see Fig. 4.4) based on the known time series. To obtain a new set of AR parameters each time a new sample is available, time-variant (or adaptive) algorithms must be used (Bianchi, 2011; Bianchi et al., 1993). These allow maintenance of the already known information and recursive estimation of only the innovation that the new sample is carrying to the model. Different methods for recursive parametric identification are available (Bianchi, 2011; Fortescue, Kershenbaum, & Ydstie, 1981). Using a proper forgetting factor makes the updating more dependent on the recent samples, while the older information fades, allowing the model to track changes in the signal each time the hypothesis of stationarity is not met. The vector of the model parameters is time-dependent $\boldsymbol{a}(t)$, and the signal of interest can be represented as follows:

$$y(t) = \varphi^T(t)\boldsymbol{a}(t-1) + e(t) \tag{4.8}$$

where $\varphi(t)$ is the observations vector containing p past samples and $e(t)$ is the prediction error. To update the vector of the model parameters, the recursive least squares (RLS) algorithms can be used; it is among the most used in the literature (see Bittanti and Campi (1994) for an exhaustive description of the applicable algorithms).

In RLS the model parameters are updated as follows:

$$\boldsymbol{a}(t) = \boldsymbol{a}(t-1) + \boldsymbol{K}(t)e(t) \tag{4.9}$$

where the coefficients at the current time $\boldsymbol{a}(t)$ are obtained by the sum of the ones at the previous time step and a correction term proportional to the prediction error $e(t)$ balanced by a time variant gain vector $\boldsymbol{K}(t)$.

The error is given by the difference between the current measured sample and its prediction:

$$e(t) = y(t) - \hat{y}(t) = y(t) - \varphi^T(t)\boldsymbol{a}(t-1) \tag{4.10}$$

In the RLS, it can be associated a forgetting factor $0 < \lambda \leq 1$ to weight a figure of merit J according to the relation $J = \frac{1}{t}\sum_{i=1}^{t} \lambda^{t-1} e(i)^2$. The forgetting factor exponentially weights the samples of the prediction error in the calculation of J, giving importance to the more recent samples while the oldest ones are gradually damped with a time constant, $T = 1/(1-\lambda)$, which is the "memory length" of the algorithm. Finally, by combining the RLS and the forgetting factor of choice [see Cerutti and Marchesi (2011) and Fortescue et al. (1981) for different formulations of the forgetting factor], the time variant gain $\boldsymbol{K}(t)$ can be obtained as follows:

$$\boldsymbol{K}(t) = \frac{\boldsymbol{P}(t-1)\varphi(t)}{\lambda + \varphi^T(t)\boldsymbol{P}(t-1)\varphi(t)} \tag{4.11}$$

The matrix $\boldsymbol{P}(t)$ is the inversion of the autocorrelation matrix of the signal calculated at $p+1$ lags, and it is also time variant, meaning that it can be updated at each iteration as in Eq. (4.12):

$$P(t) = \frac{1}{\lambda}\left[\boldsymbol{P}(t-1) - \frac{\boldsymbol{P}(t-1)\varphi(t)\varphi^T(t)\boldsymbol{P}(t-1)}{\lambda + \varphi^T(t)\boldsymbol{P}(t-1)\varphi(t)}\right] \tag{4.12}$$

At this point, at each new time instant it is possible to obtain a new set of parameters and to estimate the frequency content of the signal varying along time (Bianchi et al., 1993; Bianchi, Mainardi, & Cerutti, 2000).

The time-frequency approach has been found extremely useful in sleep analysis. Sleep is a physiological condition that is not uniform, as

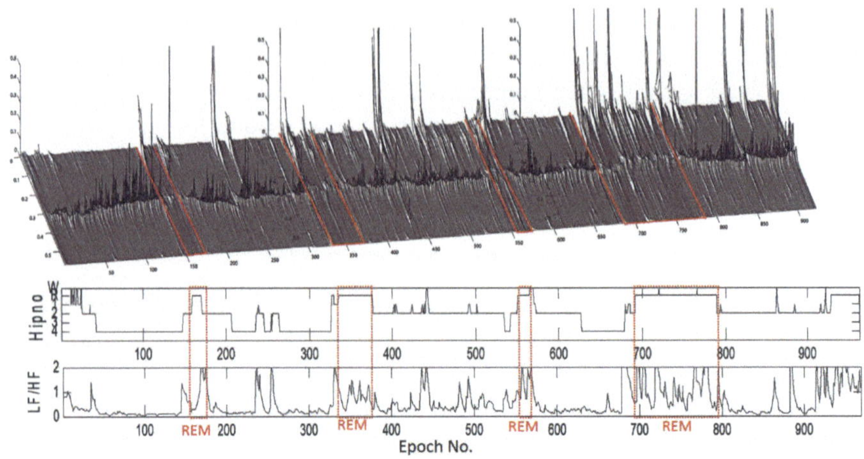

Figure 4.13 Example of time-frequency analysis of the heart rate variability signal during a night of sleep. The PSDs are obtained on a beat-to-beat bases as well as the spectral features. The low frequency (LF)/high frequency (HF) ratio is represented below the hypnogram obtained from the visual inspection of the EEG. During rapid eye movement stages, the increase in the LF/HF ratio, a marker of sympathetic activation, is clearly visible.

different sleep stages alternate and cause variations in the frequency content of the EEG and of the HRV signals. In particular, the sympathovagal balance during sleep is strongly affected by the transitions among the different sleep stages (rapid eye movement (REM) sleep and non-REM sleep classified in stages 1, 2, and 3) (Scholz, Bianchi, Cerutti, & Kubicki, 1997). Aiming for an automatic analysis, the application of TVAR methodology allows tracking changes in the frequency characteristics of the HRV signal without the need of a previous segmentation in stationary frames.

Fig. 4.13 represents the time-frequency analysis of the HRV signal recorded during a night of sleep. The PSDs are obtained on a beat-to-beat basis through the time-variant methodology, and for each cardiac beat, the spectral parameters of interest are evaluated. It is possible to recognize periods of deep sleep in which high HF is a marker of parasympathetic tone, while during REM sleep the drop in HF and the concurrent rise in LF are indices of sympathetic activation.

4.5 Conclusions

In this chapter an overview of the processing methods that are most commonly applied to biomedical signals has been presented. The applicability and pitfalls of the processing methods have also been discussed with p-health applications. Focusing on the analysis of cardiovascular-related signal methods to properly extract features from ECG, PPG, BVP, and BCG were presented, which are relevant for wearable or home monitoring devices. In particular, some common problems were presented, such as noise reduction and low sample frequency, and their effects on the extracted features were discussed. HRV parameters have been addressed with specific implementations, useful for p-health applications. This chapter provides a view of the necessary steps for correct and reliable signal analysis and the currently available procedures to reach this aim, both in a controlled clinical environment and in the patient-based health management scenario. Personal health systems are more than ever based on data acquired by using new technologies, such as wearable sensors. These inevitably introduce reliability issues that can be addressed by selecting the proper signal to be analyzed, always taking into consideration the final application, specific use cases, and clinical requirements. A key goal is to reduce as much as possible the user's intervention and create a system that can operate independently without interfering with the user's daily life while being at the same time robust and reliable. Fast or time-varying processing methods have been presented inasmuch real-time parameters extraction, in a closed-loop fashion, has become more and more required in p-health systems.

Effective continuous monitoring of physiological parameters requires the reduction of power consumption in wearable devices that are expected to uninterruptedly acquire and transmit the recorded signals. Thus also the processing procedures must be designed to operate efficiently from this point of view, and the complete system design includes choices about software and hardware related to embedded processing modules, the nature and quantity of transmitted information (sampled raw signal or extracted features), real-time or off-line processing and transmission, the amount of stored data on local devices, the amount and nature of data transmitted to the server, and local or remote processing.

There is not a general and optimal implementation for any problem. Specific solutions need to be designed for specific problems and applications, and the users' needs should be the starting point to obtain reliable and highly personalized systems to meet the requirements.

References

Aktaruzzaman, M., & Sassi, R. (2014). Parametric estimation of sample entropy in heart rate variability analysis. *Biomedical Signal Processing and Control*, *14*, 141–147. Available from https://doi.org/10.1016/j.bspc.2014.07.011.

Allen, J. (2007). Photoplethysmography and its application in clinical physiological measurement. *Physiological Measurement, 28*(3), R1−R39. Available from https://doi.org/10.1088/0967-3334/28/3/R01.

An, X., & Stylios, G. K. (2020). Comparison of motion artefact reduction methods and the implementation of adaptive motion artefact reduction in wearable electrocardiogram monitoring. *Sensors (Switzerland)*. Available from https://doi.org/10.3390/s20051468.

Anderson, B. D. O., Moore, J. B., & Eslami, M. (1982). Optimal filtering. *IEEE Transactions on Systems, Man, and Cybernetics, 12*, 235−236. Available from https://doi.org/10.1109/TSMC.1982.4308806.

Baek, H. J., Shin, J. W., Jin, G., & Cho, J. (2017). Reliability of the parabola approximation method in heart rate variability analysis using low-sampling-rate photoplethysmography. *Journal of Medical Systems, 41*. Available from https://doi.org/10.1007/s10916-017-0842-0.

Banaee, H., Ahmed, M. U., & Loutfi, A. (2013). Data mining for wearable sensors in health monitoring systems: A review of recent trends and challenges. *Sensors (Switzerland)*. Available from https://doi.org/10.3390/s131217472.

Baselli, G., Cerutti, S., Civardi, S., Liberati, D., Lombardi, F., Malliani, A., & Pagani, M. (1986). Spectral and cross-spectral analysis of heart rate and arterial blood pressure variability signals. *Computers and Biomedical Research, an International Journal*. Available from https://doi.org/10.1016/0010-4809(86)90026-1.

Bauer, A., Malik, M., Schmidt, G., Barthel, P., Bonnemeier, H., Cygankiewicz, I., … Zareba, W. (2008). Heart rate turbulence: Standards of measurement, physiological interpretation, and clinical use. International society for holter and noninvasive electrophysiology consensus. *Journal of the American College of Cardiology*. Available from https://doi.org/10.1016/j.jacc.2008.07.041.

Bent, B., Goldstein, B. A., Kibbe, W. A., & Dunn, J. P. (2002). Investigating sources of inaccuracy in wearable optical heart rate sensors. *Npj Digital Medicine, 3*(1), 1−9. Available from https://doi.org/10.1038/s41746-020-0226-6.

Bianchi, A. M. (2011). Time-variant spectral estimation. *Advanced Methods of Biomedical Signal Processing*. Available from https://doi.org/10.1002/9781118007747.ch11.

Bianchi, A. M., Mainardi, L. T., & Cerutti, S. (2000). Time-frequency analysis of biomédical signals. *Transactions of the Institute of Measurement and Control*. Available from https://doi.org/10.1177/014233120002200302.

Bianchi, A. M., Mainardi, L., Petrucci, E., Signorini, M. G., Mainardi, M., & Cerutti, S. (1993). Time-variant power spectrum analysis for the detection of transient episodes in HRV signal. *IEEE Transactions on Bio-Medical Engineering*. Available from https://doi.org/10.1109/10.212067.

Bigger, J. T., Steinman, R. C., Rolnitzky, L. M., Fleiss, J. L., Albrecht, P., & Cohen, R. J. (1996). Power law behavior of RR-interval variability in healthy middle-aged persons, patients with recent acute myocardial infarction, and patients with heart transplants. *Circulation*. Available from https://doi.org/10.1161/01.CIR.93.12.2142.

Bittanti, S., & Campi, M. (1994). Bounded error identification of time-varying parameters by RLS techniques. *IEEE Transactions on Automatic Control, 39*, 1106−1110. Available from https://doi.org/10.1109/9.284904.

Brennan, M., Palaniswami, M., & Kamen, P. (2002). Poincaré plot interpretation using a physiological model of HRV based on a network of oscillators. *American Journal of Physiology—Heart and Circulatory Physiology*. Available from https://doi.org/10.1152/ajpheart.00405.2000.

Cerutti, S., Bianchi, A., Coelli, S., & Tacchino, G. (2016). L'elaborazione dei segnali biomedici per ottenere parametri vitali significativi per il benessere e l'invecchiamento attivo. In Patron (Ed.), *Gruppo Nazionale di Biuoingegneria*. http://hdl.handle.net/11311/1040189.

Cerutti, S., Esposti, F., Ferrario, M., Sassi, R., & Signorini, M. G. (2007). Long-term invariant parameters obtained from 24-h Holter recordings: A comparison between different analysis techniques. *Chaos (Woodbury, N.Y.)*, *17*. Available from https://doi.org/10.1063/1.2437155.

Cerutti, S., & Marchesi, C. (2011). Advanced methods of biomedical signal processing. https://doi.org/10.1002/9781118007747.

Chua, C.-P., McDarby, G., & Heneghan, C. (2008). Combined electrocardiogram and photoplethysmogram measurements as an indicator of objective sleepiness. *Physiological Measurement*, *29*, 857–868. Available from https://doi.org/10.1088/0967-3334/29/8/001.

Cohen, A. (1986). *Biomedical signal processing*, . *Time and frequency domains analysis* (Vol. 1). CRC Press.

Constantine, W. L. B., & Percival, D. B. (2017). Fractal: A fractal time series modeling and analysis package R package version 1.0-3.

Costa, M., Goldberger, A. L., & Peng, C. K. (2002). Multiscale entropy analysis of complex physiologic time series. *Physical Review Letters*. Available from https://doi.org/10.1103/PhysRevLett.89.068102.

Dias, D., & Cunha, J. P. S. (2018). Wearable health devices—Vital sign monitoring, systems and technologies. *Sensors (Switzerland)*. Available from https://doi.org/10.3390/s18082414.

Dwivedi, Y., & Subba Rao, S. (2011). A test for second-order stationarity of a time series based on the discrete Fourier transform. *Journal of Time Series Analysis*, *32*, 68–91. Available from https://doi.org/10.1111/j.1467-9892.2010.00685.x.

Fernandez-Llatas, C., Martinez-Romero, A., Bianchi, A. M., Henriques, J., Carvalho, P., & Traver, V. (2016). Challenges in personalized systems for Personal Health Care. In *3rd IEEE EMBS International Conference of Biomedical Health Informatics*, BHI, 2016. https://doi.org/10.1109/BHI.2016.7455908.

Ferrario, M., Signorini, M. G., Magenes, G., & Cerutti, S. (2006). Comparison of entropy-based regularity estimators: Application to the fetal heart rate signal for the identification of fetal distress. *IEEE Transactions on Bio-Medical Engineering*, *53*, 119–125. Available from https://doi.org/10.1109/TBME.2005.859809.

Fortescue, T. R., Kershenbaum, L. S., & Ydstie, B. E. (1981). Implementation of self-tuning regulators with variable forgetting factors. *Automatica*. Available from https://doi.org/10.1016/0005-1098(81)90070-4.

Hartmann, V., Liu, H., Chen, F., Hong, W., Hughes, S., & Zheng, D. (2019). Toward accurate extraction of respiratory frequency from the photoplethysmogram: Effect of measurement site. *Frontiers in Physiology.*, *10*. Available from https://doi.org/10.3389/fphys.2019.00732.

Henriques, T., Ribeiro, M., Teixeira, A., Castro, L., Antunes, L., & Costa-Santos, C. (2020). Nonlinear methods most applied to heart-rate time series: A review. *Entropy.*, *22*, 309. Available from https://doi.org/10.3390/e22030309.

Hurst, H. E. (1951). Long-term storage capacity of reservoirs. *Transactions of the American Society of Civil Engineers*.

Inan, O. T., Migeotte, P.-F., Park, K.-S., Etemadi, M., Tavakolian, K., Casanella, R., … Di Rienzo, M. (2015). Ballistocardiography and seismocardiography: A review of recent advances. *IEEE Journal of Biomedical and Health Informatics*, *19*, 1414–1427. Available from https://doi.org/10.1109/JBHI.2014.2361732.

Kay, S. M., & Marple, S. L. (1981). Spectrum analysis—A modern perspective. *Proceedings of the IEEE*, *69*, 1380–1419. Available from https://doi.org/10.1109/PROC.1981.12184.

Kolmogorov, A. N. (1965). Three approaches to the definition of the concept of quantity of information. *IEEE Transactions on Information Theory*.

Kortelainen, J. M., Mendez, M. O., Bianchi, A. M., Matteucci, M., & Cerutti, S. (2010). Sleep staging based on signals acquired through bed sensor. *IEEE Transactions on*

Information Technology in Biomedicine: A Publication of the IEEE Engineering in Medicine and Biology Society, 14, 776–785. Available from https://doi.org/10.1109/TITB.2010.2044797.

Lempel, A., & Ziv, J. (1976). On the complexity of finite sequences. *IEEE Transactions on Information Theory*. Available from https://doi.org/10.1109/TIT.1976.1055501.

Lázaro, J., Gil, E., Bailón, R., Mincholé, A., & Laguna, P. (2013). Deriving respiration from photoplethysmographic pulse width. *Medical & Biological Engineering & Computing, 51*, 233–242. Available from https://doi.org/10.1007/s11517-012-0954-0.

Mainardi, L. (2011). Quadratic time-frequency representation. *Advanced Methods of Biomedical Signal Processing*. Available from https://doi.org/10.1002/9781118007747.ch10.

Merri, M., Farden, D. C., Mottley, J. G., & Titlebaum, E. L. (1990). Sampling frequency of the electrocardiogram for spectral analysis of the heart rate variability. *IEEE Transactions on Bio-Medical Engineering, 37*, 99–106. Available from https://doi.org/10.1109/10.43621.

Migliorini, M., Kortelainen, J. M., Pärkkä, J., Tenhunen, M., Himanen, S. L., & Bianchi, A. M. (2014). Monitoring nocturnal heart rate with bed sensor. *Methods of Information in Medicine*. Available from https://doi.org/10.3414/ME13-02-0053.

Migliorini, M., Mendez, M. O., & Bianchi, A. M. (2012). Study of heart rate variability in bipolar disorder: Linear and non-linear parameters during sleep. *Frontiers in Neuroengineering*. Available from https://doi.org/10.3389/fneng.2011.00022.

Nason, G. (2013). A test for second-order stationarity and approximate confidence intervals for localized autocovariances for locally stationary time series. *Journal of the Royal Statistical Society Series B (Statistical Methodology)*. Available from https://doi.org/10.1111/rssb.12015.

Núñez, P., Poza, J., Bachiller, A., Gomez-Pilar, J., Lubeiro, A., Molina, V., & Hornero, R. (2017). Exploring non- stationarity patterns in schizophrenia: Neural reorganization abnormalities in the alpha band. *Journal of Neural Engineering, 14*. Available from https://doi.org/10.1088/1741-2552/aa6e05.

Pan, J., & Tompkins, W. J. (1985a). A real-time QRS detection algorithm. *IEEE Transactions on Bio-Medical Engineering*. Available from https://doi.org/10.1109/TBME.1985.325532.

Pan, J., & Tompkins, W. J. (1985b). A simple real-time QRS detection algorithm a real-time QRS detection algorithm. *IEEE Transactions on Bio-Medical Engineering*. Available from https://doi.org/10.1109/IEMBS.1996.647473.

Paparoditis, E. (2010). Validating stationarity assumptions in time series analysis by rolling local periodograms. *Journal of the American Statistical Association, 105*, 839–851. Available from https://doi.org/10.1198/jasa.2010.tm08243.

Patel, M., Asch, D., & Volpp, K. (2015). Wearable devices as facilitators, not drivers, of health behavior change. *JAMA : The Journal of the American Medical Association, 19104* (5), 2–3. Available from https://doi.org/10.1001/jama.2014.14781.

Peng, C., Hausdorff, J. M., & Goldberger, A. L. (2000). *Fractal mechanisms in neuronal control: Human heartbeat and gait dynamics in health and disease. Self-organized biological dynamics and nonlinear control* (pp. 66–96). Cambridge University Press. Available from https://doi.org/10.1017/CBO9780511535338.006.

Peng, C. K., Havlin, S., Stanley, H. E., & Goldberger, A. L. (1995). Quantification of scaling exponents and crossover phenomena in nonstationary heartbeat time series. *Chaos (Woodbury, N.Y.)*. Available from https://doi.org/10.1063/1.166141.

Peter, L., Noury, N., & Cerny, M. (2014). A review of methods for non-invasive and continuous blood pressure monitoring: Pulse transit time method is promising? *IRBM*. Available from https://doi.org/10.1016/j.irbm.2014.07.002.

Pincus, S. M. (1991). Approximate entropy as a measure of system complexity. *Proceedings of the National Academy of Sciences United States A*. Available from https://doi.org/10.1073/pnas.88.6.2297.

Pincus, S. M., & Goldberger, A. L. (1994). Physiological time-series analysis: What does regularity quantify? *American Journal of Physiology—Heart and Circulatory Physiology, 266*. Available from https://doi.org/10.1152/ajpheart.1994.266.4.h1643.

Priestley, M. B., & Rao, T. S. (1969). A test for non-stationarity of time-series. *Journal of the Royal Statistical Society: Series B, 31*, 140–149. Available from https://doi.org/10.1111/j.2517-6161.1969.tb00775.x.

Reali, P., Tacchino, G., Rocco, G., Cerutti, S., & Bianchi, A. M. (2019). Heart Rate Variability from Wearables : A Comparative Analysis Among Standard ECG, a Smart Shirt and a Wristband. *PHealth 2019*, 128–133. Available from https://doi.org/10.3233/978-1-61499-975-1-128.

Richman, J. S., & Moorman, J. R. (2000). Physiological time-series analysis using approximate and sample entropy. *American Journal of Physiology—Heart and Circulatory Physiology*. Available from https://doi.org/10.1152/ajpheart.2000.278.6.h2039.

Rivolta, M. W., Migliorini, M., Aktaruzzaman, M., Sassi, R., & Bianchi, A. M. (2014). Effects of the series length on Lempel-Ziv Complexity during sleep. In *2014 36th Annual International Conference of the IEEE Engineering in Medicine and Biology Society*. EMBC 2014 (pp. 693–696). https://doi.org/10.1109/EMBC.2014.6943685.

von Sachs, R., & Neumann, M. H. (2000). A wavelet-based test for stationarity. *Journal of Time Series Analysis, 21*, 597–613. Available from https://doi.org/10.1111/1467-9892.00200.

Sassi, R., Cerutti, S., Lombardi, F., Malik, M., Huikuri, H. V., Peng, C.-K., ... Macfadyen, R. (2015). Advances in heart rate variability signal analysis: Joint position statement by the e-Cardiology ESC Working Group and the European Heart Rhythm Association co endorsed by the Asia Pacific Heart Rhythm Society. *Europace: European Pacing, Arrhythmias, and Cardiac Electrophysiology: Journal of the Working Groups on Cardiac Pacing, Arrhythmias, and Cardiac Cellular Electrophysiology of the European Society of Cardiology, 17*, 1341–1353. Available from https://doi.org/10.1093/europace/euv015.

Scholz, U. J., Bianchi, A. M., Cerutti, S., & Kubicki, S. (1997). Vegetative background of sleepspectral analysis of the heart rate variability. *Physiology & Behavior, 62*, 1037–1043. Available from https://doi.org/10.1016/S0031-9384(97)00234-5.

Sedghamiz, H. (2014). *Complete pan tompkins implementation ECG QRS detector*. Available from ww2.mathworks.cn.

Shannon, C. E. (1948). A mathematical theory of communication. *Bell Labs Technical Journal, 27*, 379–423. Available from https://doi.org/10.1002/j.1538-7305.1948.tb01338.x.

Stoica, P., & Selen, Y. (2004). Model-order selection. *IEEE Signal Processing Magazine, 21*, 36–47. Available from https://doi.org/10.1109/MSP.2004.1311138.

Sukor, J. A., Redmond, S. J., & Lovell, N. H. (2011). Signal quality measures for pulse oximetry through waveform morphology analysis. *Physiological Measurement, 32*, 369–384. Available from https://doi.org/10.1088/0967-3334/32/3/008.

Sun, Y., Hu, S., Azorin-Peris, V., Kalawsky, R., & Greenwald, S. (2012). Noncontact imaging photoplethysmography to effectively access pulse rate variability. *Journal of Biomedical Optics, 18*, 061205. Available from https://doi.org/10.1117/1.jbo.18.6.061205.

Sörnmo, L., & Laguna, P. (2006). Electrocardiogram (ECG) signal processing. *Wiley Encyclopedia of Biomedical Engineering*. Available from https://doi.org/10.1002/9780471740360.ebs1482.

Task Force of the European Society. (1996). Heart rate variability. Standards of measurement, physiological interpretation, and clinical use. Task Force of the European Society of Cardiology and the North American Society of Pacing and Electrophysiology. *European Heart Journal, 17*, 354–381. Available from https://doi.org/10.1161/01.CIR.93.5.1043.

Tompkins, W. J. (2000). *Biomedical digital signal processing*. Available from https://doi.org/10.1007/SpringerReference_12454.

Tong, S., Li, Z., Zhu, Y., & Thakor, N. V. (2007). Describing the nonstationarity level of neurological signals based on quantifications of time-frequency representation. *IEEE Transactions on bio-medical Engineering*, *54*, 1780−1785. Available from https://doi.org/10.1109/TBME.2007.893497.

Varanini, M. (2011). Linear time-frequency representation. *Advanced Methods of Biomedical Signal Processing*. Available from https://doi.org/10.1002/9781118007747.ch9.

Woo, M. A., Stevenson, W. G., Moser, D. K., Trelease, R. B., & Harper, R. M. (1992). Patterns of beat-to-beat heart rate variability in advanced heart failure. *American Heart Journal*, *123*, 704−710. Available from https://doi.org/10.1016/0002-8703(92)90510-3.

CHAPTER 5

Models for risk assessment and stratification

Teresa Rocha[1], Simão Paredes[1], Paulo de Carvalho[2], and Jorge Henriques[2]
[1]Department of Informatics and Systems, Polytechnic Institute of Engineering; Center for Informatics and Systems of the University of Coimbra, Department of Informatics Engineering, University of Coimbra, Coimbra, Portugal
[2]Center for Informatics and Systems of the University of Coimbra, Department of Informatics Engineering, University of Coimbra, Coimbra, Portugal

5.1 Introduction

Personal health (p-health) systems are patient-centered health management systems for remote management of diseases outside of hospitals and care centers. In the next decades these systems will allow a disruptive change in healthcare provision by allowing effective implementation of preventive health management strategies, keeping patients in clinical safe zones, improving quality of life, and increasing health system sustainability.

In particular, the data that are collected by using p-health solutions, together with other sources of information (clinical evidence, electronic health records, genetics, etc.), offer new opportunities for the management of chronic diseases and their comorbidities. Appropriate data analysis algorithms and models are of particular importance. The planning of optimized interventions as well as the development and implementation of prediction models and visualization tools are important to complement the available technologies. These algorithms and models are fundamental in order to fully achieve the potential of the data and therefore to extract significant information from it. In effect, they are fundamental to implementing and validating personalized algorithms and models that are capable of supporting and improving clinical decisions and stimulating the motivation of patients not only to be compliant with treatment regimens, but also to adopt beneficial lifestyles, therefore contributing to their own quality of life.

Among chronic diseases, cardiovascular diseases (CVDs) are the world's primary cause of death. According to the World Health Organization, CVDs are the cause of 17.1 million deaths per year, and it is estimated that the number of people who die from CVDs will increase to 23.3 million by

Personalized Health Systems for Cardiovascular Disease
DOI: https://doi.org/10.1016/B978-0-12-818950-4.00003-3

2030 (WHO, 2017). On the other hand, it is recognized that a person's cardiovascular condition is strongly linked to behavior and lifestyle. Therefore the focus of modern medicine should be on prevention, recognized by clinical professionals as the right approach to avoid the disease from happening. Therefore the prompt diagnosis of CVD and the proper prognosis for populations are key factors to reduce their clinical, social, and economic costs. In this scenario the development of advanced algorithms and models for patient stratification, diagnosis, risk assessment, and prognosis, providing an effective support for clinical decision making, are of fundamental importance.

This chapter focuses on algorithms and models to determine stratification, risk assessment, and prognosis. Although these results are generic and may be applied in several fields, they have been particularly integrated into innovative solutions in p-health scenarios, with specific application to CVD management and situations of preventive medicine. The main applications have been focused on the development of stratification and short- and long-term cardiovascular risk assessment models in the context of heart failure and coronary artery disease. These applications have also addressed the development of dynamic models to support the progression and early detection of relevant clinical conditions, such as hypotensive and hypertension states and prediction of decompensation in heart failure.

5.2 Risk assessment and stratification

To adequately stratify the populations, clinical guidelines recommend the use of CVD risk assessment tools in daily clinical practice. In fact, the correct CVD risk assessment, that is, the evaluation of the probability of occurrence of an event given the patient's past and current risk factors, is acknowledged as a decisive contributor to support clinical decision making.

Clinical risk scores that are currently available in clinical practice were created on the basis of long-term surveillance of populations. By means of this monitoring, it is possible to create stratification models to estimate the likelihood of developing a CVD over a period of time (typically months or years) according to the person's risk variables. Two main types of risks can be commonly computed: absolute and relative. The first (absolute) estimates the probability of developing an event for an individual over a given period of time. The second (relative) estimates the risk based on the comparison with a healthy person (with no risk) of the same age and gender over a given period of time (D'Agostino et al., 2008; Tang et al., 2007).

Although there are several ways to classify risk scores, a common approach includes two types: long-term and short-term risk scores. Long-term risk tools consider a period of years; short-term risk tools consider a period of months. For both cases, these risks can be applied to numerous CVDs and clinical conditions, such as risk of death, risk of a new myocardial infarction event, or risk of rehospitalization. Examples of long-term risk tools are the Framingham study (D'Agostino et al., 2008), SCORE (Conroy et al., 2003), Qrisk (Cox et al., 2007), ASSIGN (Woodward, 2006), PROCAM (Assmann, Cullen, & Schulte, 2002), UKPDS (Stevens et al., 2001), Joint British charts (British Cardiac Society, 2000), New Zealand (Jackson, 2002), and Sheffield (Wallis et al., 2000). Examples of short-term risk scores are GRACE (Tang et al., 2007), TIMI (Antman et al., 2000), and PURSUIT (Boersma, Pieper, & Steyerberg, 2000). These risk score schemes also vary according to the patient's clinical condition (e.g., coronary artery disease, heart failure), prediction of occurrences (e.g., death, myocardial infarction, unstable angina, hospitalization), type of prevention (primary or secondary), and the particular situation of the patient (e.g., diabetes).

While these tools are helpful, they have some significant drawbacks: (1) They are general models; therefore low performance results can be obtained when applied to a specific patient. (2) They present limitations in dealing with missing risk variables. (3) They do not allow inclusion of complementary clinical knowledge, such as new risk factors. (4) They ignore the information that was available in earlier developed risk assessment tools. (5) They do not allow the simultaneous use of several risk tools, thus forcing clinicians to select a specific tool in clinical practice. As result, some methodologies have been recently introduced to defeat some of the identified problems (Caruana et al., 2015; Damen et al., 2016; Paredes, Rocha, de Carvalho, Henriques, Mendes, et al., 2015). This chapter addresses two innovative approaches: grouping of patients to achieve a personalized stratification and combination methodologies using different sources (individual models, clinical evidence) to achieve global models.

The patient grouping approach is based on the evidence that risk assessment tools perform differently between distinct populations, suggesting that the best model (stratification) can be found for each group if the patients are correctly grouped. The personalization of CVD risk assessment based on grouping of patients involves mainly two procedures: clustering patients and similarity measures. Essentially, the clustering process involves the creation of a set of clusters (groups of patients) based on the values of respective risk factors and using a suitable measure of pattern similarity to assess patients with related characteristics.

The combination approach deals with the problem of the CVD risk assessment from a different perspective. In this approach, the combination of existent knowledge (risk tools) is considered more important than the creation of a new stratification tool. In effect, by combining in a global model some existing models (e.g., risk assessment models validated in clinical practice), some of the main disadvantages of current tools can be overcome: few risk factors (considering tools individually), problems in dealing with incomplete data (lack of risk variables), and inadequacy to incorporate clinical expertise. Moreover, this approach avoids the selection of a particular risk assessment model by professionals; the approach enables simultaneous use of several risk models, thereby increasing the confidence and satisfaction of professionals. This methodology is based on two main assumptions: (1) It is possible to create a common representation of individual risk assessment tools to facilitate their combination, and (2) it is possible to combine the obtained common individual models in a global model.

5.3 Risk progression and prognosis

Hospitals and healthcare centers accumulate numerous datasets with patients' data, such as physiological time series routinely collected in intensive care units by the continuous monitoring of patients or resulting from telemonitoring systems. This context creates new opportunities to the development of algorithms and models not only for the automatic evaluation of a clinical condition but, principally, to assess their progression, allowing the detection of forthcoming clinical severe events and the prompt intervention of clinicians in order to avoid critical situations for the patients.

From the clinical perspective it is assumed that similarities between physiological temporal series can be used to detect and predict specific clinical conditions that contribute to the global cardiovascular assessment of the patient. For this effect it is recognized that a relevant source of information could be the patient's historical data or, as an alternative, the historical data of other patients who have similar behaviors in their health data. From the scientific perspective the main goal is the development of predictive models capable to forecast the evolution of biosignals or the early detection of clinical conditions on the basis of the temporal trajectories of related physiological signals and/or on interpatient similarities.

Important advances in methodologies for similarity searches in time series have been presented in recent years. The computation of Euclidean distance between raw time series of the same length is one such algorithm. Alternatively, for time series of different lengths, a possible approach is dynamic time warping techniques (Park et al., 2000). Considering the common high dimensionality of time series, many methods have been proposed to decrease data dimensionality. These include discrete Fourier transform (Agrawal et al., 1993), principal component analysis (Karhunen-Loève transform) (Yang & Shahabi, 2004), and wavelet transform (Saeed & Mark, 2006). Rocha et al. (2012) suggested an innovative approach in this context to assess, in an effective manner, the similarity between two physiological time series. The method combines the Haar wavelet with the Karhunen-Loève transform to describe signals as an optimal linear combination of reduced base functions. The method's computational complexity is considerably reduced through an iterative algorithm for computing the coefficients of the linear bases.

Relating to prediction methods, linear regression techniques, in particular autoregressive schemes, have been used recurrently in practice. However, linear models are not always appropriate for biosignals, since they are not able to deal with the nonlinear nature of biosignals. In terms of nonlinear techniques, founded on their universal approximation characteristics, neural networks have become very popular. Many distinct kinds of neural networks, such as time delay and recurrent neural networks, have been shown to be efficient in modeling and predicting time series (Haykin, 2008). On the other hand, a global stationarity assumption cannot be guaranteed in most clinical time series, leading to the use of time-frequency methods. Wavelet transformation has been commonly implemented among time-frequency techniques, as it guarantees a good local representation of the signal in both time and frequency domains, providing a suitable scheme for dealing with nonstationarities. Although the wavelet transform itself is not a predictive scheme, it can be incorporated efficiently into hybrid predictive structures involving the multiresolution decomposition of the signal (Fryzlewicz et al., 2003).

This chapter addresses the development of predictive methodologies to estimate the future values of biosignals. The approach uses trend analysis of blood pressure values to forecast the patient's hypertension risk (whether blood pressure evolves to high values or, on the contrary, blood pressure values decreases to or maintain normal values). The strategy is based on the assumption that the estimation of the future evolution of biosignals can be supported by present and past historical measurements obtained from historical data. As a consequence, two main subjects are discussed from the research and practical perspectives: how to assess and compare time series trends and how to apply these trends in the prediction mechanism.

5.4 Assessment of patients' similarity

The proper identification of groups of patients could be very useful for performing a correct CVD risk assessment and the respective patient risk stratification. These groups should be created on the basis of the similarity or dissimilarity of a set of features (e.g., age, clinical history, symptoms, clinical exams) that are considered relevant to characterize a specific patient condition (e.g., CVD). According to this perspective, distinct groups (classes) of patients can be created on the basis of the hypothesis that individuals with similar characteristics present a similar outcome. However, the assessment of similarity among real patients' data is neither obvious nor simple, as it involves multiple aspects.

Clustering algorithms are particularly important in this context. Directly related with clustering, dimensionality reduction techniques assume an important role as they are applied to maximize the efficiency of those algorithms.

5.4.1 Dimensionality reduction

Dimensionality reduction techniques aim at the creation of a low-dimensional representation of high-dimensional data. This reduction has to retain most of the intrinsic information, that is, the minimum number of parameters needed to explain the observed properties of data derived from the original data. This means that a set of representative uncorrelated variables should be found while the remaining ones are discarded without losing significant information. This reduction of dimensionality is very important in many domains, since it reduces the number of data samples required to estimate a function, avoiding the curse of dimensionality and other undesired properties of high-dimensional spaces, which facilitates the data's classification (Sugiyama, 2010).

Actually, given a p-dimensional data vector $x = \left[x_1 \ldots x_p\right]^T$, a lower-dimensional representation $y = \left[y_1 \ldots y_q\right]^T$ is obtained, with $p < q$, such that it retains the content (intrinsic information) of the original data (Fodor, 2002). There are several possible qualifications of dimensionality reduction methods (e.g., hard/soft, supervised/unsupervised, continuous/discrete, layered/stand-alone embedding). However, the most frequently adopted classifications of dimensionality reduction methods are linear methods and nonlinear methods (Fodor, 2002; Lee, 2007; Maaten, 2009; Sugiyama, 2010). Linear techniques ensure that each one of the $q \leq p$ elements of the new data space is a linear combination of the original variables. Nonlinear techniques, assuming nonlinear relationships, are able to deal with complex nonlinear data (Maaten, 2009).

5.4.1.1 Linear methods

Linear methods assume that each of the $q \leq p$ components $y_i, i = 1, \ldots, q$, of the new instance y is a linear combination of the original variables:

$$y_i = w_{i,1}x_1, + \ldots + w_{i,p}x_p, \quad i = 1, \ldots, q \tag{5.1}$$

considering the following matrix operation:

$$\boldsymbol{Y}_{q \times N} = \boldsymbol{W}_{q \times p}\mathbf{X}_{p \times N} \tag{5.2}$$

where p is the dimension of original data, q denotes the dimension of the lower-dimensional representation, and N is the number of instances. The best-known linear methods are the principal component analysis (PCA), independent component analysis, and factor analysis (Fodor, 2002; Maaten, 2009). PCA is possibly the most common linear technique applied in dimensionality reduction. It reduces the original dimension of data by finding a few orthogonal linear combinations with the largest variance. The first principal component $y_1 = \mathbf{x}^T\mathbf{w}_1$ is the linear combination with the largest variance, the second principal component is the linear combination with the second largest variance, and the same reasoning is applied to the remaining components. There are as many principal components as the number of original variables. However, for the majority of the applications the first components explain most of the variance. This allows the elimination of the remaining principal components with minimal loss of information (Fodor, 2002). The covariance matrix $\sum_{p \times p}$ of $\mathbf{X}_{p \times N}$ is assumed to be decomposed as follows:

$$\sum = \mathbf{U}\Lambda\mathbf{U}^T \tag{5.3}$$

where $\Lambda = \text{diag}(\lambda_1, \ldots, \lambda_p)$ is the diagonal matrix of the ordered eigenvalues $\lambda_1 \leq \ldots \leq \lambda_p$ and $\mathbf{U}$ is a $p \times p$ orthogonal matrix containing the eigenvectors. The final data (dimensionality reduction) is obtained through the following expression:

$$\mathbf{Y}_{p\times N} = \mathbf{U}^{T}_{p\times p}\mathbf{X}_{p\times N} \tag{5.4}$$

The q first elements (rows) of $\mathbf{Y}$ are considered, while the remaining $(p-q)$ are discarded, which permits a reduction from p to q dimensions.

5.4.1.2 Nonlinear methods

Nonlinear methods are applied when a linear transformation weight matrix $\mathbf{W}$ between dimensional spaces p and $q \leq p$ cannot be created. Three main categories can be identified: global techniques, local techniques, and global alignment of linear models (Maaten, 2009).

Global techniques aim to preserve the global properties of the data. Multidimensional scaling retains the pairwise distances between the original and the respective reduced data space. The target is the minimization of the error between the pairwise distances in the two dimensional data spaces. The following equation shows a possible criterion to be minimized:

$$\phi = \sum \left(x_i - x_j - \mathbf{y}_i - \mathbf{y}_j \right)^2 \tag{5.5}$$

In some specific situations, Euclidean distance may lead to biased results. The Isomap algorithm intends to circumvent this difficulty by considering the geodesic[1] (curvilinear) distances between data points. In this case, geodesic distances between the data instances $\mathbf{x}_i, i = 1, \ldots, N$, are determined on the basis of the construction of a neighborhood graph in which every point is connected with its k nearest neighbors in the dataset. The geodesic distance between two points is given by the shortest path between them. Global techniques category comprises other methods, such as maximum variance unfolding, diffusion maps, and neural networks.

Local nonlinear techniques for dimensionality reduction intend to preserve properties of small neighborhoods around the data instances (consider the nearest neighbors). Local linear embedding, Laplacian

[1] The geodesic distance is the distance between two points measured over the manifold, which is an abstract mathematical space in which every point has a neighborhood. This neighborhood resembles the geometry spaces described by Euclidean geometry.

Eigenmaps, and Hessian local linear embedding are examples of local techniques.

Global alignment of linear models techniques combines global and local techniques. Locally linear coordination and manifold charting are included in this category (Maaten, 2009).

5.4.2 Clustering

Clustering techniques group data instances into clusters such that $\Upsilon \in R^{N \times p}$ represents a set of N instances $\mathbf{x}_i \in R^p$, the goal is to partition Υ into K groups $G = \{G_1, \ldots, G_K\}$, where data that belong to the same group are more similar than data that belong to the other groups (Han, Kamber, & Pei, 2011).

This capability to find similarities between data instances based on the underlying structure of the dataset can be very useful in the context of risk assessment and stratification. The discovery of similarities between patients (creation of groups of patients) can be important not only to discover unknown patterns contained in the dataset (knowledge discovery) but also to identify the risk or stratification models that presents the best performance within a specific group of patients (Table 5.1).

Table 5.1 Distance between data instances.

Interval scaled attributes	Euclidean	$d(\mathbf{u},\mathbf{v}) = \sqrt{\sum_{i=1}^{p}(u_i - v_i)^2}$
	Minkowsky	$d(\mathbf{u},\mathbf{v}) = \sqrt[r]{\sum_{i=1}^{p}\lvert u_i - v_i\rvert^r}$
	Manhattan	$d(\mathbf{u},\mathbf{v}) = \sum_{i=1}^{p}\lvert u_i - v_i\rvert$
	Chebychev	$d(\mathbf{u},\mathbf{v}) = max_{i=1}^{n}\lvert u_i - v_i\rvert$
	Camberra	$d(\mathbf{u},\mathbf{v}) = \sum_{i=1}^{p}\frac{\lvert u_i - v_i\rvert}{\lvert u_i + v_i\rvert}$
Binary attributes {0, 1}	Simple matching coefficient	$d(\mathbf{u},\mathbf{v}) = \frac{n_1 + n_2}{p}$
	Jaccard similarity coefficient	$d(\mathbf{u},\mathbf{v}) = \frac{n_1}{n_1 + n_3 + n_4}$
	Hamming distance	$d(\mathbf{u},\mathbf{v}) = n_3 + n_4$
Nominal scaled attributes	Dissimilarity coefficient	$d(\mathbf{u},\mathbf{v}) = \frac{p + o}{p}$
Ordinal scaled attributes	Similar to interval-based attributes	$= \frac{u_i - 1}{U_k - 1}$

5.4.2.1 Distance metrics

The concepts of similarity and dissimilarity are defined on the basis of the resemblance between data instances, which can be assessed on the basis of different distance metrics applied to different types of data. All the distance metrics, $d(\bullet)$, should verify the following conditions:

$$d(\mathbf{u},\mathbf{v}) \geq 0$$

$$d(\mathbf{u},\mathbf{v}) = 0 \text{ifandonlyif} \mathbf{u} = \mathbf{v}$$

$$d(\mathbf{u},\mathbf{v}) = d(\mathbf{v},\mathbf{u})$$

$$d(\mathbf{u},\mathbf{z}) \leq d(\mathbf{u},\mathbf{v}) + d(\mathbf{v},\mathbf{z}) \tag{5.6}$$

$$\mathbf{u} = \left[u_1 \ldots u_p\right]^T; v = \left[u_1 \ldots u_p\right]^T; \mathbf{z} = \left[z_1 \ldots z_p\right]^T$$

$\mathbf{u}$, $\mathbf{v}$ data vectors, $\mathbf{u} = \left[\mathrm{u}_1 \ldots \mathrm{u}_p\right]^T, \mathbf{v} = \left[\mathrm{v}_1 \ldots \mathrm{v}_p\right]^T$
p: number of attributes
n_1: 1's in both vectors $\mathbf{u}$, $\mathbf{v}$
n_2: 0's in both vectors
n_3: 1's in $\mathbf{u}$ and 0's in $\mathbf{v}$
n_4: 0's in $\mathbf{u}$ and 1's in $\mathbf{v}$
0: number of matches
U_k: maximum value that attribute u_i can assume

5.4.2.2 Algorithms

Ideally, a clustering algorithm should verify some characteristics: scalability, that is, the ability to deal with a large number of instances; ability to group mixed attributes; handling of outliers; immunity to attributes order in data instances; and ability to deal with a large number of attributes (Han et al., 2011). Addressing the unsupervised learning problem, clustering algorithms can be divided in three main groups: partitional algorithms, hierarchical algorithms, and density-based algorithms (Han et al., 2011).

Partitional clustering can be defined as a class of algorithms that construct k partitions of the data. A clustering criterion, for example, the minimization for the sum of squared distance from the mean within each cluster, is applied. K-means is a classic algorithm that belongs to the category of partitional clustering. It considers a set of N vectors

$\mathbf{x}_i, i = 1, \ldots, N$, that may be partitioned into K groups $G_j, j = 1, \ldots, K$, that contain the respective cluster centers $\mathbf{c}_j, j = 1, \ldots, K$, such that

$$Q_j \sum_{r:x_r \in G_j} \mathbf{x}_r - \mathbf{c}_j^2 \tag{5.7}$$

where Q_j is the objective function to be minimized, that is, the distance between the instances $\mathbf{x}_r \in G_j$ and the respective cluster center $\mathbf{c}_j$.

The partitioned groups G_j are defined by a $K \times N$ binary membership matrix, K clusters, N instances, where the respective elements $u_{ji} = 1$ if the instance $\mathbf{x}_i$ belongs to group G_j, as presented in Eq. (5.8):

$$u_{ji} \begin{cases} 1 \text{if} \mathbf{x}_i - \mathbf{c}_j^2 \leq \mathbf{x}_i - \mathbf{c}_k^2, \text{for} k \neq j \\ 0, \text{otherwise} \end{cases} \tag{5.8}$$

The centers of the different clusters can be updated to optimize the separation of instances. K-means is extensively used in cluster analysis, although it has several drawbacks, including (1) the difficulty in choosing the proper number of clusters centers, (2) that the accuracy of the algorithm depends directly on the initialization of the clusters centers that must be a priori defined, and (3) that the algorithm is sensitive to outliers (Hammouda, 2000). There are several extensions to the original k-means to minimize these flaws, such as k-means++ (Arthur & Vassilvitskii, 2007) and k-medoids (Han et al., 2011).

Hierarchical algorithms create a multilevel hierarchy in which clusters at one level are joined as clusters in the next level. The graphical representation of this hierarchical decomposition of the data instances is designated as a dendrogram. The methods that are used to decompose data instances hierarchically can be agglomerative (bottom-up) or divisive (top-down). The former assumes that each instance is a separate cluster that must be merged according to a specific distance measure. The stop condition is achieved when all the clusters belong to the same cluster. The divisive method works in reverse mode, assuming that all data instances belong to the same cluster, which must be split in disjoint clusters. The process iterates until each data instance belongs to a separate cluster or reaches a stopping condition (Hammouda, 2000).

Density-based algorithms group data instances on the basis of their density, that is, the number of data instances that exist in a specific neighborhood. Subtractive clustering is one of the best-known density-based algorithms (Chen, Qin, & Jia, 2008). All data instances are viewed as candidates for cluster centers, being assessed the respective density through the following formula:

$$\rho_i = \sum_{j=1}^{N} \exp\left(- \frac{\mathbf{x}_i - \mathbf{x}_j{}^2}{(\chi/2)^2} \right) \tag{5.9}$$

where χ is a neighborhood radius. If a data point has many neighboring data points, it will have a high density value. The data point with the highest density value, ρ_i, is the first cluster center. Then the density values are updated as follows:

$$\rho_i = \rho_i - \rho_{\mathbf{c}_1} \exp\left(- \frac{\mathbf{x}_i - \mathbf{c}_1{}^2}{(\chi_d/2)^2} \right) \tag{5.10}$$

where the parameter $\rho_{\mathbf{c}_1}$ is the density value of the previous cluster center $\mathbf{c}_1$ and χ_d is a positive constant that decreases the density in the neighborhood of $\mathbf{x}_i$. This density reduction is directly proportional to the proximity between the several data instances and the selected cluster center $\mathbf{c}_1$. The process iterates in order to find the next cluster center until an adequate number of clusters has been identified. Data instances are assigned to the several clusters centers (Hammouda, 2000).

All of the algorithms that have been presented have advantages and disadvantages. Considering the partitioning algorithms, *k*-means is a very simple algorithm to implement and can run efficiently in linear time. Its downside is the sensitivity to outliers as well as to the initial randomly generated centers. In regard to some of its extensions, *k*-medoids is more robust, since it is not as sensitive to outliers, and fuzzy *c*-means is able to deal with fuzzy logic and create rules to put new instances on a cluster. However, they still have the disadvantages of *k*-means: They cannot discover clusters with nonconvex shapes, they cannot handle noise, and the number of clusters has to be decided a priori. Besides, they do not scale well for large datasets.

The classical hierarchical approaches are very robust in terms of outliers, although they do not handle well missing values, and there are a lot of possible measures for them, which means that choosing a good measure may not be trivial.

The density-based algorithms can handle noise easily as well as outlier and missing values; they also have the ability to discover clusters of arbitrary shape. However, they also have drawbacks. Subtractive clustering, for instance, is not very efficient in terms of time complexity (Hammouda, 2000; Han et al., 2011).

5.5 Risk assessment

Clinical guidelines recognize the importance of risk assessment tools and models in daily clinical practice and recommend their incorporation in clinical decision support systems to aid the medical decision. In spite of their importance, some challenges persist, and some of them are particularly relevant. Specifically, these models must ensure high performance, be suitable for a specific individual (personalization), combine or incorporate new knowledge, and be clinically interpretable. Owing to the complexity of real data, these aspects have to be addressed on the basis of innovative approaches, frequently taking advantage of hidden patterns or knowledge that is present in the clinical datasets.

5.5.1 Personalization strategies

Risk assessment models perform differently among different populations. In fact, a specific risk assessment model may be suitable (high performance) for a given group of patients and useless (poor performance) for other groups. This evidence leads to the hypothesis that if patients are properly grouped, it would be possible to find the best classifier for each group.

5.5.1.1 Clustering of models outputs

The derivation of groups may be constrained by two aspects: heterogeneity of risk factors (quantitative data, qualitative data, binary data) and high dimensionality (number of risk factors). Fig. 5.1 presents a possible strategy based on a dimensionality reduction procedure (nonlinear) followed by a clustering procedure.

Assuming that a set of risk assessment models can be applied to a real patient dataset (e.g., acute coronary syndrome (ACS) patients and secondary prevention), all instances $\mathbf{x}_i = \left[x_p^i \dots x_p^i\right]^T \in \mathbf{X}_{p\times N}$ that correspond to the N patients are mapped into $\mathbf{y}_i \in \mathbf{Y}_{Q\times N}, i = 1, \dots, N$, where y_q^i denotes the output of model q to classify the patient i (e.g., $\mathbf{y}_i = \left[y_G^i \quad y_P^i \quad y_T^i\right]$).[2] This reduction of dimensionality is possible as a specific model q considers J risk factors (subset of the p risk factors). Then an instance $\mathbf{x}_i^q$ containing the J risk factors (values) of patient i is applied to

[2] Assuming g**R**ace, **P**ursuit, and **T**imi risk assessment models in the context of secondary prevention.

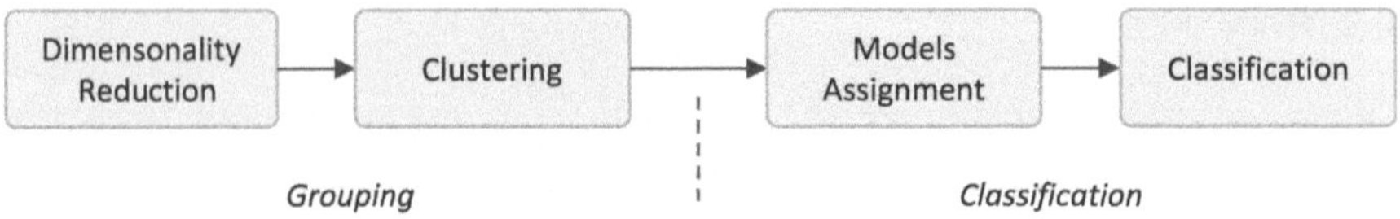

Figure 5.1 Proposed approach to derivation of groups.

the q model to obtain the respective $y_q^i \in \mathbf{y}_i$. All the y_q^i should be normalized into the interval [0, 1].

This procedure allows the creation of clusters based on the outputs of the risk models instead on the initial risk factors. Actually, K disjoint groups (clusters) $G = \{G_1, \ldots, G_K\}$ of patients are created based on $\mathbf{Y}_{Q \times N}$ that represents a set of N patients.

The global set of patients $D = \{(\mathbf{x}_1, c_1), \ldots, (\mathbf{x}_N, c_N)\}$ is clustered in K clusters G_i, where a given patient belongs to only one cluster G_i.

The dimension of the clusters must ensure the concept of patient grouping. Therefore it has to be adjusted. If the clusters are too big, they may not characterize the behavior of the different tools; if the clusters are too small, they will block the creation of groups. Subtractive clustering is particularly useful, as it allows the control of the clusters dimension.

The third phase concerns the identification of the most suitable model to classify patients from a given cluster. Each of the considered individual risk assessment models is tested within each cluster. Thus each y_q^i is converted to a risk class c_q^i according to the original specifications of each model. The output (class) of each model q is compared with the real data (occurrence of an event) within a given period of time. This procedure is repeated for each patient i of each cluster $G_k, k = 1, \ldots, K$, which allow the assessment (e.g., sensitivity or specificity) of each model in the different clusters.

Classification is the final step of this approach, and it can be depicted as follows: (1) An instance $\mathbf{y}_i$ is obtained based on $\mathbf{x}_i$ (the different risk assessment tools assess the risk of a new patient). (2) Based on $\mathbf{y}_i$ the cluster G_k to which this new patient i belongs is identified. (3) Considering G_k, the best model q to classify the patient is selected. (4) Model q provides the final classification.

This strategy, depicted in Fig. 5.2, was validated in a dataset composed of $N = 460$ consecutive patients who were admitted to the Santa Cruz Hospital (in Portugal) with ACS with non-ST segment elevation and an event rate (30 days, death or myocardial infarction) of 7.2% (33 events). Bootstrapping validation ($N_B = 1000$) was applied to the original dataset

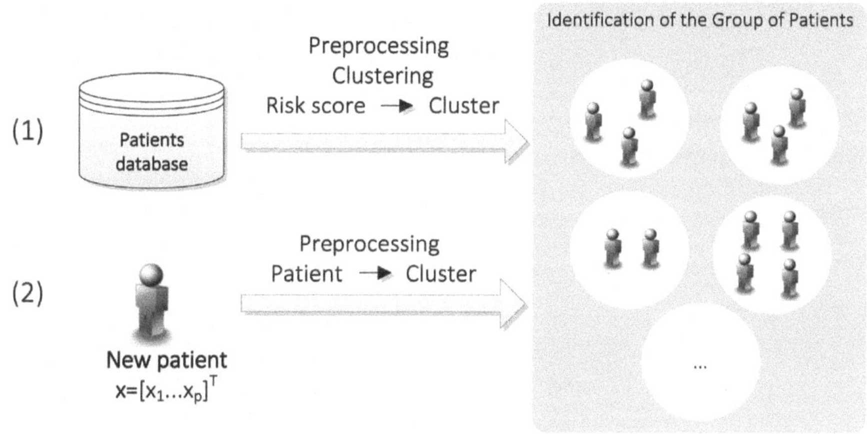

Figure 5.2 Clustering patients based on $\mathbf{y}_i = [y_G^i \quad y_P^i y_T^i]$.

(Paredes, Rocha, Mendes, et al., 2015). This approach allowed a sensitivity (SE) of 72.9% and a specificity (SP) of 75.1%, which corresponds to a geometric mean (GM) of 73.9%. A more comprehensive explanation of this methodology can be found in the work of Paredes and colleagues (Paredes, Rocha, de Carvalho, Henriques, Morais, et al., 2015).

5.5.1.2 Identification of the best risk assessment models

The identification of the best risk assessment models can be systematized as shown in Fig. 5.3.

The classification of new patients can be based on similarities between patients. This strategy avoids the complexity of the clustering process and explores the hypothesis that if a new patient is closest to one that is correctly classified by a CVD risk assessment model, it is probable that the same model will also be able to classify the patient accurately.

However, the calculation of this similarity is not obvious, as several distances may be applied, depending of the dataset specificities, such as the type of data (interval-scaled, nominal, binary). Fig. 5.4 depicts the proposed strategy (Marques et al., 2015).

The first phase is composed of two steps: group creation using risk scores and preprocessing of the data. Instances that are correctly classified by a risk score are grouped together. By using this procedure, a set of initial groups is created.

On the other hand, similarity assessment, that is, the identification of the group to which a new instance belongs, is not trivial and may involve

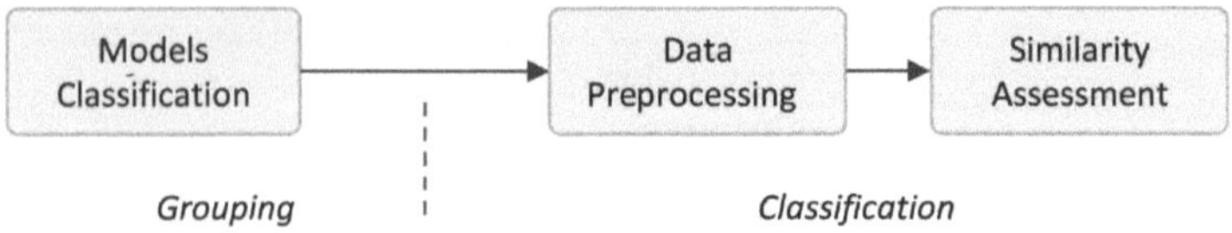

Figure 5.3 Proposed approach for identifying the best risk assessment models.

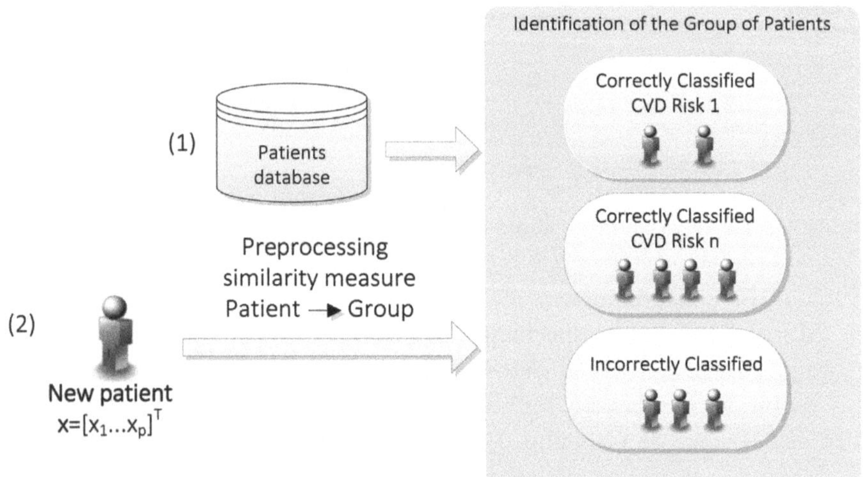

Figure 5.4 Classification of risk assessment models.

some data preprocessing. This preprocessing includes dealing with missing data, which can be addressed by using different approaches (e.g., deletion, mean/median substitution, multiple imputation) (Sterne et al., 2009). The mean substitution was particularly important in the proposed approach. Normalization is also very useful in this phase, as it may minimize the problems that arise from the different types of data (interval-scaled, nominal, binary). A possible solution to deal with all these types of values relies on the normalization of the attributes to adjust their scales and use of an interval-scaled distance such as the Euclidean distance to assess similarity. This normalization can be performed through the z-score, where μ is the mean of the population and σ is the standard deviation:

$$z = \frac{x - \mu}{\sigma} \tag{5.11}$$

An alternative to normalization is based on a mixed distance, such as the one proposed by Andritsos et al. (2002), in which the interval-based attributes use Euclidean distance and the nominal and binary ones use

Hamming distance. However, even in this case, it is important to use the *z*-score in the interval-based attributes to adjust the scale.

Imbalanced data is another important issue that must be addressed in the data preprocessing; otherwise, it can potentially produce a classifier with worse accuracy for the minority class. Thus balancing data is an option that may improve classification. There are several methods for imbalanced data. In this approach, the random minority oversampling and random majority undersampling have been applied (He & Stevens, 2009).

Features selection can also be applied in this preprocessing phase to enhance the assessment of similarity among the several instances. In this particular case, a weight has been assigned to each variable, giving more importance to the relevant features or even eliminating the irrelevant ones. Genetic algorithms were applied to adjust those weights (optimization procedure). More details about this strategy are described in the work of Marques et al. (2015). Groups that were created in the training phase are used in the validation phase to assign new patients to the most adequate risk score. First, the new data must be preprocessed, as these were the training data. Then the similarity measures identify the most similar instance of the training set for each new instance. This is done by comparing all the training set instances to the new instance, using a similarity measure. The closest one is considered the most similar. Basically, it is assumed that similar patients are correctly classified by the same model. Then the new patient belongs to the group that contains the most similar instance. One of the main drawbacks of this strategy is its obvious exposure to outliers.

This approach was also validated in the Santa Cruz Hospital, using data from 460 patients with ACS with non-ST segment elevation. However, a different validation procedure was followed, as 10 subsets of 46 patients were created. Then in each run, 9 subsets were used as training data, and the remaining subset was used as the testing dataset. A SE of 78% and SP of 63% were obtained, which corresponds to a GM of 70%. A more comprehensive explanation of this methodology can be found in the work of Marques et al. (2015).

5.5.2 Combination strategies

The combination approach relies on the hypothesis that a combination of individual risk assessment tools and current clinical knowledge allows the implementation of optimization methodologies to increase the CVD risk

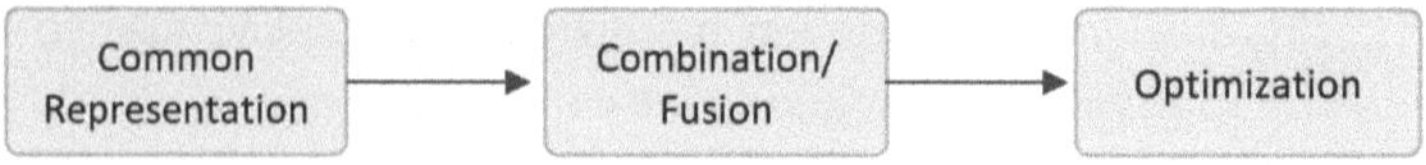

Figure 5.5 Combination of risk assessment models.

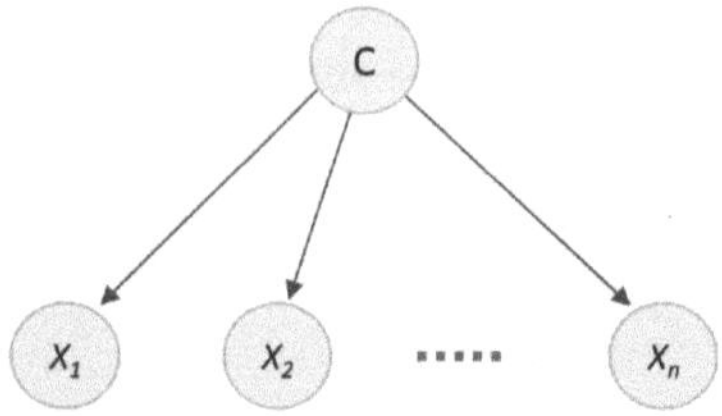

Figure 5.6 Naive Bayes structure.

prediction performance. This approach includes three main steps, as depicted in Fig. 5.5.

Because current risk assessment tools are diversely represented (charts, equations, etc.), the first step is the creation of a common representation of the individual sources of knowledge or information. The naïve Bayes classifier was applied to enable this common representation, as it:

- has a very simple structure, which facilitates the creation of a proper combination scheme (Fig. 5.6). In effect, it is composed of only one parent (unobserved node: C) and several children (observed nodes: $X_1, \ldots, X_p$).
- has an acceptable performance when compared with other classifiers.
- has an inherent ability to deal with missing risk factors. The inference mechanism of naive Bayes is given by

$$P(C|\mathbf{X}) = P\left(C|X_1, \ldots, X_p\right) = \alpha P(C)\prod^{p} P(X_i|C) \tag{5.12}$$

- allows that the conditional probability table of a missing risk factor $P(X_i|, C)$ is set to one that disables its influence in the final classification.
- ensures the clinical interpretability. The naive Bayes parameters $P(X_i|, C), P(C)$ provide information about the probabilistic relationship between the several attributes X_i and the class of risk $c \in C$ as well as the prior probability of the different risk classes.
- matches the reasoning required to establish a clinical diagnosis. Actually, it implies that the physician makes an inference that involves assessing the probability that a patient has a disease on the basis of the revealed symptoms.

The final classification c is achieved on the basis of the following equation:

$$c = \underset{c_j}{\text{argmax}} \left(\alpha P(c_j) \prod_{i=1}^{p} P\left(x_i|, c_j\right) \right) \tag{5.13}$$

where c_j is a mutually exclusive class of C and x_i is the value of attribute X_i that belongs to the query instance $\mathbf{x}_q = \left[x_1, \ldots, x_p\right]$. Thus an instance $\mathbf{x}$ contains values of the attributes or risk factors (e.g., age, sex) of a particular patient, c_j encodes a level of risk (e.g., low/high), and α is a normalization constant.

Since the structure of the naïve classifier Bayes is fully described, the learning method is limited to the learning parameters ($P(X_i\,|\,C)$, $P(C)$). Thus the representation of a given individual risk assessment tool as a naive Bayes classifier can be systematized as follows:

- A training dataset (N instances $\mathbf{x} - [x_1 \ldots x_p\,]$ composed of p attributes) is applied to a risk assessment model for obtaining a full labeled dataset.
- $J = \{(\mathbf{x}_1, c_1), \ldots, (\mathbf{x}_N, c_N)\}$.
- Conditional probabilities can be calculated based on J through the use of the following formula:

$$P(X_i = x_i|, C = c) = \frac{\sum_{1}^{N} (X_i = x_i \Lambda C = c)}{\sum_{1}^{N} (C = c)} \tag{5.14}$$

- Laplace smoothing[3] is applied to avoid conditional probabilities with value 0. Although the assessment of these probabilities is accurate only if the attributes are categorical, the discretization of numerical attributes can have a major effect. To enhance the clinical interpretability of the model, a discretization based on intervals with clinical significance was also applied to some attributes.[4]

[3] $\frown \theta_l = \frac{n_i + \alpha}{n + \alpha k}$; n_i is the number of instances that assume the value i, where n is the total number of instances, α is the constant value (usually the value 1), and k is the number of the possible values of θ.

[4] Clinical guidelines identify limit values for certain risk factors (e.g., systolic blood pressure, where <120 corresponds to normal values, $121-140$ refers to the prehypertension category, and >140 refers to hypertension stages I and II.

- The prior probability $P(C)$ results directly from the class value distribution.
- This process must be repeated for each of the individual risk assessment models that integrate the combination scheme.

The second step of this methodology is the combination of individual naive Bayes classifiers. This combination methodology is intended to create a classification system based on the integration of those individual sources of information. It takes advantage of the probabilistic reasoning as well as of the specific structure of the naïve Bayes classifier to implement the fusion of the individual models' parameters.

Thus several individual classifiers $M_i \in M = \{M_1, \ldots, M_l\}$ are regarded; each classifier is described by a particular conditional probability table $P\left(X_i^j|, C_j\right)$ and by their corresponding prior output class probability $P\left(C_j\right).P\left(X_i^j|, C_j\right)$ represents the conditional probability table of attribute i of model j, $P\left(C_j\right)$, the prior probability distribution of model j regarding a specific number of mutually exclusive classes, is the input instance considered by the model j (risk factors considered by j that are a subset of the p risk factors).

The combination methodology that is created assigns distinct weights for the individual models depending on their results in a particular dataset. Therefore this weighted combination of the individual models is performed on the basis of the following expressions:

$$P(C) = \sum_{j=1}^{l} P\left(C_j\right) \times \frac{w_j}{\Gamma}, \text{where} \Gamma = \sum_{j=1}^{l} w_j$$

$$P(X_i|, C) = \sum_{j=1}^{b} P\left(X_i^j|, C_j\right) \times \frac{w_j}{\vartheta}, \text{where} \vartheta = \sum_{j=1}^{b} w_j \qquad (5.15)$$

where l is the number of individual models, b is the number of individual models that contain the attribute $X_i \in \left\{X_1, \ldots, X_p\right\}$, C_j denotes each individual model, and w_j is the weight of model j. Some risk factors (model inputs) may be considered by more than one model, while other inputs belong only to a single model. In this case, the global CPT table must match the respective individual CPT.

The last stage is an optimization method that aims to modify the parameters of the model resulting from the combination approach to enhance the global model's performance. It seemed appropriate to apply genetic algorithms, as they are suitable to both constrained and unconstrained optimization problems in which the objective function $f(x)$ is nondifferentiable or highly nonlinear.

Genetic algorithms implementation focuses on $P(X_i | C)$, $P(C)$, the parameters of global model. The optimization procedure, however, cannot distort the information provided by the individual risk assessment models, therefore the adjustment of the global model's parameters must be constrained to the neighborhood of the initial values:

$$-\varphi \times P\left(X_i = x_i^k |, C = c_j\right) \leq \delta_{kj} \leq \varphi \times P\left(X_i = x_i^k |, C = c_j\right) \qquad (5.16)$$

The parameters to be optimized δ_{kj} denote the permitted variation in the probability of the category k of attribute X_i given the output class c_j (risk level), φ is the neighborhood value.

Individuals are represented as real numbers that codify each parameter's variation. Population size (number of individuals) is generally set to a value greater than an individual's size (number of parameters to optimize). A multiobjective optimization was implemented, where the objective functions f_1, f_2 were defined to transform the specificity/sensitivity maximization into a minimization problem.

$$f_1 = 1 - \frac{TP}{TP + FN}; f_2 = 1 - \frac{TP}{TP + FN} \qquad (5.17)$$

TP, True positive; *TN*, true negative; *FN*, false negative; *FP*, false positive.

The parents selection function was implemented through the roulette wheel algorithm, while the variation operators were uniform crossover and a Gaussian mutation operator. Variation operators are also very important for the operation of genetic algorithms. The chosen crossover operator in this optimization is the uniform crossover. To ensure the needed mutation, a Gaussian mutation operator was implemented.

The Survival selection is carried out based on the fitness of individuals of current generation as well as on the fitness of individuals of the respective offspring (fitness based replacement). Finally, several termination conditions have been tested. In this optimization the condition that checks whether the fitness improvements stay below a threshold value over a specified period of time is implemented.

This approach was also validated with the Santa Cruz Hospital dataset where Bootstrapping validation ($N_B = 1000$) was applied. Performance was improved, achieving a maximum value of SE, SP, and GM of 79.8%, 83.8%, and 80.9%, respectively.

5.5.3 Conclusion

The methodologies that are depicted in this section address two different weaknesses of the current CVD risk assessment strategies. The correct stratification of patients has to involve a personalization perspective, in which the best classifier for a specific patient must be provided. Owing to the complexity of real data, innovative approaches have been developed in which clustering and similarity assessment are key elements. The low performance of risk assessment is also addressed through and innovative combination strategy merging the knowledge provided by individual models and sources. In both cases, the results obtained throughout the respective validation using a dataset made available by Santa Cruz Hospital ($N = 460$) suggest the potential of the proposed approaches.

5.6 Risk progression

5.6.1 Hypertension risk

One of the greatest risk variables connected with CVDs is high blood pressure (hypertension). In effect, keeping blood pressure under control is vital for preserving health and reducing the risk of alterations in the myocardial structure, coronary vasculature, and conduction system of the heart, which can lead to the development of left ventricular hypertrophy, coronary artery disease, myocardial infarction, cardiac arrhythmias, heart failure, among others (Riaz and Ahmed, n.d.).

This chapter deals with a predictive methodology for estimating future values of biosignals, particularly applied to blood pressure signals in order to manage the hypertension condition. In fact, by means of a trend analysis the objective is to predict whether a patient's blood pressure evolves to hypertension values. For this purpose the strategy assumes that the future evolution of this signal can be determined on the basis of current and past measurements taken from the historical data of a group of patients, including the patient being studied. Essentially, it involves three major phases, as depicted in Fig. 5.7.

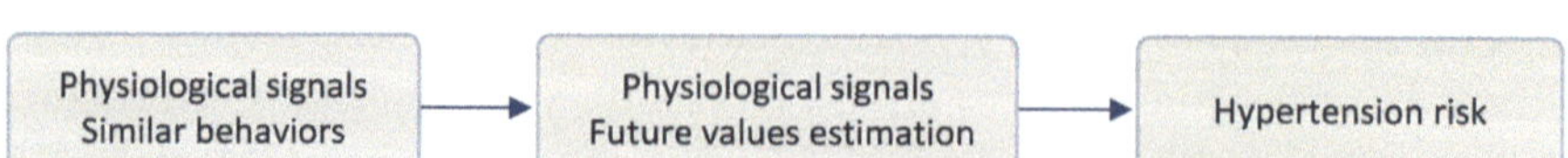

Figure 5.7 Predictive methodology for estimating future biosignal values.

The first phase consists of the selection of patients whose physiological time series show comparable behaviors through a similarity analysis process. The second phase includes the prediction of future values of the biosignal based on the analogous time series found in the first phase. Finally, the hypertension risk of the patient under study is assessed by using values that were previously estimated.

The approach combines the Haar wavelet with the Karhunen-Loève transforms, which enables signals to be represented as a linear combination of an optimal reduced set of basic functions. Then the method's computational complexity is considerably reduced through an iterative algorithm that computes the expansion coefficients. The presented approach aims not to predict the signal accurately but rather to estimate its future trend. Essentially, from the wavelet decomposition of similar signals selected from historical data, the most representative trends at the various levels of decomposition are identified and combined through an optimization process, providing a direct estimate of the current signal evolution.

5.6.2 Trend progression

The main idea behind the proposed prediction methodology is illustrated in Fig. 5.8. Essentially, the approach considers the signal to be predicted as the template, $X(t) \in R^{1,N}$. Then, by using this template and through a

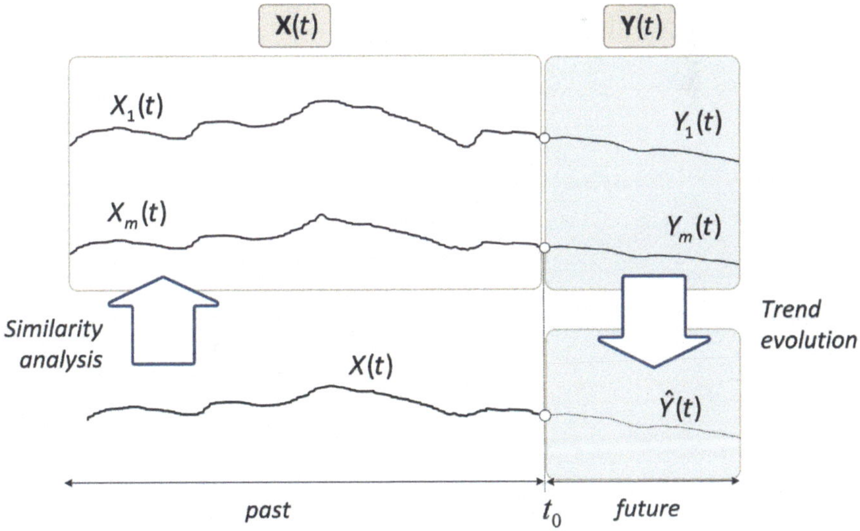

Figure 5.8 Prediction strategy based on similar signals.

similarity analysis process, the set of the M most similar conditions (patterns), $X(t) \equiv \{X_m(t) \in R^{1,N}\}, m = 1, \ldots, M$, is determined.

According to the scheme, the subsequent P future values corresponding to the selected patterns, $\mathbf{Y}(t) \equiv \{Y_m(t) \in R^{1,P}\}$, are easily obtained (since past values from the historic dataset are known). At that point, the evolution of the current template, $\hat{Y}(t)$, can be estimated by using the known "future" evolution of the identified patterns, $\mathbf{Y}(t) \equiv \{Y_m(t)\}$. The global set of patterns, $\mathbf{Z}(t) \in R^{M,N+P}$, is therefore composed of two components, $\mathbf{X}(t)$ and $\mathbf{Y}(t)$, in the form of Eq. (5.18):

$$\mathbf{Z}(t) = [\mathbf{X}(t) \quad \mathbf{Y}(t)] \tag{5.18}$$

By using a wavelet decomposition scheme, the assessment of $\hat{Y}(t)$ based on the similar patterns $\mathbf{Z}(t)$ involves the steps illustrated in Fig. 5.9.

5.6.2.1 Template decomposition

The first step is to decompose the template $X(t)$ by using the shift-invariant Haar à trous wavelet transform (Renaud et al., 2003). For example, assuming three levels of decomposition, the template can be obtained at the time instant t_0 as the sum of details $d^l X(t)$, for scales 1 to 3, plus the trend $a^3 X(t)$, as given by Eq. (5.19):

$$x\{t_0\} = d^1x(t_0) + d^2x(t_0) + d^3x(t_0) + a^3x(t_0) \tag{5.19}$$

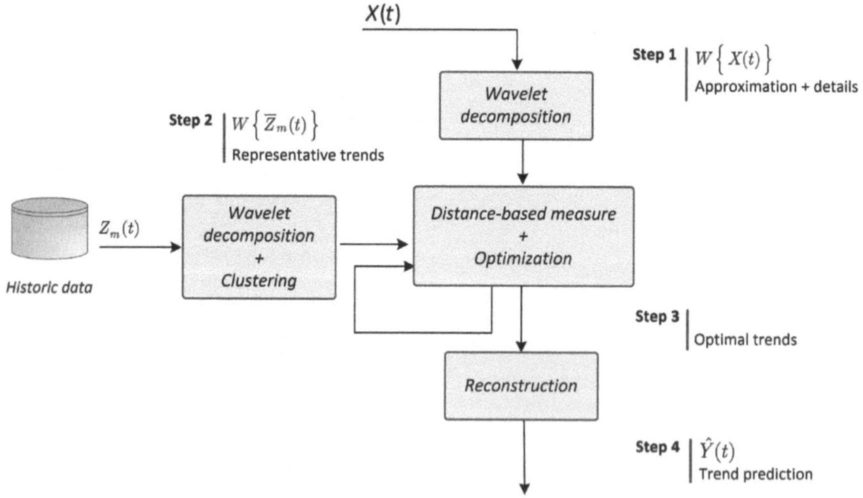

Figure 5.9 Prediction methodology.

For a general case considering L decomposition levels, the wavelet decomposition is described by $W\{X\} \in R^{L+1,N}$, according to Eq. (5.20):

$$W\{X\} = \left\{d^l X(t), a^L X(t)\right\}, l = 1, \ldots, L \tag{5.20}$$

5.6.2.2 *Representative trends*

In the second step, the most representative time series (trends) from the retrieved similar historic signals are determined. For this purpose the historic signals are in a first phase decomposed using the à trous wavelet, according to Eq. (5.21), where $a^L Z\ (t)$ and $d^l Z(t)$, $m = 1, \cdots, M$, represent the approximation and the details, respectively:

$$W\{Z_m\} = \left\{d^l X(t), a^L X(t)\right\}, l = 1, \ldots, L \tag{5.21}$$

It is important to note that in this case, the decomposition can be extended to the "future" (time instants from $N+1$ to $N+P$), with length $N+P$, that is, $WZ_{\mathrm{m}} \in R^{L+1,N+P}$.

After that, in a second phase, the representative decomposition trend at each level is determined through a subtractive clustering method (Kriegel et al., 2003), according to Eqs. (5.22) and (5.23), where variables $d^l\overline{Z}(t) \in R^{1,N+P}$ and $a^L\overline{Z}(t) \in R^{1,N+P}$ denote the representative details and approximation, respectively:

$$d^l\overline{Z}(t) = \text{subCustering}\left\{d^l Z_m(t)\right\}, m = 1, \ldots, M, l = 1, \ldots, L \tag{5.22}$$

$$d^l\overline{Z}(t) = \text{subCustering}\left\{d^l Z_m(t)\right\}, m = 1, \ldots, M \tag{5.23}$$

5.6.2.3 *Optimal trends*

In the third step, the optimal trends are determined by reducing the representative trends to a set of trends (decomposition levels) that have the potential to contribute to a consistent prediction. For this effect, a combination process is implemented, which consists of minimizing a group of distance-based measures that assess the probability of a representative trend contributing to a correct estimate.

5.6.2.3.1 Distance-based measures

The distance-based measures are computed for each decomposition level $l = 1, \ldots, L+1$, where $L+1$ stands for the approximation by using (1) the template $X(t) \in {}^{1,N}$; (2) the corresponding wavelet decomposition at l

level, $d^l X(t) \in R^{1,N}$; (3) the wavelet decomposition of similar patterns at the same level, $d^l Z_m(t) \in R^{1,N+P}, m = 1, M$; and (4) the corresponding clustering, that is, the representative trends $d^l \overline{Z}(t) \in R^{1,N+P}$. Based on these signals, a set of distance-based measures θ_i^l is computed as follows for $m = 1, \ldots, M$:

$$\theta_1^l = S\big(X(t), d^l X(t)\big), t = 1, \ldots, N \tag{5.24}$$

$$\theta_2^l = S\big(d^l X(t), d^l \overline{Z}(t)\big), t = 1, \ldots, N \tag{5.25}$$

$$\theta_3^l = \text{mean}\big[S(d^l X(t), d^l Z_m(t))\big], t = 1, \ldots, N \tag{5.26}$$

$$\theta_4^l = \exp\big[-\text{std}\big\{S(d^l X(t), d^l Z_m(t))\big\}\big], t = 1, \ldots, N \tag{5.27}$$

$$\theta_5^l = \text{mean}\big[S\big(d^l \overline{Z}(t), d^l Z_m(t)\big)\big], t = 1, \ldots, N + P \tag{5.28}$$

$$\theta_6^l = \exp\big[-\text{std}\big\{S\big(d^l \overline{Z}(t), d^l Z_m(t)\big)\big\}\big], t = N + 1, \ldots, N + P \tag{5.29}$$

As a consequence, a six-measure vector is generated, $\boldsymbol{\theta}^l = \left[\theta_1^l, \theta_2^l, \ldots, \theta_6^l\right]$, where each $\theta_i^l \in 0, 1$. The similarity measure $S(X_1(t), X_2 \ (t)) \in [0, 1]$ is a normalized measure, so a value of 1 means a total match between the signals. The operators mean$(\cdot)$ and std$(\cdot)$ represent the mean and standard deviation operators, respectively.

5.6.2.4 Selection of the optimal trends

The optimization approach assumes that each of the measures θ_i^l enables evaluation of the quality of each representative trend. Consequently, the decision to include or exclude a particular representative trend in the optimal set is taken on the basis of the measures obtained. To this end, operators maximum$(\cdot)$ and product$(\cdot)$ are used as aggregation and conjunction operators, respectively, being the quality of a particular forecast evaluated in accordance with Eq. (5.30):

$$p(\boldsymbol{\theta}) = \text{maxp}(\boldsymbol{\theta}\sigma_1), \ldots, \text{p}(\boldsymbol{\theta}\sigma_\text{i}), \ldots, \text{p}(\boldsymbol{\theta}\sigma_\text{n}) \tag{5.30}$$

Each variable $p(\Theta\sigma_i)$ in Eq. (5.30) represents the possible combinations of decomposition levels resulting from the operator $C(nL, nN)$ (combinations of nL taken nN at a time). In this procedure the product$(\cdot)$

operation Eq. (5.31) provides the combination of the metrics corresponding to a particular level:

$$p(\Theta) = \max p(\Theta\sigma_1), \ldots, p(\Theta\sigma_i), \ldots, p(\Theta\sigma_n) \tag{5.31}$$

For example, the combination of two levels L_i and L_j, corresponds to aggregation $p(\Theta\sigma_1)$ obtained by Eq. (5.32):

$$p(\Theta\sigma_1) = \max\{p(\Theta^{Li}), p(\Theta^{Lj})\} \tag{5.32}$$

5.6.2.5 Trend prediction

Finally, the future trend prediction of the template $X(t)$ is obtained by combining the optimal trends that resulted from the optimization process, according to Eq. (5.33), where the subscript σ denotes these optimal trends:

$$\hat{Y}(t) = a^{\upsilon} Z(t) + \sum \sigma \overline{Z}(t) \quad t = N+1, \ldots, N+P \tag{5.33}$$

5.6.3 Hypertension risk evaluation

The created methodology was applied to blood pressure signals to evaluate the risk of hypertension using the TEN-HMS (Cleland et al., 2005) and MyHeart datasets (Habetha, 2006).

5.6.3.1 Experiments

A group of experiments were conducted mostly involving patients with critical blood pressure values (around the hypertension threshold). The primary aim was to determine whether a patient's blood pressure signal, as illustrated in Fig. 5.10, would evolve toward hypertension values during the following week or whether it would be maintained or decrease to regular values.

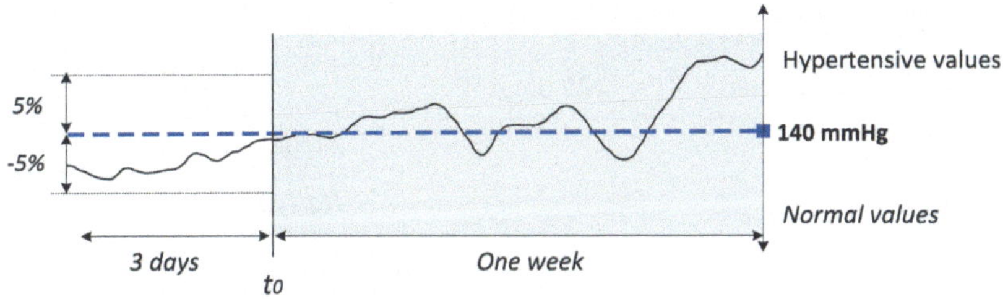

Figure 5.10 Assessment of hypertension risk.

The procedure began by identifying patients who had lately exhibited blood pressure values in a critical range, that is, who during three successive days had shown blood pressure values in the range [− 5%, +5%] of the limit value of 140 mmHg.

For these patients the following week's blood pressure values were then estimated by using the methodology presented, and depending on the proportion of values above the limit threshold (140 mmHg), the risk of the patient was calculated. In effect, if the proportion was greater than 75%, the patient was deemed to be in danger of developing hypertension; in the other situation (less than 75%) the patient was deemed not to have any risk of hypertension.

5.6.3.2 Results with the TEN-HMS dataset

The validation of the methodology began by choosing those from a collection of 600 random templates that verified the necessary condition (to be within the critical range). In fact, a total of 68 templates met this requirement; in 19 situations the patient had a risk of developing a disease of hypertension, and in 49 situations the patient did not have any risk. The method's capacity to discriminate is shown in Table 5.2.

The SE and SP were calculated to quantify the effectiveness of the methodology, with values of 84.2% and 75.5%, respectively. Taking into account that prediction was made to fully random templates, the SE and SP values that were obtained were very acceptable. In fact, these metrics demonstrate the potential of the trend prediction strategy.

5.6.3.3 Results with the MyHeart dataset

With respect to the second dataset, 500 templates were chosen in a random way. From these a total of 95 exhibited values in the critical range; in 21 situations the patient revealed risk of developing an hypertension condition, while in 74 situations the patient revealed no risk. Table 5.3 shows the discrimination capability of the method for this dataset.

Table 5.2 Confusion matrix (TEN-HMS dataset).

		Actual class	
		No risk	**In risk**
Predicted class	No risk	37	3
	In risk	12	16

Table 5.3 Confusion matrix (MyHeart dataset).

		Actual class No risk	In risk
Predicted class	No risk	68	3
	In risk	6	18

In this second group of experiments, the SE and SP were 85.71% and 91.89%, respectively, demonstrating the potential of the trend prediction methodology.

The sensitivity and specificity in this second group of experiments were 85.71% and 91.89% respectively, demonstrating the potential of the methodology to predict trends.

5.6.4 Conclusions

The presented methodology, based on a wavelet decomposition to predict biosignals, aims not to perform accurate predictions, but rather to reasonably estimate the future evolution trend of the signal. The ability of the proposed strategy was tested in evaluating the hypertension risk of patients whose blood pressure values were in a critical range (around the threshold of hypertension). For this purpose, real data collected by two telemonitoring platforms, TEN-HMS and MyHeart, were used. The values of SE and SP resulting from the performed experiments demonstrated the capacity of the methodology.

5.7 Conclusions

The stratification, risk assessment, and prognosis of a patient's condition are challenging tasks that physicians have to deal with in their daily clinical practice. The development and implementation of innovative algorithms and models that are able to process and analyze the available information are undoubtedly decisive for supporting the decision of professionals in a more proactive manner.

This chapter addresses these issues, through the research and implementation of models following three distinct approaches. The first proposes a personalization approach, based on the evidence that the performance of risk assessment models differs among different groups of patients. Therefore the creation of groups of patients for whom it is possible to identify a specific risk tool that ensures a good performance is the main foundation of this methodology. The second approach proposes the development of a generic risk assessment model that is capable of simultaneously integrating a set of individual well-established risk models. This approach makes it possible to obtain a robust solution that is able to deal with the lack of information by using of several models simultaneously, avoiding the selection of a particular risk model and increasing the clinical confidence. The last approach addresses the development of solutions to dynamically assess the progression and the early detection of relevant clinical conditions, in particular hypertension states. Basically, the proposed strategy is founded on a case-based reasoning approach. It compares current trends of vital signals with historical data and uses the similar behaviors that have been identified in the historical data in the prediction of current events.

Experimental results, carried out by using three clinical datasets (a dataset of patients admitted to the emergency unit of Santa Cruz Hospital and data collected during two telemonitoring studies, MyHeart and TEN-HMS) have shown the potential of the proposed strategies.

References

Agrawal, R., et al. (1993). Efficient similarity search in sequence databases. *Proceeding of the International Conference on Foundations of Data Organizations and Algorithms*, 69–84.

Andritsos, P., et al. (2002). Data clustering techniques, Toronto, University of Toronto *Department of Computer Science*, *1*(1), 3–2.

Antman, E., et al. (2000). The TIMI risk score for unstable angina/non-st elevation MI—A method for prognostication and therapeutic decision making. *JAMA: The Journal of the American Medical Association*, *284*, 835–842.

Arthur, D., & Vassilvitskii, S. (2007). "k-means++: The advantages of careful seeding" (PDF). In *Proceedings of the eighteenth annual ACM-SIAM symposium on discrete algorithms* (pp. 1027–1035). Philadelphia, PA: Society for Industrial and Applied Mathematics.

Assmann, G., Cullen, H., & Schulte, H. (2002). Simple scoring scheme for calculating the risk of acute coronary events based on the 10-year follow-up of the Prospective Cardiovascular Münster (PROCAM). *Circulation*, *105*, 310–315.

Boersma, E., Pieper, K., & Steyerberg, E. (2000). Predictors of outcome in patients with acute coronary syndromes without persistent ST-segment elevation. Results from an international trial of 9461 patients. *Circulation*, *101*, 2557–2567.

British Cardiac Society. (2000). Joint British recommendations on prevention of coronary heart disease in clinical practice. *BMJ (Clinical Research ed.)*, *320*.

Caruana, R., et al. (2015). Intelligible models for healthcare: Predicting pneumonia risk and hospital 30 days readmission. In *Proceedings of the 21th ACM SIGKDD international conference on knowledge discovery and data mining*.

Chen, J. Y., Qin, Z., & Jia, J. (2008). A weighted mean subtractive clustering algorithm. *Information Technology Journal*, 7, 356–360.

Cleland., et al. (2005). Noninvasive home telemonitoring for patients with heart failure at high risk of recurrent admission and death. *Journal of the American College of Cardiology*, *45*, 1654–1664.

Conroy, R., Pyorala, K., Fitzgerald, A., et al. (2003). Estimation of ten-year risk of fatal cardiovascular disease in Europe: The SCORE project. *European Heart Journal, 24*, 987–1003.

Cox, J., Coupland, C., Vinogradova, Y., Robson, J., May, M., & Brindle, P. (2007). Derivation and validation of QRISK, a new cardiovascular disease risk score for the United Kingdom: Prospective open cohort study. *BMJ (Clinical Research ed.)*.

D'Agostino, R., Vasan, R., Pencina, M., Wolf, A., Cobain, M., & Massaro, J. K. (2008). *General cardiovascular risk profile for use in primary care: The Framingham heart study. American Heart Association.*

Damen, J., et al. (2016). Prediction models for cardiovascular disease risk in the general population: Systematic review. *BMJ (Clinical Research ed.), 353*, i2416.

Fodor, I. (2002). A survey on reduction techniques. UCRL-ID-148494. *Lawrence Livermore National Laboratory*.

Fryzlewicz., et al. (2003). Forecasting non-stationary time series by wavelet process modeling. *ISM, 55*(4), 737–764.

Habetha, J. (2006). MyHeart—A new approach for remote monitoring and management of cardiovascular diseases. *IEEE*.

Hammouda, K. (2000). A comparative study of data clustering. *Techniques, SYDE 625: Tools of Intelligent Systems Design*, Course Project. University of Waterloo.

Han, J., Kamber, M., & Pei, J. (2011). *Data mining: Concepts and techniques, ISBN: 9780123814791* (3rd ed.). Morgan Kaufmann.

Haykin, S. (2008). *Neural networks and learning machines* (3rd ed.). Prentice Hall.

He, H., & Stevens, E. (2009). Learning from imbalanced data. *IEEE Transactions on Knowledge and Data Engineering Archive, 21*(9).

Jackson, R. (2002). Updated New Zealand cardiovascular disease risk-benefit prediction guide. *BMJ (Clinical Research ed.), 320*, 709–710.

Kriegel., et al. (2003). Density-based clustering. *WIREs Data Mining and Knowledge Discovery, 1*(3), 231–232.

Lee, D. (2007). *Nonlinear dimensionality reduction*. Springer.

Maaten, L. (2009). Dimensionality reduction: A comparative review. *TiCC TR 2009–005*, Tilburg University.

Marques, T., Henriques, J., Carvalho, P., Paredes, S., Rocha, T., & Morais, J. (2015). Personalization based on grouping strategies for short-term cardiovascular event risk assessment. *Cardiovascular Engineering and Technology*. Available from https://doi.org/10.1007/s13239-015-0228-8.

Paredes, S., Rocha, T., de Carvalho, P., Henriques, J., Mendes, D., Cabete, R., ... Morais, J. (2015). The cardiorisk project: Improvement of cardiovascular risk assessment. *The Journal of Computational Science*. Available from https://doi.org/10.1016/j.jocs.2015.04.025.

Paredes, S., Rocha, T., de Carvalho, P., Henriques, J., Morais, J., & Ferreira, J. (2015). Integration of different risk assessment tools to improve stratification of patients with coronary artery disease. *Medical & Biological Engineering & Computing (MBEC)*. Available from https://doi.org/10.1007/s11517-015-1342-3.

Paredes, S., Rocha, T., Mendes, D., de Carvalho, P., Henriques, J., Morais, J., ... Mendes, D. (2015). New approaches for improving cardiovascular risk assessment. *Revista Portuguesa de Cardiologia*. Available from https://doi.org/10.1016/j.repc.20150.10.006.

Park, S., et al. (2000). Efficient searches for similar subsequences of different lengths in sequence databases. *Proceeding of the International Conference of Data Engineering*, 23–32.

Renaud., et al. (2003). Prediction based on a multiscale decomposition. *International Journal of Wavelets, Multiresolution and Information Processing, 1*(2), 217–232.

Riaz, K., & Ahmed, A. *Hypertensive heart disease*. Department of Internal Medicine, Section of Cardiology, Wright State University. http://emedicine.medscape.com/article/162449-overview.

Rocha, T., et al. (2012). An efficient strategy for evaluating similarity between time series based on Wavelet/Karhunen-Loève transforms. *IEEE EMBS*, 6216–6219, San Diego.

Saeed, M., & Mark, R. (2006). A novel method for the efficient retrieval of similar multiparameter physiologic time series using wavelet-based symbolic representations. *AMIA Symposium*.

Sterne, J., et al. (2009). Multiple imputation for missing data in epidemiological and clinical research: Potential and pitfalls. *BMJ (Clinical Research ed.)*. Available from https://doi.org/10.1136/bmj.b2393.

Stevens, R., et al. (2001). The UKPDS risk engine: A model for the risk of coronary heart disease in Type II diabetes. *Clinical Science*, *101*, 671–679.

Sugiyama, M. (2010). Semi-supervised local Fisher discriminant analysis for dimensionality. *Machine Learning*, *78*, 35–61.

Tang, E., et al. (2007). Global registry of acute coronary events(GRACE) hospital discharge risk scores accurately predicts long term mortality post acute coronary syndrome. *American Heart Journal*.

Wallis, E., Ramsay, L., Haq, I., Ghahramani, P., Jackson, P., Rowland, K., & Yeo, W. (2000). Coronary and cardiovascular risk estimation for primary prevention: Validation of a new Sheffield table in the 1995 Scottish health survey population. *BMJ (Clinical Research ed.)*, *320*, 671–676.

WHO. (2017). *World Heart Day*. Fact sheet 2017. http://www.who.int/cardiovascular_diseases/world-heart-day-2017/. Accessed February 2018.

Woodward, M. (2006). *Adding social deprivation and family history to cardiovascular risk assessment—The ASSIGN score from the Scottish Heart Health Extended Cohort*. Available from http://heart.bmj.com/cgi/rapidpdf/hrt0.2006.108167v1

Yang, K., & Shahabi, C. (2004). A PCA-based similarity measure for multivariate time series. *Proceeding of the 2nd ACM International Workshop on Multimedia Databases*.

CHAPTER 6

Connected health technologies for knowledge extraction and knowledge-based medicine in cardiac care

Ioanna Chouvarda
Lab of Computing, Medical Informatics, and Biomedical Imaging Technologies, School of Medicine, Aristotle University of Thessaloniki, Thessaloniki, Greece

6.1 Introduction

Connected health technologies (CHT) have been advancing during the last 15 years and have brought the promise for a paradigm shift in care, entailing timely technology-based information and better decisions (Caulfield & Donnelly, 2013). This is widely needed in chronic care, including cardiovascular diseases (CVDs). As has been reported by the World Health Organization (WHO),[1] 71% of all yearly deaths globally are due to chronic noncommunicable diseases (NCDs). CVDs account for most NCD deaths, or more than 17 million people annually, followed by cancer, respiratory diseases, and diabetes. Between the ages of 30 and 69 years, this is disproportionately prevalent in low- and middle-income countries. The statistics of CVD as the leading global cause of death are expected to increase in the next decades.

Multiple factors, genetic, physiological, environmental, and behavioral, play a role in the NCDs in general and CVDs in particular. Among others, an unhealthy lifestyle (smoking, alcohol, poor diet, and inactivity) increases mortality risk; therefore reducing these modifiable risk factors is a significant primary and secondary prevention aim in which both policy-makers and technology providers have been engaged. A second major challenge is disease management, specifically how to optimize health and quality of life for this population and decrease hospitalizations along with medical costs. With heart failure as the endpoint of a variety of CVDs

[1] https://www.who.int/news-room/fact-sheets/detail/noncommunicable-diseases

Personalized Health Systems for Cardiovascular Disease
DOI: https://doi.org/10.1016/B978-0-12-818950-4.00001-X

among elderly populations (Guha & McDonagh, 2013), providing optimal therapy and decreasing the burden of disease remain significant challenges.

While technology has dramatically advanced toward supporting new cardiac care services, there is still a need for technological integration for more combined and contextualized sensing. Different point-of-care devices have been proposed, from lab-on-a-chip (LoC) biological testing (Wu et al., 2017) to biomarkers in body fluids (Hu et al., 2016), such as brain natriuretic peptide (Sarangadharan et al., 2018), and physiological measurement systems. These are still treated as separate solutions or as promises for new and better biomarkers. The lack of persuasive evidence has hindered their wider adoption. Generating evidence on integrated approaches that put together different sensing and point-of care-technologies can result in new knowledge within a systems medicine context.

Among the still unmet challenges for the point-of-care devices for chronic diseases and cardiac care is the lack of knowledge about the behaviors and diversity of measurements in a continuous real-life setting. Questions such as "What is the day-to-day fluctuation in biosignals?" and "What do these fluctuations mean or what can be inferred from them?" need to be investigated, and knowledge must be built before such systems can be used for advanced decision making. The ambition is to leverage knowledge in a manner that speaks about personal dynamics and thus customize medical intervention for the individual patient.

Multiparametric data integration and analytics analysis in personal cloud platforms is foreseen as the cornerstone for understanding chronic conditions and their relationship to patient's life and specific events and interventions, for more safely predicting adverse events, for exploring interventions, and for making smarter closed-loop systems with more realistic feedback loops. These would include physiological measurements in daily life, lifestyle data (e.g., nutrition, activity, behavior, environment) via the inclusion of consumer electronics and smart environmental sensors, point-of-care and LoC sensors for biological information, such as extracellular vesicles (Chistiakov, Orekhov, & Bobryshevy, 2016) and biomarkers, clinical information, and intervention-related data.

This chapter discusses first the connected health technologies in cardiac care, along with the needed technological building blocks for advanced cardiac care services, including data acquisition and point-of-care devices, big data analytics, health behavior informatics, interventions, and knowledge-based medicine. Then CHT in the scope of knowledge-based medicine and the concepts of learning health systems are presented. Finally, challenges and future directions are discussed.

6.2 Enabling technologies and building blocks: The connected health technologies in cardiac care

6.2.1 Connected health technologies and mobile health

Connected health technologies has been described as "a paradigm shift looking after the individual and community health in a process that speaks to the health journey of the person, through the entire lifespan, leveraging a variety of technologies to do so" (Mountford et al., 2016). In view of the WHO priorities for prevention and disease management of chronic diseases, the role of CHT in support of integrated care (Chouvarda, Goulis, Lambrinoudaki, & Maglaveras, 2015) and new models of cardiac care (Forman et al., 2011) is an important one.

Connected health technologies can make available the relevant information in a timely fashion and thus help all involved stakeholders make better decisions (Caulfield & Donnelly, 2013). As a conceptual model for health management, CHT deploys devices, services, and interventions that are designed around the patient's needs. The health-related data are shared among the involved stakeholders, and the patient can receive care in the most proactive and efficient manner possible.

A pivotal development in CHT is the generation of personal health systems (PHS) as an alternative to centralized clinically driven data management. The aims of PHS are to provide better access to information and to enlist the active participation of patients in the management of their own health. The concept of PHS was introduced in the 1990s as a target activity of the European Commission research agenda (Gatzoulis & Iakovidis, 2007). Its core is the personal health record, "an electronic application through which individuals can access, manage and share their health information, and that of others for whom they are authorized, in a private, secure, and confidential environment" (Tang, Ash, Bates, Overhage, & Sands, 2006). Around this concept, a loosely connected ecosystem of sensor systems and applications for all stakeholders—patients and citizens, healthcare professionals, other informal caregivers, and health policymakers—can grow (Chouvarda et al., 2015).

Within CHT, mobile applications and remote technologically enhanced heart failure (HF) monitoring have been proposed and studied in terms of earlier identification of decompensation, better adherence to lifestyle changes, and medication and interventions (such as diuretic dosage changes) that reduce the need for hospitalization.

The impact of mobile health (mHealth) interventions on HF outcomes (mortality, hospitalizations, NYHA class, quality of life) is yet inconclusive (Cajita, Gleason, & Han, 2016).

In a review by Brahmbhatt and Cowie, two issues were raised with respect to the effectiveness of CHT: (1) While remote data collection is facilitated, the transformation to better decisions has not yet been accomplished, and (2) despite the technology-driven potential for digital health, evidence and knowledge are not yet consistent (Brahmbhatt and Cowie, 2019).

As Woods, Duff, Roehrer, Walker, and Cummings (2019) suggested, a significant barrier for the adoption of consumer mobile health interventions for chronic conditions is the lack of integration of technology into everyday life in combination with already established disease self-management routines.

6.2.2 Point-of-care diagnostics and sensor systems

The majority of the studies for remote monitoring of HF typically included a blood pressure (BP)—measuring device, a weighing scale, and an electrocardiogram (ECG) recorder (Cajita et al., 2016). However, from the technology side, a variety of devices have been studied for diagnostic and monitoring purposes in cardiological connected health applications. In an attempt to map the sensing devices employed in the domain, the following classification can be applied.

6.2.2.1 Physiological monitoring

In CVDs, continuously monitoring the ECG signals, combined with activity status, is vital for understanding within context arrhythmias and other adverse events. To overcome practical issues of Holter monitors for routine use (weight, attached electrodes, and gel), wearable sensors have been proposed for these continuous measurements.

In the work of Miao et al., a wearable, low-power context-aware ECG monitoring system integrated with built-in kinetic sensors of the smartphone with a self-designed ECG sensor, incorporating a commercial microcontroller unit, a secure digital (SD) card, and a Bluetooth module (Miao, Cheng, He, He, & Li, 2015). The proposed system can monitor the user's physical activity and thus identify the most common abnormal ECG patterns in different activities.

A more sophisticated solution has been proposed in the WELCOME project (https://www.csem.ch/Doc.aspx?id = 45291) to address the needs of complex multimorbid patients in whom either cardiac or pulmonary decompensations may occur (e.g., heart failure, diabetes, anxiety, depression). The monitoring system proposes the integration of medical devices (a BP meter) with a light vest including a large number of noninvasive chest sensors for monitoring ECG, lung sounds, electrical impedance tomography, and activity (Chouvarda, Philip et al., 2014).

Pulse transit time (PTT)—based BP measurement devices promise accurate and continuous cuffless BP estimation, so they have attracted active research. PTT-based BP estimations have mainly combined ECG information, while other solutions are also being sought, including measuring PTT through plethysmography between two distal points, ballistocardiography (heart sound) sensors, radar technologies, and tonometry. The review of PTT devices by Bard, Joseph, and van Helmond (2019) concludes that the promising developments and preliminary data suggest the need for further validation, addressing potential issues of motion artifacts, calibration procedures, and the stability of measurements over time, before the deployment of clinical studies for concrete clinical knowledge establishment, along with reimbursement structures.

6.2.2.2 Ambient monitoring

In conjunction with wearable sensors, effort has been given to developing sensors embedded in the patient's environment that can continuously and unobtrusively measure relevant signals, for example, signals relating to the patient's sleep or frailty.

A characteristic example is the use of a bed pressure sensor for heart rate (HR) and respiration rate estimation during sleep, which is useful in detecting bradycardia and apnea, among other conditions. In a study by Kortelainen et al., a bed sensor with multiple pressure-sensitive noncontacting electrodes was applied for unobtrusive monitoring during sleep, and multichannel algorithms were applied to extract the HR and respiration signal from the recorded ballistocardiographic data (Kortelainen, Van Gils, & Parkka, 2012). To determine the reliability of the estimated nocturnal HR recorded through a bed sensor, a matrix of piezoelectric sensors integrated into the mattress was assessed and compared with polysomnography; differences in heartbeat detection were found to be minor (Migliorini et al., 2014).

When it comes to fall and fainting (syncope) detection, most technological solutions rely on wearables and intelligent algorithms (Cotechini et al., 2019). However, to address the needs of people who have limited ability to maintain and use wearable devices, Tyrer and Muheidat (2016) proposed the use of a prototype smart carpet, which uses 128 sensors, and the sensors output a voltage due to a person walking or falling on the carpet. Employing computational intelligence techniques, they detected falls with high accuracy (96.2%) and a real-time display.

6.2.2.3 Lab on a chip

A different category of measurements includes devices that can detect multiple biomarkers in biological fluids for CVD. LoC biosensors have shown high diagnostic potential by measuring relevant blood biomarkers such as interleukin-6 and C-reactive protein (Wu et al., 2017). Other targets may include cholesterol and lipid components and protein biomarkers for inflammation (e.g., apolipoprotein A1) and heart attack (e.g., cardiac troponin, fibrinogen, plasminogen activator inhibitor-1). Extracellular vesicles, exosomes, have attracted interest in microfluidic research as an ideal resource for specific multibiomarker detection. Within CHT there is an emerging trend to use smartphones as the detection tools to read the signals from the LoC biosensors, the so-called Ms^2 technology (i.e., mobile sensing based on microfluidic devices and smartphones).

6.2.3 Health behavior informatics

Health-related behaviors are actions taken by a person to maintain, attain, or regain good health and prevent illness or the opposite: actions not taken that would have had an impact on health and quality of life.

Health behavior informatics has been introduced as an emerging transdisciplinary research domain, with "the potential to optimize interventions through monitoring, assessing, and modeling behavior in support of providing tailored and timely interventions" (Pavel, Jimison, Korhonen, Gordon, & Saranummi, 2015) and the ambition to create closed-loop health behavior interventions based on multiscale models of behavior change.

As highlighted by Ansary, Azuma, Komatireddy, and Barrett (2013), the American Heart Association has outlined seven key health metrics, including physical activity, adequate BP control, weight, and healthy diet, at the core of CVD management for a substantial reduction in cardiovascular mortality. In the review on cardiovascular risks and behaviors by

Winter, Sheats, and King (2016), the main CVD risk behaviors and indicators were physical activity (46%), weight loss (38%), healthy eating (29%), tobacco cessation (26%), health promotion (14%), BP (12%), glucose monitoring (9%), lipid monitoring (5%), and sitting (2.5%). The same review suggested the following as important patient behaviors that can mediate positive or negative outcomes: self-management (15%), reducing alcohol consumption (6%), stress management (2%), reducing risks (2%), and healthy coping and support (1%). These metrics are well suited to a connected health management strategy.

Health behavior monitoring and change support has to take into account behaviors that are overt and directly measurable or observable, such as talking or running, and behaviors that are covert and not directly viewable, such as stressful thoughts. The latter may either be reported by the subjects or detected by inference or through the use of special techniques and devices. Because behaviors are intertwined, it is crucial to take into account the full range of behaviors and influences upon these behaviors. The revolution of smart wearable devices has provided opportunities and means for developing objective and unobtrusive behavior detection methods in real-life settings that can replace or be combined with the more biased and inaccurate self-reporting of various behaviors.

6.2.3.1 Monitoring

Physical activity monitoring and support is a major issue in CVD, and it is systematically focused on cardiac rehabilitation (CR) programs to slow or reverse the progression of CVD. Nevertheless, uptake of community-based CR and the required physical activity is low. Buys et al. (2016) explored the suitable technology usage for CVD patients and their needs and interests for technology-enabled CR. A technology usage questionnaire was developed and completed by 298 patients (mean age: 61.7 years) from a supervised ambulatory CR program, an adult congenital heart disease clinic, and two community-based CR programs. Results suggest that most patients had a mobile phone and used the Internet. A high percentage were familiar with HR monitors, especially when exercising at home, and they were interested in CR support through the Internet and their mobile phone, while many patients were interested in game-based CR and virtual rehabilitation.

Focusing on physical activity for CVD patients, the work of Chatzitofis, Zarpalas, and Daras (2018) proposes a computerized system for monitoring exercise performance and e-coaching in exercise-based rehabilitation and training. The system acquires and fuses motion capture data from different modalities (Kinect and IMUs) and performs real-time anthropometric measurements and analysis. The system can capture, monitor, and evaluate physical exercises, detect and evaluate exercise repetitions, and e-coach the subjects through real-time feedback. Using less sophisticated and more affordable approaches, digital self-monitoring of physical activity after the CR program can enhance activity maintenance after the completion of a CR program (Vogel et al., 2017).

Maramis, Kilintzis, Scholl, and Chouvarda (2018) addressed the objective monitoring of smoking behavior using smart watch inertial sensory data (three-axis gyroscope) that are routinely acquired by any Android Wear smartphone and the detection of smoking instances and the constituting puffs with machine learning. The feasibility of the method with actual real-life data yielded very promising preliminary results.

Estimation of medication adherence is a necessary piece of information before decisions can be made about treatment optimization, especially as adherence is not always high among CVD patients. In an effort to unobtrusively estimate medication incompliance of HF and hypertensive patients, Chouvarda, Mabote, et al. (2014) analyzed vital signs data to detect differences due to medication incompliance, taking into account physiological fluctuations introduced by different factors of daily life, such as medication timing, diet, and activity. Classification models based on machine learning trained with a pair of features (systolic BP and HR in a semirecumbent position) achieved over 97% accuracy in a cross-validation setup, in detecting 48-hour incompliance, a promising step towards a CHT application of vital signs measurement and analysis for detection and monitoring of medication incompliance.

6.2.3.2 Interventions

Regarding dieting behavior, a systematic review of salt consumption reduction by mHealth interventions (Ali et al., 2019) revealed only a few interventions, and limited study resources. Most interventions employed short message services, had a primary focus of improving awareness of dietary salt consumption, and provided dubious outcome evidence to evaluate the effectiveness of salt reduction interventions. Overall, salt reduction and dietary behaviors in mHealth initiatives remain relatively unexplored, although they have high potential.

The use of games, including augmented reality technologies, has been employed for increasing patient engagement. A serious digital game was developed for improving knowledge and self-management behaviors of community-dwelling HF patients (Radhakrishnan et al., 2016). Testing suggested that it was both satisfying and acceptable, and, more important for participants with lower education levels and ages, it was the preferred medium for receiving information.

In a later scoping study of the use of digital games to improve self-management behaviors of CVD patients, mostly toward activity, the results were conflicting, and barriers appeared (loss of interest, poor perception through games, sensor problems, lack of social aspects), which have to be taken into account in designing and personalizing approaches (Radhakrishnan, Baranowski, Julien, Thomaz, & Kim, 2019).

Overall, the most frequently used behavior change techniques were self-monitoring and feedback on performance (Winter et al., 2016). To better target CVD behavioral risk factors and to optimize technology-enabled interventions, a variety of health behavior change theories and techniques and related evidence need to be better integrated.

6.2.4 Data management and analytics

An overview of big data methods in cardiology addressed issues of data management for different types of data (Chouvarda & Maglaveras, 2019). Remote patient monitoring employing ECG and relevant biosignals is expected to vastly increase the amount of data to be managed and analyzed as well as reused; this makes electrocardiology a big-data domain (Deserno & Marx, 2016) in terms of data management and analytics. Cloud computing and new analysis methods, such as deep learning, are emerging in the field, while edge computing and privacy-preserving designs also gain attention.

6.2.4.1 Data integration and management

Cloud computing has been the dominant model for organizing data management and analytics infrastructures in recent years (Navale & Bourne, 2018). According to the National Institute of Standards and Technology (NIST):

> *Cloud computing is a model for enabling convenient, on-demand network access to a shared pool of configurable computing resources (e.g., networks, servers, storage applications and services) that can be rapidly provisioned and released with minimal management effort or service provider interaction.*

Cloud computing promises advantages in dynamic resources such as computing power and storage capacities, ubiquitous access to resources at any time from any place, and high flexibility and scalability of resources. A review of cloud computing in healthcare can be found in (Griebel et al., 2015). However, the term "cloud" often means just "using virtual machines" or "web-based" rather than being part of a true cloud paradigm. On one hand, involving external cloud partners brings data safety and security issues; on the other hand, elasticity, pay-per-use, and broad network access are the main favorable features.

The software-as-a-service model has offered several cloud-deployed software tools for public use, mostly in the "omics" domain but also in biosignal analysis. In the case of a PHS, private or hybrid approaches have been followed as well. For example, a cloud computing–based ECG teleconsultation service has been implemented on the Microsoft Azure platform that enables a 12-lead ECG to be transmitted via mobile phones and interpreted accordingly in a convenient, efficient, and inexpensive manner (Hsieh & Hsu, 2012).

The idea of a personal data cloud has been introduced that aggregates the heterogeneous personal data scattered in different clouds into one cloud so that a person could effectively store, acquire, and share their data, based on semantic and linked data concepts for data integration, and adaptive service collaboration could be deployed (Wang & Wang, 2014). As regards methods for PHS data management and integration, the issues of managing health data for integrated care is tackled in the work of Kilintzis, Chouvarda, Beredimas, Natsiavas, and Maglaveras (2019). To account for the data heterogeneity and volume, a semantic framework based on HL7 FHIR (https://www.hl7.org/fhir/) resources is proposed that follows Linked Data principles (https://www.w3.org/wiki/LinkedData) and is combined with a NoSQL persistent storage approach using the Virtuoso Triple Store engine (http://vos.openlinksw.com/owiki/wiki/VOS).

6.2.4.2 Analytics and artificial intelligence

A review of multiomics analysis for CVDs focused on the integration of genomics, epigenomics, transcriptomics, and proteomics for the investigation of novel mechanisms and plasma biomarkers involved in CVDs (Leon-Mimila, Wang, & Huertas-Vazquez, 2019). To provide a platform for further studies in the field, Fernandes, Patel, and Husi (2018) developed a CVD database, an integrated information resource that covers multiomic studies (microRNA, genomics, proteomics, and metabolomics) of cardiovascular-related traits with particular emphasis on coronary artery disease. The resource is based on a specific ontology for data harmonization and offers a dedicated interactive web interface to access the data search and export functionality (www.padb.org/cvd).

The ECG is an affordable signal that is well established in clinical practice and has been traditionally employed as input to biosignal analysis and machine learning techniques for diagnostic purposes. Its acquisition via portable and wearable technologies is feasible. Therefore its analysis continues to be essential in the CHT field, exploring noisy data, nonstandard leads, and different contexts, to leverage quality to medical standards.

An overview of ECG analysis methods along with the main clinical application areas focused on time-domain methods (Chouvarda, Filos, & Maglaveras, 2019). As highlighted, a group of methods, which is actually very relevant to CHT and continuous ECG recordings, focuses on the temporal variability of ECG characteristics, wave intervals, or morphologies. Better understanding and modeling of the underlying phenomena will undoubtedly be of great value in decision making. This review highlights the barriers that have to be surmounted for better adoption of ECG analytics; the standardization, including the reproducibility and validation, of analytic methods as well as of public ECG databases; and the availability of analytics resources in clinical practice.

Advanced machine learning methods have been proposed for ECG analysis, addressing different problems. Deep neural network (DNN)–based ECG classification, in normal or arrhythmic beats, has drawn the attention of numerous researchers, employing mostly convolutional neural networks (CNNs) and recurrent neural networks (RNNs). These methods can automatically learn complex representative features directly from the data, thereby eliminating the need for manual feature extraction. They are end-to-end learning systems that take ECG signals as input and provide arrhythmia class prediction as output while extracting the "deep features" autonomously. In the presence of enough data, they can deliver higher accuracy and better classification results. In most cases, the well-known Physionet MIT-BIH Arrhythmia Database is used, owing to its high availability of data. Among the interesting options is the transformation of the one-dimensional ECG signal into a two-dimensional image using spectrograms or time scale representations and shifting the problem to the image classification and object recognition domain.

Li et al. (2019) addressed the detection of a ventricular ectopic beat, often mixed with artifacts, in a method combining the wavelet transform with a deep learning network. ECG waveforms are transformed into two-dimensional time-frequency images and fed into a CNN. Independent testing resulted in an F1 score of 84.96% and accuracy of 97.36%, showing a good generalization.

Focusing on the classification of ECG acquired with wearable devices, Saadatnejad, Oveisi, and Hashemi (2019) proposed a solution that employs wavelet transform and multiple long short-term memory (LSTM) recurrent neural networks, providing a high classification performance with low computational resources, suitable for continuous and real-time use in wearable devices. Screening of hyperkalemia, a severe condition associated with fatal arrhythmias, is proposed by Galloway et al. (2019), based on a deep-learning model that uses ECG as input. The model was trained and tested with chronic kidney disease patients and achieved an area under the curve of 0.853−0.883.

Photoplethysmography (PPG) combined with accelerometer data has been used and provides the time-frequency spectra of synchronized PPG and accelerometer signals as input to various convolutional neural network architectures with estimated HR as output (Reiss, Indlekofer, Schmidt, & Van Laerhoven, 2019). The deep learning model performed significantly better than previous methods. A single wrist-worn PPG in ambulant setup has been used to estimate HR information and perform biometric identification in a DNN that combines CNN with LSTM and output layers (Biswas et al., 2019). The system, named CorNet, performs both tasks successfully in realistic environments.

Aiming at the screening of atrial fibrillation (AF) via wearable devices and mobile technology, an AF detection algorithm was developed, based on PPG signal, and two DNN architectures, 1D-CNN and RNN (Kwon et al., 2019). The algorithm worked in the presence of premature atrial complexes and in both cases outperformed previously developed AF detectors.

A significant issue and criticism in such efforts, besides the need for generalization and more extensive validation, is that users need to trust the artificial intelligence (AI) model and understand the result and the mechanisms behind it. The concepts of explainability (Holzinger, Langs, Denk, Zatloukal, & Müller, 2019) and interpretation (London, 2019) are gaining attention and leading to hybrid approaches with human and AI in the loop (Holzinger, Plass, et al., 2019).

6.3 Knowledge-based cardiovascular disease medicine in the context of connected health technologies

Knowledge-based medicine (KBM) integrates the pathophysiological vision with evidence-based medicine (EBM) and evaluates the applicability to the individual patient of the evidence acquired as the average derived from pure clinical groups. KBM looks into tools to customize medical intervention for the individual patient, relying on available and dynamically acquired knowledge, also beyond the classical controlled clinical trials [see the concept introduced by Bertolini (2014)]. These concepts are highly suitable in the context of CHT-based care services, which can serve in deriving further patient knowledge and in customizing care based on this knowledge.

An important step is to organize better and to disambiguate concepts while extending them from the clinical setting to the daily life continuum. An example has been given related to lifestyle adherence (Livitckaia et al., 2018). Adherence to a physical activity regimen in both daily life and rehabilitation programs is an important aspect and a challenge. The concept of adherence is complex. Adherence to CR physical exercise in several studies is defined through program attendance (irrespective of content execution), as the number of exercise sessions attended divided by the number of sessions scheduled, with nonadherence thresholds varying (50% or 66%) (Hawley-Hague, Horne, Skelton, & Todd, 2016). The criteria for dropout are equally varying.

Organizing knowledge to enhance decision making can involve semantic approaches. Following the previous line of work on concept disambiguation that focuses on patient adherence, Livitckaia et al. (2019) addressed two aspects: the need to span knowledge and adherence factors in multiple dimensions, enhancing personalization of approaches, and the heterogeneity of the available medical research evidence regarding factors affecting patients' adherence, which is a significant challenge for knowledge reusability. The OPTImAL ontology was proposed, focusing on CVD patient adherence to physical activity and exercise training. OPTImAL ontology encodes domain knowledge based on published studies. Further, the semantic model was conceptualized, formalized, and implemented, while the developed ontology was validated for its consistency, and externally evaluated for appropriateness and usefulness. The formal model describes the relationships of different factors of CVD patient profile with adherence and adherence quality, as well as the associated types and dimensions of physical activity and exercise. The formal model can serve as a knowledge tool in the practice of cardiac rehabilitation experts, supporting the process of activity regimen recommendations for better patient adherence. Besides extending to other aspects of behavior, a further enhancement of this approach is the addition of relation weights, derived from data analysis, and quantitative inferencing mechanisms. Fuzzy cognitive maps have been adopted in this direction (Papageorgiou, Roo, Huszka, & Colaert, 2012).

Clinical decision support is considered in a complex multimorbidity scenario, based on PHS data (Chouvarda et al., 2016). A multitude of data is employed, along with a semantic description of data and features (Carvalho et al., 2016) and the implementation of rules within the semantic framework, using SPIN (http://spinrdf.org/) and SPARQL technologies (Kilintzis, Beredimas, & Chouvarda, 2014). The scope of decision support is broad, and it aims at detecting changes in patient state originating from a number of disease comorbidities and recommending the appropriate action and the users involved. Decision support system (DSS) knowledge is heavily based on expert knowledge and medical evidence, which involve high-level definitions of medical conditions and medical intervention, requiring actual day-to-day data for patient classification and abnormality detection and complex rules, involving mandatory and optional features for diagnostic and intervention purposes. An overview is presented in Fig. 6.1. Among the issues raised in this work are the

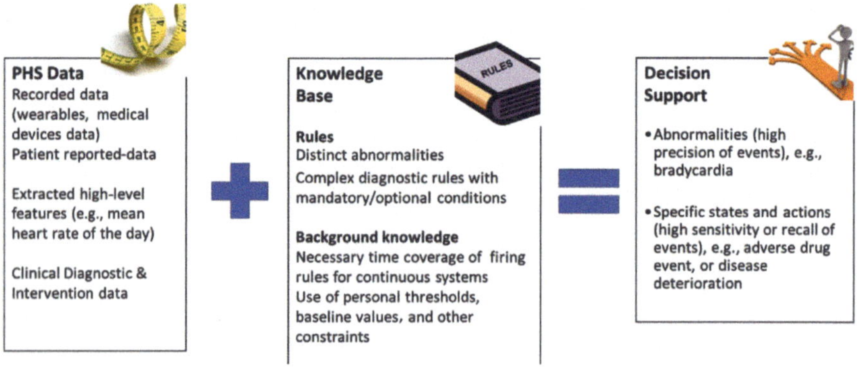

Figure 6.1 Overview of a personal health systems-related decision support system. Of note, precision is the number of correct events divided by the number of all detected events. Recall (or sensitivity) is the number of correct events divided by the number of actual events, events that should have been detected It can be viewed as the probability that an actual event is detected.

following: the guideline gaps in home-based comorbidity management, the increased need for information and measurements, the quality of measurements, and the sparseness of knowledge about the day-to-day or continuous measurements and their normal fluctuation, requiring the definition of personalized thresholds. Some of the conditions that affect quality of measurements, and correspondingly of the DSS, have been investigated (Vogt et al., 2016).

A different aspect of decision support in CVD aims to directly support patients. The work of (Triantafyllidis et al., 2018) presents the development and evaluation of a computerized DSS for unsupervised exercise rehabilitation at home and demonstrates the potential of patient decision support to improve the benefits of rehabilitation programs. The DSS, accessible via a RESTful web service, is based on international guidelines and expert knowledge. It employs data from a prescribed exercise program, HR from a wrist band device, and motion accuracy from a depth camera and subsequently generates personalized adaptations to the exercise program. It was evaluated in simulation and real-world studies with CVD patients, showing the improvement introduced by the DSS. This work demonstrates the use of personalized predictions of HR response during CR exercise programs (Filos et al., 2017).

6.3.1 From enabling technologies and research to a next-generation cardiac care platform and back

When cloud analytics platforms are involved, they may be regarded as research platforms (RP), decision support platforms (DP), or both. In seeking a continuum between knowledge discovery and knowledge-based decisions, it is considered useful to sharpen the two concepts, RP and DP.

A DP supports a CHT-service user (clinician or patient) in their daily routine challenges by synthesizing, summarizing, combining, and presenting information in a useful and actionable manner and providing predictions based on machine learning. A DP is locally accessible (at the user space) but can use cloud-based functionality; for example, it may run cloud-based machine learning. An RP enables data-driven research, in terms of selection, exploration, and visualization of data, along with analytics, and exploration of descriptive and predictive analytics specialized for different types of data. An RP is seen basically as a cloud service.

Regarding the similarities and differences between the two platforms, some important points are as follows:

- The users of the two platforms are different. A DP is used in routine practice by CHT users, patients, and healthcare professionals, while an RP is used by a multidisciplinary biomedical research team.
- The scope of use may differ: local in a DP versus multiple organizations in an RP. Different data governance and sharing policies may apply.
- The types of questions that are explored may differ: for the generation of new knowledge in an RP and to directly support clinical practice in a DP.
- The relevant methods differ, forming a more extensive range of analytics in an RP and adopting mature analytics in a DP.
- Data literacy is more demanding for an RP.
- Human-computer interaction and the level of interaction and presentation differ. In an RP, user interaction is extensive (exploratory analysis options, analytics pipelines). In a DP, efficiency is the priority (fast, simple, and straightforward access to information), direct crystallized views and direct answers to predefined questions without much interaction and need for user input.
- The level of time response in a DP is critical, and immediate response is needed in clinical practice. In an RP the volume of data for research, rather than the real-time response, can be the challenge.

The RP and DP are both parts of the health digital data economy. An RP establishes the data-driven research paradigm and data repurposing, while a DP produces value and impact from the mature data analytics and further promotes data-driven research and exploration. Both can be regarded as parts of a continuously learning health system, in which knowledge is extracted in an RP and integrated in a DP while the impact of the DP further refuels and leverages collaborative data-driven research.

6.3.2 A cardiovascular disease personal health system as part of a learning health system

Knowledge-based medicine needs to dynamically obtain and incorporate new knowledge, especially when the new domain of CHT-based services for the patients is in focus. The concept of a learning health system (LHS) is a very relevant one and can be seen at different organizational levels of care. An LHS can be defined as "an integrated ecosystem ... in which progress in science, informatics, and care culture align to generate new knowledge as an ongoing, natural by-product of the care experience, and seamlessly refine and deliver best practices for continuous improvement in health and healthcare" (Rubin et al., 2018). As stated by Delaney et al. (2015), "the LHS describes linking routine healthcare systems directly with both research translation and knowledge translation as an extension of the evidence-based medicine paradigm, taking advantage of the ubiquitous use of electronic health record (EHR) systems". A set of core values are attributed to an LHS, among which are that it should be person-focused, privacy-preserving, inclusive and participatory, transparent, and trustworthy; that it should have sustainability-oriented governance; and that it should have has scientific integrity.

Friedman, Rubin, and Sullivan (2017) highlights that LHSs embrace the secondary use of health data, envisioning complete cyclical processes, that is, successive iterations of learning cycles, in which information is essential. These mobilize health data, analyze it to create new knowledge (D2K), and apply that new knowledge to improve the health of individuals and populations and influence performance of the healthcare system (K2P). Changes in performance are documented and generate new data, which sees the next iteration of the cycle (P2D). A conceptualization in the context of CHT and PHS is provided in Fig. 6.2.

This iterative procedure can be supported and materialized by enabling infrastructures, mostly data-intensive and information-intensive ones, that

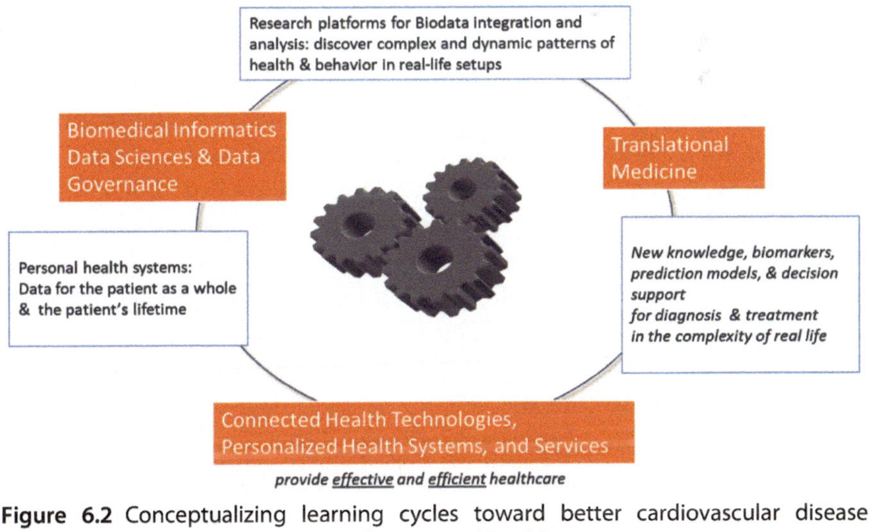

Figure 6.2 Conceptualizing learning cycles toward better cardiovascular disease knowledge, with the involvement of a personal health systems.

should be compatible with or transferable to CHT-based services. An example is the project work of TRANSFoRm concerning the infrastructure for the LHS in European primary care (Delaney et al., 2015). One of the project's use cases is a diagnostic DSS for chest pain, abdominal pain, and shortness of breath, and four directions were studied, clinical research, clinical data, provenance, and diagnosis, with the goal of creating an approach to interoperability. The project employs ontologies and archetypes to address the problem of data heterogeneity in the LHS. On the technological side, the infrastructure to ensure closing the D2K-K2P-P2D loop in a CHT context would require, beyond data harmonization methods, standardization activities in applying new decision rules and validating their performance and in dynamically updating all data acquisition and management services.

6.4 Discussion

Cardiovascular CHT is devoted to changing the management and prevention of CVD, a worldwide leading cause of death. As more patients and healthcare providers adopt CHT that allows for self-monitoring and point-of-care diagnostics, more data about patients' health and how best to influence it become available, allowing for more dynamic iterations of new knowledge and new services. In this path toward medicine that is both knowledge-based and CHT enabled, several enabling technologies are in place, but a series of challenges still need to be faced.

Table 6.1 highlights some of the experiences and challenges that are recognized in the field of establishing CHT and PHS in healthcare.

In investigating the path from new technological methods for data acquisition to analysis and then to new knowledge and the path from patient knowledge to better interventions, new visions can be helpful.

Vision 1: A new paradigm for combining technology with KBM. While several remarkable new sensing technologies are in place, approaches still tend to follow a single path, for example, focusing solely on genetic biomarkers or on physiological measurements. There is a need to work more on integrated approaches that combine such technologies. In addition, there is a need to bring closer the medical knowledge, data-driven models, and systems medicine approaches (Bousquet et al., 2011). As regards the health behavior, a need for knowledge elicitation, standardization, and fusion in the systems medicine realm of health behavior is more than evident. In this direction it is essential to bridge the gap between consumer electronics and

Table 6.1 An overview of connected health technologies-related challenges to wider adoption in healthcare.

Theme	Challenges
Difficulty in using connected health technologies	How to leverage digital health literacy? How could we educate the elders? Automate more procedures without user interaction?
Need for mature electronics	Are consumer electronics enough? Can experimental devices be trusted? Wearables energy and communication robustness
ICT robustness	Interoperability and standardization among services and devices How easily can new sensors be added? How to trust and interpret artificial intelligence
How to pass from observation to intervention	Data quality: difficulties for the health professional Lack of guidelines: how to decide interventions based on home data New knowledge on which patient segments can benefit more and when How deteriorations can be predicted and prevented: which information and what rules?

medical devices by combining them, expanding interoperability in wearable platforms, and using AI to extract value from this fusion. Extending data availability will benefit the much more comprehensive evaluation needed before the predictive tools can be applied in real-life DSSs. Human-like interaction with technology can be sought; virtual agents are already gaining attention as components of CHT interfaces.

Vision 2: From EBM to KBM iterations in a CHT setting. Gaining new knowledge from CHT-based services can gradually help to fulfill the needs for knowledge on which patient segments can benefit most from which services and when; this will aid in personalizing healthcare services. This is especially true for multimorbid patients or those with complex health needs. Insights into how parts of the "expert" decisions and actions can be delegated to patients can be gained, and this may translate to new service paradigms with an enhanced role of the patient in health coproduction. In this participatory effort, the role of all users is also revisited.

To better involve users, there is a need to teach them and leverage medical technology mentality and digital data literacy and to work toward more personalized methods beyond EBM. The level of validation of new devices and new services faces barriers and obstacles in moving beyond laboratory studies. To advance these concepts, some flexibility is required without compromising safety. Thus even partial sharing of data and knowledge in open data schemes is crucial. Knowledge production and sharing must move beyond classical EBM. The reuse of PHS data is one aspect, but repositories for sharing of methods and knowledge are also needed, and multiinstitutional RPs can play a role in this. Finally, in the foreseen LHS cycle, how to really measure and assess the impact is a crucial question. Moving beyond typical services and trials, which are typically monothematic, there is a need to approach the impact of CHT in new and dynamic ways, also extending the domain of health technology assessment within the CHT services and iterative KBM context.

References

Ali, S. H., Luo, R., Li, Y., Liu, X., Tang, C., & Zhang, P. (2019). Application of mobile health technologies aimed at salt reduction: Systematic review. *Journal of Medical Internet Research*. Available from https://doi.org/10.2196/13250.

Ansary, A., Azuma, A., Komatireddy, R., & Barrett, P. M. (2013). The connected health of cardiovascular medicine: Current status and future directions. *QJM: Monthly Journal of the Association of Physicians*, *106*(11), 979–982. Available from https://doi.org/10.1093/qjmed/hct159.

Bard, D. M., Joseph, J. I., & van Helmond, N. (2019). Cuff-less methods for blood pressure telemonitoring. *Frontiers in Cardiovascular Medicine*. Available from https://doi.org/10.3389/fcvm.2019.00040.

Bertolini, G. (2014). [The SIAARTI consensus document on the management of patients with end-stage chronic organ failure. From evidence-based medicine to knowledge-based medicine]. *Recenti Progressi in Medicina*, *105*(1), 7–8. Available from https://doi.org/10.1701/1398.15553.

Biswas, D., Everson, L., Liu, M., Panwar, M., Verhoef, B. E., Patki, S., & Van Helleputte, N. (2019). CorNET: Deep learning framework for PPG-based heart rate estimation and biometric identification in ambulant environment. *IEEE Transactions on Biomedical Circuits and Systems*. Available from https://doi.org/10.1109/TBCAS.2019.2892297.

Bousquet, J., Anto, J. M., Sterk, P. J., Adcock, I. M., Chung, K. F., Roca, J., & Auffray, C. (2011). Systems medicine and integrated care to combat chronic noncommunicable diseases. *Genome Medicine*. Available from https://doi.org/10.1186/gm259.

Brahmbhatt, D. H., & Cowie, M. R. (2019). Remote management of heart failure: An overview of telemonitoring technologies. *Cardiac Failure Review*. Available from https://doi.org/10.15420/cfr.2019.5.3.

Buys, R., Claes, J., Walsh, D., Cornelis, N., Moran, K., Budts, W., & Cornelissen, V. A. (2016). Cardiac patients show high interest in technology enabled cardiovascular rehabilitation. *BMC Medical Informatics and Decision Making*. Available from https://doi.org/10.1186/s12911-016-0329-9.

Cajita, M. I., Gleason, K. T., & Han, H. R. (2016). A systematic review of mhealth-based heart failure interventions. *Journal of Cardiovascular Nursing*. Available from https://doi.org/10.1097/JCN.0000000000000305.

Carvalho, P., Henriques, J., Teixeira, C. A., Couceiro, R., Rocha, T., Mendes, L., & Paiva, R. P. (2016). Biodata analytics for COPD. *3rd IEEE EMBS International Conference on Biomedical and Health Informatics, BHI 2016*, 469–472. Available from https://doi.org/10.1109/BHI.2016.7455936.

Caulfield, B. M., & Donnelly, S. C. (2013). What is connected health and why will it change your practice? *QJM: Monthly Journal of the Association of Physicians, 106*(8), 703–707. Available from https://doi.org/10.1093/qjmed/hct114.

Chatzitofis, A., Zarpalas, D., & Daras, P. (2018). A computerized system for real-time exercise performance monitoring and e-coaching using motion capture data. *In IFMBE Proceedings*. Available from https://doi.org/10.1007/978-981-10-7419-6_40.

Chistiakov, D. A., Orekhov, A. N., & Bobryshevy, Y. V. (2016). Cardiac extracellular vesicles in normal and infarcted heart. *International Journal of Molecular Sciences*. Available from https://doi.org/10.3390/ijms17010063.

Chouvarda, I., Filos, D., & Maglaveras, N. (2019). Time-domain analysis of the electrocardiogram. In S. Golemati, & K. S. Nikita (Eds.), *Cardiovascular Computing—Methodologies and Clinical Applications* (pp. 81–102). Singapore: Springer Singapore. Available from https://doi.org/10.1007/978-981-10-5092-3_4.

Chouvarda, I., Kilintzis, V., Beredimas, N., Natsiavas, P., Perantoni, E., Vogiatzis, I., & Maglaveras, N. (2016). Clinical flows and decision support systems for co-ordinated and integrated care in COPD. In *3rd IEEE EMBS International Conference on Biomedical and Health Informatics, BHI 2016* (pp. 477–480). https://doi.org/10.1109/BHI.2016.7455938.

Chouvarda, I., & Maglaveras, N. (2019). Title cardiovascular big data analytics. In S. Golemati, & K. S. Nikita (Eds.), *Cardiovascular Computing—Methodologies and Clinical Applications* (pp. 303–313). Singapore: Springer Singapore. Available from https://doi.org/10.1007/978-981-10-5092-3_15.

Chouvarda, I., Philip, N. Y., Natsiavas, P., Kilintzis, V., Sobnath, D., Kayyali, R., & Maglaveras, N. (2014). WELCOME—Innovative integrated care platform using wearable sensing and smart cloud computing for COPD patients with comorbidities. *Conference Proceedings:... Annual International Conference of the IEEE Engineering in Medicine and Biology Society. IEEE Engineering in Medicine and Biology Society. Annual Conference*. Available from https://doi.org/10.1109/EMBC.2014.6944298.

Chouvarda, I. G., Goulis, D. G., Lambrinoudaki, I., & Maglaveras, N. (2015). Connected health and integrated care: Toward new models for chronic disease management. *Maturitas*. Available from https://doi.org/10.1016/j.maturitas.2015.03.015.

Chouvarda, I. G., Mabote, T., Torabi, A., Caffarel, J., van Gils, M., Cleland, J., & Maglaveras, N. (2014). Medication incompliance and vital signs in heart failure patients. *IFMBE Proceedings, 42*, 51–54. Available from https://doi.org/10.1007/978-3-319-03005-0_14.

Cotechini, V., Belli, A., Palma, L., Morettini, M., Burattini, L., & Pierleoni, P. (2019). A dataset for the development and optimization of fall detection algorithms based on wearable sensors. *Data in Brief*. Available from https://doi.org/10.1016/j.dib.2019.103839.

Delaney, B. C., Curcin, V., Andreasson, A., Arvanitis, T. N., Bastiaens, H., Corrigan, D., & Wagner, P. (2015). Translational medicine and patient safety in Europe:

TRANSFoRm—Architecture for the learning health system in Europe. *BioMed Research International*. Available from https://doi.org/10.1155/2015/961526.

Deserno, T. M., & Marx, N. (2016). Computational electrocardiography: Revisiting holter ECG monitoring. *Methods of Information in Medicine, 55*(4), 305–311. Available from https://doi.org/10.3414/ME15-05-0009.

Fernandes, M., Patel, A., & Husi, H. (2018). C/VDdb: A multi-omics expression profiling database for a knowledge-driven approach in cardiovascular disease (CVD). *PLoS One*. Available from https://doi.org/10.1371/journal.pone.0207371.

Filos, D., Triantafyllidis, A., Manolios, V., Livitckaia, K., Claes, J., Buys, R., & Chouvarda, I. (2017). *Predictive modeling of exercise response in CVD patients under rehabilitation, IFMBE Proceedings* (Vol. 65, pp. 201–204). Singapore: Springer. Available from https://doi.org/10.1007/978-981-10-5122-7_51.

Forman, D. E., Rich, M. W., Alexander, K. P., Zieman, S., Maurer, M. S., Najjar, S. S., & Wenger, N. K. (2011). Cardiac care for older adults: Time for a new paradigm. *Journal of the American College of Cardiology*. Available from https://doi.org/10.1016/j.jacc.2011.02.014.

Friedman, C. P., Rubin, J. C., & Sullivan, K. J. (2017). Toward an information infrastructure for global health improvement. *Yearbook of Medical Informatics*. Available from https://doi.org/10.15265/IY-2017-004.

Galloway, C. D., Valys, A. V., Shreibati, J. B., Treiman, D. L., Petterson, F. L., Gundotra, V. P., & Friedman, P. A. (2019). Development and validation of a deep-learning model to screen for hyperkalemia from the electrocardiogram. *JAMA Cardiology*. Available from https://doi.org/10.1001/jamacardio.2019.0640.

Gatzoulis, L., & Iakovidis, I. (2007). Personal health systems: How can successful research reach implementation? *Annual International Conference of the IEEE Engineering in Medicine and Biology - Proceedings*. Available from https://doi.org/10.1109/IEMBS.2007.4353753.

Griebel, L., Prokosch, H. U., Köpcke, F., Toddenroth, D., Christoph, J., Leb, I., & Sedlmayr, M. (2015). A scoping review of cloud computing in healthcare. *BMC Medical Informatics and Decision Making*. Available from https://doi.org/10.1186/s12911-015-0145-7.

Guha, K., & McDonagh, T. (2013). Heart failure epidemiology: European perspective. *Current Cardiology Reviews*. Available from https://doi.org/10.2174/1573403x11309020005.

Hawley-Hague, H., Horne, M., Skelton, D. A., & Todd, C. (2016). Review of how we should define (and measure) adherence in studies examining older adults' participation in exercise classes. *BMJ Open, 6*(6), e011560. Available from https://doi.org/10.1136/bmjopen-2016-011560.

Holzinger, A., Langs, G., Denk, H., Zatloukal, K., & Müller, H. (2019). Causability and explainability of artificial intelligence in medicine. *Wiley Interdisciplinary Reviews: Data Mining and Knowledge Discovery*. Available from https://doi.org/10.1002/widm.1312.

Holzinger, A., Plass, M., Kickmeier-Rust, M., Holzinger, K., Crişan, G. C., Pintea, C.-M., & Palade, V. (2019). Interactive machine learning: Experimental evidence for the human in the algorithmic loop. *Applied Intelligence*. Available from https://doi.org/10.1007/s10489-018-1361-5.

Hsieh, J., & Hsu, M.-W. (2012). A cloud computing based 12-lead ECG telemedicine service. *BMC Medical Informatics and Decision Making, 12*(1), 77. Available from https://doi.org/10.1186/1472-6947-12-77.

Hu, J., Cui, X., Gong, Y., Xu, X., Gao, B., Wen, T., & Xu, F. (2016). Portable microfluidic and smartphone-based devices for monitoring of cardiovascular diseases at the point of care. *Biotechnology Advances*. Available from https://doi.org/10.1016/j.biotechadv.2016.02.008.

Kilintzis, V., Beredimas, N., & Chouvarda, I. (2014). *Evaluation of the performance of open-source RDBMS and triplestores for storing medical data over a web service. Conference Proceedings: ... Annual International Conference of the IEEE Engineering in Medicine and Biology Society. IEEE Engineering in Medicine and Biology Society. Annual Conference* (pp. 4499–4502). IEEE. Available from https://doi.org/10.1109/EMBC.2014.6944623.

Kilintzis, V., Chouvarda, I., Beredimas, N., Natsiavas, P., & Maglaveras, N. (2019). Supporting integrated care with a flexible data management framework built upon Linked Data, HL7 FHIR and ontologies. *Journal of Biomedical Informatics, 94*, 103179. Available from https://doi.org/10.1016/j.jbi.2019.103179.

Kortelainen, J. M., Van Gils, M., & Parkka, J. (2012). *Multichannel bed pressure sensor for sleep monitoring. Computing in Cardiology*. IEEE.

Kwon, S., Hong, J., Choi, E.-K., Lee, E., Hostallero, D. E., Kang, W. J., & Yi, Y. (2019). Deep learning approaches to detect atrial fibrillation using photoplethysmographic signals: Algorithms development study. *JMIR MHealth and UHealth*. Available from https://doi.org/10.2196/12770.

Leon-Mimila, P., Wang, J., & Huertas-Vazquez, A. (2019). Relevance of multi-omics studies in cardiovascular diseases. *Frontiers in Cardiovascular Medicine*. Available from https://doi.org/10.3389/fcvm.2019.00091.

Li, Q., Liu, C., Li, Q., Shashikumar, S. P., Nemati, S., Shen, Z., & Clifford, G. D. (2019). Ventricular ectopic beat detection using a wavelet transform and a convolutional neural network. *Physiological Measurement*. Available from https://doi.org/10.1088/1361-6579/ab17f0.

Livitckaia, K., Koutkias, V., Kouidi, E., van Gils, M., Maglaveras, N., & Chouvarda, I. (2019). "OPTImAL": An ontology for patient adherence modeling in physical activity domain. *BMC Medical Informatics and Decision Making, 19*(1), 92. Available from https://doi.org/10.1186/s12911-019-0809-9.

Livitckaia, K., Koutkias, V., Maglaveras, N., Kouidi, E., van Gils, M., & Chouvarda, I. (2018). *Adherence to physical activity in patients with heart disease: Types, settings and evaluation instruments. Precision Medicine Powered by pHealth and Connected Health* (pp. 255–259). Springer.

London, A. J. (2019). Artificial intelligence and black-box medical decisions: Accuracy vs explainability. *Hastings Center Report*. Available from https://doi.org/10.1002/hast.973.

Maramis, C., Kilintzis, V., Scholl, P., & Chouvarda, I. (2018). *Objective smoking: Towards smoking detection using smartwatch sensors. Precision Medicine Powered by pHealth and Connected Health* (pp. 2–5). Springer.

Miao, F., Cheng, Y., He, Y., He, Q., & Li, Y. (2015). A wearable context-aware ECG monitoring system integrated with built-in kinematic sensors of the smartphone. *Sensors (Switzerland)*. Available from https://doi.org/10.3390/s150511465.

Migliorini, M., Kortelainen, J. M., Pärkkä, J., Tenhunen, M., Himanen, S. L., & Bianchi, A. M. (2014). Monitoring nocturnal heart rate with bed sensor. *Methods of Information in Medicine*. Available from https://doi.org/10.3414/ME13-02-0053.

Mountford, N., Kessie, T., Quinlan, M., Maher, R., Smolders, R., Van Royen, P., Caulfield, B. (2016). *Connected health in Europe: Where are we today?* Retrieved from https://www.researchgate.net/profile/Roman_Lewandowski2/publication/311666177_Connected_Health_in_Europe_Where_are_We_Today/links/5852dce008aef7d030a51915/Connected-Health-in-Europe-Where-are-We-Today.pdf?origin = publication_list&ev = srch_pub_xdl.

Navale, V., & Bourne, P. E. (2018). Cloud computing applications for biomedical science: A perspective. *PLoS Computational Biology*. Available from https://doi.org/10.1371/journal.pcbi.1006144.

Papageorgiou, E. I., Roo, J. D., Huszka, C., & Colaert, D. (2012). Formalization of treatment guidelines using Fuzzy Cognitive Maps and semantic web tools. *Journal of Biomedical Informatics*. Available from https://doi.org/10.1016/j.jbi.2011.08.018.

Pavel, M., Jimison, H. B., Korhonen, I., Gordon, C. M., & Saranummi, N. (2015). Behavioral informatics and computational modeling in support of proactive health management and care. *IEEE Transactions on Biomedical Engineering*. Available from https://doi.org/10.1109/TBME.2015.2484286.

Radhakrishnan, K., Baranowski, T., Julien, C., Thomaz, E., & Kim, M. (2019). Role of digital games in self-management of cardiovascular diseases: A scoping review. *Games for Health Journal*. Available from https://doi.org/10.1089/g4h.2018.0011.

Radhakrishnan, K., Toprac, P., O'Hair, M., Bias, R., Kim, M. T., Bradley, P., & MacKert, M. (2016). Interactive digital e-health game for heart failure self-management: A feasibility study. *Games for Health Journal*. Available from https://doi.org/10.1089/g4h.2016.0038.

Reiss, A., Indlekofer, I., Schmidt, P., & Van Laerhoven, K. (2019). Deep PPG: Large-scale heart rate estimation with convolutional neural networks. *Sensors*. Available from https://doi.org/10.3390/s19143079.

Rubin, J. C., Silverstein, J. C., Friedman, C. P., Kush, R. D., Anderson, W. H., Lichter, A. S., & Rockhold, F. W. (2018). Transforming the future of health together: The learning health systems consensus action plan. *Learning Health Systems*. Available from https://doi.org/10.1002/lrh2.10055.

Saadatnejad, S., Oveisi, M., & Hashemi, M. (2019). LSTM-based ECG classification for continuous monitoring on personal wearable devices. *IEEE Journal of Biomedical and Health Informatics*. Available from https://doi.org/10.1109/jbhi.2019.2911367.

Sarangadharan, I., Wang, S. L., Tai, T. Y., Pulikkathodi, A. K., Hsu, C. P., Chiang, H. H. K., & Wang, Y. L. (2018). Risk stratification of heart failure from one drop of blood using hand-held biosensor for BNP detection. *Biosensors and Bioelectronics*. Available from https://doi.org/10.1016/j.bios.2018.02.036.

Tang, P. C., Ash, J. S., Bates, D. W., Overhage, J. M., & Sands, D. Z. (2006). Personal health records: Definitions, benefits, and strategies for overcoming barriers to adoption. *Journal of the American Medical Informatics Association*. Available from https://doi.org/10.1197/jamia.M2025.

Triantafyllidis, A., Filos, D., Buys, R., Claes, J., Cornelissen, V., Kouidi, E., & Chouvarda, I. (2018). Computerized decision support for beneficial home-based exercise rehabilitation in patients with cardiovascular disease. *Computer Methods and Programs in Biomedicine*. Available from https://doi.org/10.1016/j.cmpb.2018.04.030.

Tyrer, H. W., & Muheidat, F. (2016). Adding intelligence to a floor-based array personnel detector. *Alzheimer's & Dementia*. Available from https://doi.org/10.1016/j.jalz.2016.06.1182.

Vogel, J., Auinger, A., Riedl, R., Kindermann, H., Helfert, M., & Ocenasek, H. (2017). Digitally enhanced recovery: Investigating the use of digital self-tracking for monitoring leisure time physical activity of cardiovascular disease (CVD) patients undergoing cardiac rehabilitation. *PLoS One*. Available from https://doi.org/10.1371/journal.pone.0186261.

Vogt, B., Mendes, L., Chouvarda, I., Perantoni, E., Kaimakamis, E., Becher, T., & Frerichs, I. (2016). Influence of torso and arm positions on chest examinations by electrical impedance tomography. *Physiological Measurement*, *37*(6), 904–921. Available from https://doi.org/10.1088/0967-3334/37/6/904.

Wang, J., & Wang, Z. (2014). A survey on personal data cloud. *Scientific World Journal*. Available from https://doi.org/10.1155/2014/969150.

Winter, S. J., Sheats, J. L., & King, A. C. (2016). The use of behavior change techniques and theory in technologies for cardiovascular disease prevention and treatment in adults: A comprehensive review. *Progress in Cardiovascular Diseases*. Available from https://doi.org/10.1016/j.pcad.2016.02.005.

Woods, L. S., Duff, J., Roehrer, E., Walker, K., & Cummings, E. (2019). Patients' experiences of using a consumer mhealth app for self-management of heart failure: Mixed-methods study. *Journal of Medical Internet Research*. Available from https://doi.org/10.2196/13009.

Wu, J., Dong, M., Santos, S., Rigatto, C., Liu, Y., & Lin, F. (2017). Lab-on-a-chip platforms for detection of cardiovascular disease and cancer biomarkers. *Sensors (Switzerland)*. Available from https://doi.org/10.3390/s17122934.

CHAPTER 7

Increasing and standardizing quality of care using computerized guidelines for clinical decision support

Fedor Lehocki[1,2], Erez Shalom[3], Silvia Putekova[4], Jozef Beňačka[4], Alexandra Krištúfková[5], Timotej Matak[1], and Marek Mydliar[2,4]
[1]Slovak University of Technology in Bratislava, Bratislava, Slovakia
[2]National Center of Telemedicine Services, Bratislava, Slovakia
[3]Medical Informatics Research Center, Ben-Gurion University of the Negev, Beer-Sheva, Israel
[4]Faculty of Health Care and Social Work, University of Trnava, Trnava, Slovakia
[5]Faculty of Medicine, Comenius University in Bratislava, Bratislava, Slovakia

7.1 Introduction

Closing the loop and providing the correct feedback to the patient or user is a fundamental step in any reliable personalized health (p-health) solution. The user is not only made aware of her or his health conditions or risks, but also proper advices and suggestions are provided for improving health status and lifestyle. Automatic advice can be generated through algorithms based on specific clinical guidelines used for screening, diagnosis, management, treatment, or referral of patients. Critical situations may include the direct advice of the general practitioner or of the specialist who is part of the loop. Help is provided for a better compliance with therapy and for more informed management of any alerts.

Clinical decision support systems (CDSS) are information systems that are designed to support clinicians' decision making about individual patients. These systems have a significant impact on how medicine is delivered if they are used at the point of care. How active or passive this support is may differ. In an active approach, the CDSS actively provides alerts and reminders; in a passive approach, it passively generates responses based on the physician's input or patient-specific information (Berner, 2016). Decision support can be provided also to nonclinical users, such as patients, to facilitate prevention and to suggest proper activities to maintain the patient's health status (Peleg et al., 2017).

Personalized Health Systems for Cardiovascular Disease
DOI: https://doi.org/10.1016/B978-0-12-818950-4.00004-5

Knowledge-driven systems store the expertise in a knowledge base that is derived from medical literature, clinical guidelines, or experts' skills. Then an inference engine applies the rules from knowledge base on patient data. A communication module is responsible for interfacing with patient data (inputs) and user (outputs), who then makes relevant decisions related to matters such as laboratory test ordering, diagnoses (diagnostic decision support systems), medication orders, or care plans. Non-knowledge-based systems, such as data-driven systems, are based on an artificial intelligence approach, such as machine learning, that provides pattern recognition from clinical data. Other approaches include artificial neural networks and genetic algorithms. Advantages of this type of decision support system relate to processing of incomplete data stored in datasets that do not need to be large. Examples of applications of such systems include diagnosis of appendicitis, back pain, myocardial infarction, prediction of pulmonary embolisms (Berner, 2016).

Enablers for using CDSS in clinical practice are easing the integration of these systems into culture and process of care with pervasive mobile technologies, more effective management, and prevention of medical errors; using knowledge from guidelines thus increases patient safety, standardization, and quality of care. Challenges associated with CDSS implementation include integration with existing information systems used by healthcare providers and electronic medical or health records, development and maintenance of knowledge, selection and use of controlled vocabularies, and design of a usable user interface.

In this chapter we present implementation of clinical guidelines as repositories of standardized knowledge for purposes of computerized clinical decision support. Section 7.2 briefly introduces diagnosis and treatment of preeclampsia and heart failure. In Section 7.3 we introduce the domain of clinical guidelines and life cycle of their transformation into computerized format for use in CDSSs. We also illustrate the application of a CDSS in the management of preeclampsia. Section 7.4 describes the use case of computerized guidelines in a CDSS for management of patients with heart failure. The chapter closes with discussion and conclusion in Sections 7.5 and 7.6.

7.2 Diagnosis and treatment of preeclampsia and heart failure

7.2.1 Preeclampsia

Preeclampsia is a hypertensive disorders in pregnancy and one of the most frequent complications in pregnancy. This complication has a great influence on maternal and newborn health in pregnancy, during labor, and also in life after delivery. Hypertension is defined as systolic blood pressure (BP) ≥140 mmHg and diastolic BP ≥90 mmHg (ACOG, 2019). The BP measurements should be repeated to confirm true hypertension and to determine the exact diagnosis. According to the time of occurrence, clinical signs, and other symptoms, the classification of hypertensive disorders is used (Table 7.1) (ACOG, 2013; Brown, Magee, & Kenny, 2018; ESC Guidelines, 2013).

The global incidence of hypertensive disorders in pregnant women during 2002–12 was 6%, and the worldwide incidence rate of preeclampsia was approximately 16% (Kongwattanakul, Saksiriwuttho, & Chaiyarach, 2018). The most important risk factors are obesity, higher age of the pregnant woman, preeclampsia or hypertensive disease in the past, and pregnancy after use of an assisted reproduction technique.

The determination of an exact diagnosis (Table 7.2) is very important for proper management of the pregnant woman and the child and for prevention of future complications arising from untreated or insufficiently treated preeclampsia.

Prevention is the most important if the woman has risk factors. In the treatment we use magnesium sulfate and antihypertensive drugs in

Table 7.1 Definition and classification of hypertensive disorders in pregnancy (ACOG, 2013; Brown et al., 2018; ESC Guidelines, 2013).

Time period	Type
Hypertension known before pregnancy or present in the first 20 weeks of pregnancy	Chronic hypertension Essential Secondary White-coat hypertension Masked hypertension
Newly diagnosed hypertension at or after the 20th week of pregnancy	Transient gestational hypertension Gestational hypertension **Preeclampsia** De novo (newly diagnosed) Superimposed on chronic hypertension ! HELLP syndrome: one of the manifestations of preeclampsia ! Eclampsia: tonic-clonic convulsions Postpartum hypertension: after 2 weeks until 6 months after labor

cooperation with internal medicine specialists (Brown et al., 2018). Besides the proper treatment of preeclampsia, good compliance and self-monitoring are also needed to prevent serious complication, such as eclampsia, HELLP syndrome, cardiac failure, brain damage (e.g., posterior reversible encephalopathy syndrome), fetal damage, and long-lasting complications or consequences after the pregnancy and puerperium for mother and her child (Brown et al., 2018; Kongwattanakul et al., 2018).

7.2.2 Congestive heart failure

Congestive heart failure (CHF) occurs when the heart muscle does not pump blood as well as it should (ESC Guidelines, 2016). The heart works less efficiently than normal. Blood moves through the heart and body at a slower rate, and pressure in the heart increases. As a result, the heart cannot pump enough oxygen and nutrients to meet the body's needs. The heart chambers may respond by stretching to hold more blood to pump through the body or by becoming stiff and thickened. This helps to keep the blood moving, but the heart muscle walls may eventually weaken and

Table 7.2 Diagnostic criteria for preeclampsia.

Preeclampsia is defined as hypertension with proteinuria:	
Hypertension	BP ≥ 140/90 mmHg 2 measurements within 4 h, after 20th week of pregnancy BP ≥ 160/110 mmHg, confirmed by more measurements (interval between measurements in minutes to speed up the treatment)
Proteinuria (protein in urine)	≥ 300 mg in 24-h collected urine Ratio of proteins to creatinine > (0.3) Labstick 1 + (if another method of measurement of proteinuria is not available)
Preeclampsia can be diagnosed also without proteinuria. However, at least one of the following signs has to be present:	
Thrombocytopenia	Number of thrombocytes <100,000/μL
Renal insufficiency	Creatinine concentration in serum >1.1 mg/dL, or double concentration of creatinine in serum without occurrence of another renal disease
Impairment of liver function	Double concentration of liver enzymes in serum
Pulmonary edema	
Defect of vision and cerebral function	

become unable to pump as efficiently. As a result, the endocrine system and kidney may respond by causing the body to retain fluid and salt, the body then becomes congested, and CHF results. Heart failure signs and symptoms may include shortness of breath (dyspnea) during exercise or in repose caused by congested lungs; fatigue and weakness; swelling (edema) in the legs, ankles, and feet; rapid or irregular heartbeat; reduced ability to exercise; persistent cough or wheezing; increased need to urinate at night; swelling of the abdomen (ascites); very rapid weight gain from fluid retention; lack of appetite and nausea; and difficulty concentrating or decreased alertness. Although these signs and symptoms may be due to heart failure, there are many other possible causes, including other life-threatening heart and lung conditions.

The reasons for CHF (etiology) include any of the following conditions: coronary artery disease, high blood pressure (hypertension), faulty heart valves, cardiomyopathy, myocarditis, abnormal heart rhythms (arrhythmias), or other chronic diseases, such as diabetes, HIV, hyperthyroidism, or hypothyroidism.

For the purposes of diagnosis, a detailed history should always be obtained. CHF is unusual in an individual with no relevant medical history (e.g., a potential cause of cardiac damage), whereas certain features, particularly previous myocardial infarction, greatly increase the likelihood of CHF in a patient with appropriate symptoms and signs. A variety of tests are used to diagnose heart conditions, such as the plasma concentration of natriuretic peptides (NPs). The plasma concentration of NPs can be used as an initial diagnostic test, especially in the nonacute setting when echocardiography is not immediately available. Elevated NPs help to establish an initial working diagnosis, identifying patients who require further cardiac investigation. Patients with values below the cut point for the exclusion of important cardiac dysfunction do not require echocardiography. Patients with normal plasma NP concentrations are unlikely to have CHF. The use of NPs is recommended for ruling out CHF but not to establish the diagnosis.

An abnormal electrocardiogram (ECG) increases the likelihood of a diagnosis of CHF but has low specificity. CHF is unlikely in patients presenting with a completely normal ECG (sensitivity: 89%). Echocardiography is the most useful, widely available test for patients with suspected CHF to establish the diagnosis. It provides immediate information about wall thickness, valve function, chamber volumes, and ventricular systolic and diastolic function. An ejection fraction is used to help classify heart failure and guide treatment. In a healthy heart, the ejection fraction is 50% or higher, meaning that more than half of the blood that fills the ventricle is pumped out with each beat.

The goals of treatment in patients with CHF are to decrease the likelihood of disease progression (thereby decreasing the risk of death and the need for hospitalization) and to improve the patients' clinical status, functional capacity, and quality of life. CHF therapy is based on lifestyle changes, heart medications, and permanently monitoring. There are more treatment options available for heart failure than ever before. The key to preventing heart failure is to reduce the risk factors by stopping smoking, controlling high blood pressure and diabetes, staying physically active, eating healthy foods, maintaining a healthy weight, and reducing and managing stress.

7.3 What are clinical guidelines?

Since the 1990s there has been growing interest in clinical guidelines (GLs). These guidelines are related to the emphasis on evidence-based medicine, in which the best available evidence gained from scientific methods, such as research studies, metaanalyses and reviews, is applied to support better clinical decision making (Peleg et al., 2017).

Using clinical GLs has the potential to reduce adverse events (e.g., administration of the wrong procedure, or acquisition of a preventable infections), medical mistakes, and costs. The U.S. Department of Health and Human Services reported adverse medical events in at least 13.5% of Medicare-funded hospitalizations. These amounted to 3.5% of Medicare costs or $4.4 billion in 2009. Approximately 44% of all these events were considered to be preventable (Levinson & General, 2010). A more recent Johns Hopkins study found that more than 250,000 people in the United States die every year from medical errors, which are the third-leading cause of death after heart disease and cancer (Makary & Daniel, 2016).

7.3.1 Automated support for clinical guideline application

Most clinical GLs are text-based and are not easily accessible to healthcare providers who need to match them to their patients and apply them at the point of care. This creates a dilemma for practitioners: the information is impractical for most healthcare providers because they must cope with a great amount of data to read, interpret, and apply in the very short time span of a patient-doctor visit. Therefore there is low adherence in trying to translate them into daily practice (Shalom, Shahar, Parmet, & Lunenfeld, 2015).

Some progress has been made by publishing some clinical GLs in an electronic format, such as HTML or PDF files that can be accessed via the Internet. Even so, healthcare providers, overloaded with information, rarely have the time or computational means to assist themselves in utilizing the valuable knowledge encoded in the GLs during treatment. Therefore healthcare providers, healthcare managers, and patients would highly benefit from automated computerized GL-based CDSSs that support electronic, formal machine-comprehensible specifications and representations of GLs, as well as their automated dissemination, runtime application at the point of care, and retrospective quality assessment (Hansen et al., 2018; Isern & Moreno, 2008).

There are multiple approaches to the task of provision of automated support for GL application; however, one subtask common to all frameworks is the acquisition and formal representation, in a fashion understandable by machines, of an appropriate medical knowledge base (KB). The reason is that all of the benefits of providing automated support to GL-based care cannot be achieved without an appropriate computerized infrastructure. Since analyzing unstructured text-based GLs is not operative solution yet, such an infrastructure should include a formal specification language (i.e., formal representation) of clinical GLs that can be parsed and executed by machines. This representation is often called machine comprehensible (the term "comprehensible" is used here in a strictly formal sense, not a cognitive one). Thus the need to automate GLs implies, in practice, a need to convert the mass of free-text GLs gradually into machine-comprehensible representations in order to apply them (Combi, Keravnou-Papailiou, & Shahar, 2010; Tso et al., 2017).

A computerized GL-based CDSS infrastructure requires a central database (DB), a central medical knowledge base (KB) that stores the knowledge used during the task (sometimes modifying it), and a CDSS engine that applies the knowledge to the data. Fig. 7.1 shows an abstract view of a typical knowledge-based DSS architecture. The medical knowledge of the GLs is stored and retrieved from a central KB library (examples of knowledge items stored in the KB are the medical definition of high BP or definition of a plan to take a specific drug) (Shalom, Shahar, & Lunenfeld, 2016).

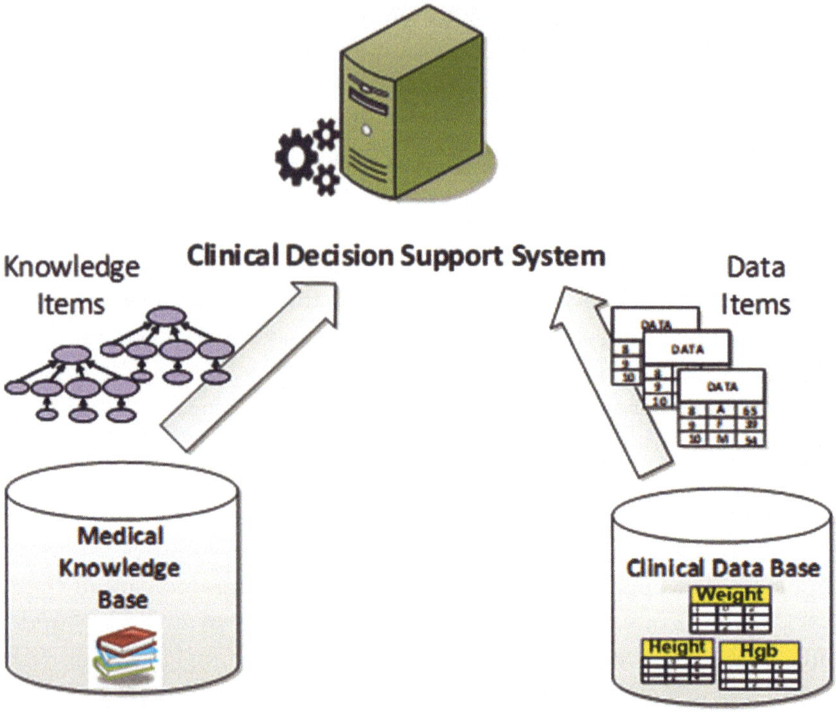

Figure 7.1 An abstract view of the architecture of a knowledge-based medical decision-support systems.

The patient data are stored and retrieved from an electronic medical record (EMR). The CDSS engine applies the medical knowledge to the data to provide alerts and recommendations at the point of care to health-care providers (e.g., physicians or nurses), to the patient (e.g., through messages sent to the patient's cell phone), or even to knowledge engineers (KEs) to debug or simulate the CDSS engine.

7.3.2 Clinical guideline application frameworks: A brief overview

In the last two decades comprehensive work was conducted regarding GL application frameworks. In the United States the ONCOCIN project led to many GL-based application framework projects, such as EON, GLIF3, which supports computer-interpretable format, and SAGE. During this period, significant research among European research groups was also being carried out. Italian groups developed the Guide and GLARE frameworks; and in England, Prestige, ProForma, and PRODIGY were developed.

One of the main languages for GL representation is Asbru, which was developed as part of the Asgaard project. The Vienna group in Austria and the Netherlands focused on developing Asbru interpreters, while the Ben-Gurion University team in Israel initially focused on developing the Digital Electronic Guideline Library, along with its tools. Multiple comparisons of the various GL-based support frameworks and GL application engines can be found in a work by Peleg and González-Ferrer (2014).

7.3.3 The digital electronic guideline library

One of the main frameworks that was developed as distributed, web-based architecture to support all of the design time and runtime tasks involved in GL-based care is the Digital Electronic Guideline Library (DeGeL) (Furberg, Williams, Bagwell, & LaBresh, 2017; Shahar, 1997). The DeGeL framework's guideline KB and various task-specific tools were designed to handle all of the hybrid GL representation levels, enabling incremental specification in collaborative fashion between the expert physician (EP) and the KE. There are three main components in DeGeL's conceptual architecture: (1) a permissions and authorizations manager component responsible for generating user-profiles and controlling user access to DeGeL's GL repository; (2) a GL content manager responsible for performing create, retrieve, update, and delete (CRUD) operations on all knowledge entities (e.g., guidelines) stored in DeGeL's repository; and (3) a search and retrieval engine responsible for performing text indexing and storing semantic classification of GLs as well as handling search queries processing.

To support the specification of a GL in one or more different GL specification languages, the DeGeL architecture includes a hybrid GL metaontology ("meta" is used here in the sense of "above"). The metaontology is composed of two components: (1) a documentation ontology, which specifies knowledge roles that are common to all target GL ontologies and defines the ontologies of the sources of the GLs and of the marked-up GLs, and (2) a specification metaontology for describing a new target ontology in order to enable adding it into the DeGeL (meta) knowledge base. Thus DeGeL provides an XML schema that describes how to generate XML documents that conform to the DeGeL expected structure for designers of existing or new GL ontologies. These documents are instances of the specification metaontology and describe particular target ontologies, such as GLIF or Asbru. Implementing the hybrid metaontology in DeGeL enables uploading and structuring in more than one ontology. Fig. 7.2 shows the gradual conversion process in the DeGeL framework.

7.3.4 The life cycle of a computerized clinical guideline

Once an appropriate declarative and procedural KB exists, the goal is to apply it to the patient's data to provide support to healthcare providers and other users.

De Clercq has identified four areas involved in the development of GL-based decision support systems (De Clercq, Blom, Korsten, & Hasman, 2004):

1. *Guideline modeling and representation*, which includes the representation of the GL, including the determination of the complexity of and level of abstraction, the knowledge types used, such as declarative knowledge (which should be modeled separately), the GL documentation, the GL specification formal language, and local adaptation methods for implantation at different institutes.
2. *Guideline knowledge acquisition*, which includes the tools that facilitate the knowledge acquisition process by helping domain experts to formulate and structure the knowledge used in the GL according to some specification language.
3. *Guideline verification and testing*, which includes the performance of verification tests to detect various types of logical and procedural errors and the testing of the GL in a simulation environment to increase the nonambiguity, syntactic correctness, and semantic correctness of the GL.

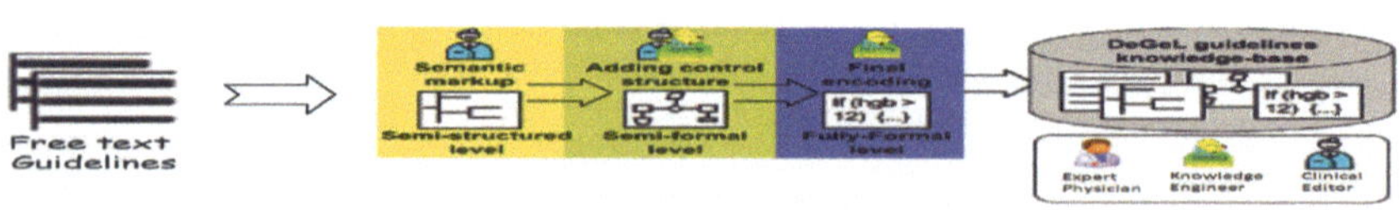

Figure 7.2 The incremental conversion process in the DeGeL architecture. Input free-text GLs are loaded into a markup editor. The EPs' index and markup (structure) portions of the GLs by semantic labels from a chosen target ontology create semi-structured and, in collaboration with a KE, semiformal GL representations. KEs use an ontology-specific tool to add executable expressions in the formal syntax of that ontology.

4. *Guideline execution* (application), which includes providing decision support by interpreting the formal representation of a GL by the automatic GL application engine.

The first three tasks are related to the preexecution phases and are performed by GL authors and KEs before GL application. The last task supports healthcare providers and is performed by the GL application engine during GL application.

Based on our experience gained within DeGeL implementation, Fig. 7.3 describes our view of the life cycle of a computerized, machine-comprehensible GL: all tasks use a central DB and KB to save and retrieve clinical data and knowledge, respectively. The clinical DB usually contains patient data. This guarantees consistency, synchronization, and orchestration among all of the tasks.

7.3.4.1 Guideline knowledge acquisition

The process of acquiring the knowledge is called knowledge acquisition (KA). Musen et al. defined KA as "transformation of knowledge from the forms in which it is available in the world into forms that can be used by a knowledge system" (Musen, Fagan, Combs, & Shortliffe, 1987) and

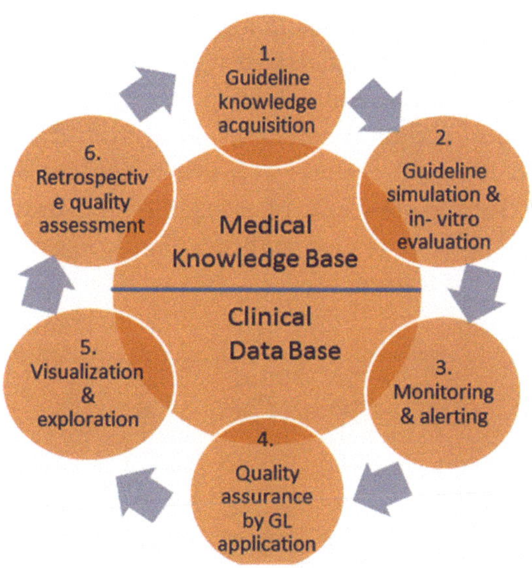

Figure 7.3 An idealized view of the life cycle of a computerized guideline. All tasks use the shared medical knowledge base and the longitudinal patient clinical database, reading and possibly modifying them, except for the first task (knowledge acquisition or specification), which modifies only the knowledge base.

make a distinction between tacit knowledge (knowing how) and conscious, explicit knowledge (knowing that). When experts first solve a task, they have declarative knowledge about the application area of the task (e.g., the definition of high blood pressure), but as they become experienced with the application, the knowledge becomes procedural knowledge (e.g., defining taking a drug plan or a daily workup plan). Consequently, the tacit knowledge is the kind we would most likely want to incorporate into our KB. An example for this process was implemented within DeGeL by using KA tools and a three-phase, nine-step KA methodology for specification of GLs by EPs, clinical editors (CEs), and KEs and conducting quantitative and qualitative evaluation. The results showed that given an ontology-specific consensus and a textual representation of a GL, any EP with some ontological training (not necessarily a domain expert) can structure and specify its knowledge in a semi-formal representation completely. An ontology-specific consensus is a structured document that describes schematically the interpretation of the GL agreed upon by both the EPs and the KE and includes the clinical directives of the GL and the semantic logic of the specification language (Shalom et al., 2006). However, to structure and specify it correctly, an EP with good computational skills should be selected (Shalom et al., 2008). Fig. 7.4 depicts this methodology. Subjective research was conducted as well to test the GL editor's perception of the KA process (Shalom et al., 2009). The results showed that aspects considered important for formation of a clinical consensus differ from those for structuring of GLs. Understanding the features of a structuring ontology is positively correlated with the reported ease of using these features, but neither of these subjective reports correlated with the actual objective quality of the structuring using these features.

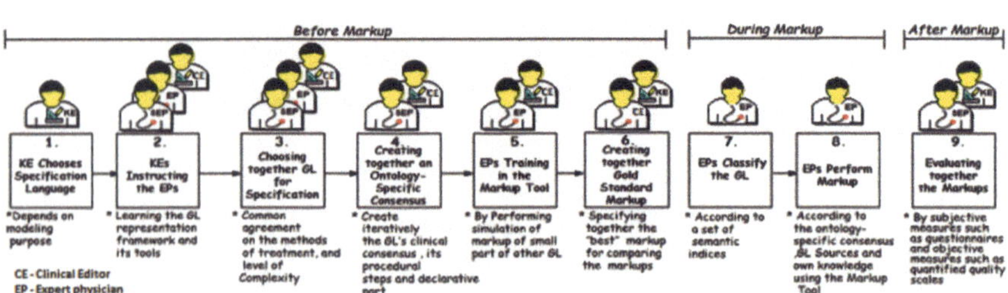

Figure 7.4 The three main phases of the methodology before, during, and after the markup, and the activities in each phase. Note the descriptions under each activity. Note the participants in each activity.

The same results were shown in a later study, which tested specification quality in Gesher, a new graphical framework for GL KA by (Hatsek et al., 2010), shown in Fig. 7.5. Gesher is a client application designed to support the process of incremental GL specification at multiple representation levels according to multiple target specification ontologies.

To achieve a high-quality specification in a reasonable time, Gesher supports the collaboration of the EPs, CEs and KEs. Gesher supports this gradual specification process through all of the steps of creating a formal representation of the GL. Note that the capability for effective gradual specification also supports maintenance and modification of the clinical GL's knowledge. Although Gesher supports specification into multiple

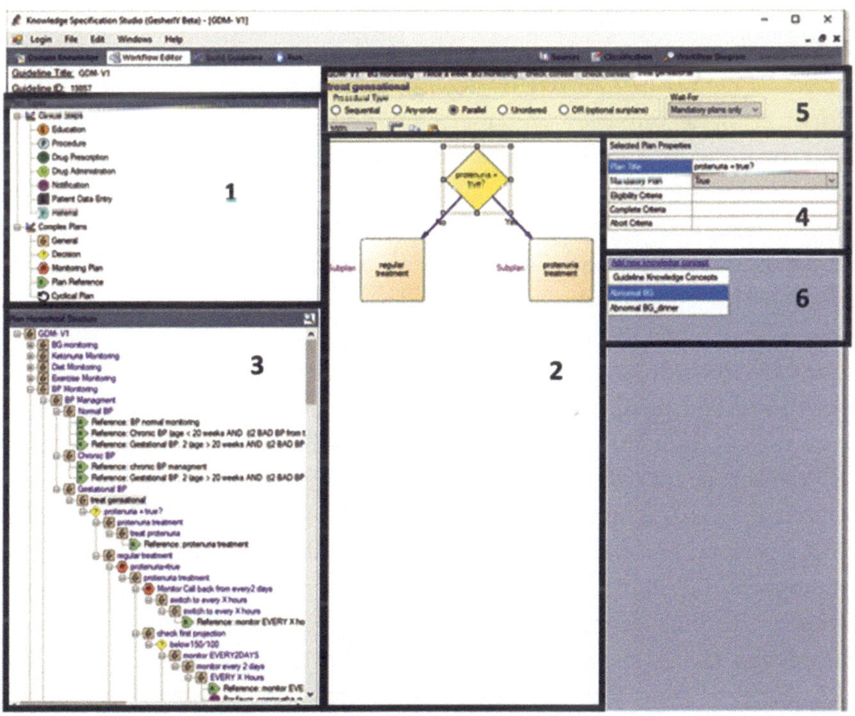

Figure 7.5 The hierarchical plan builder in Gesher that the expert physicians use for specifying the procedural aspects of the GL—in this case the "checking proteinuria" plan of the gestational diabetes mellitus (GDM) GL. The user selects plans from different types (frame 1) and drags them into the hierarchical flow chart (frame 2). The plan is added and displayed in a hierarchical tree-view display (frame 3). For each plan, several properties can be defined (frame 4); for composite plans the procedural aspect are specified (frame 5). In this phase the expert also defines a list of declarative concepts that will be further specified in the following phases (frame 6).

target ontologies and is not restricted to a specific one, we used the Asbru ontology for the formal level of representation, and the components we developed for this level are used to generate a representation according to the Asbru language. The evaluation of Gesher showed high levels of completeness and correctness of the GL specification process by both the clinicians and the KEs, although the best results, in the case of declarative knowledge specification, were achieved by teams that included a clinician and a KE. The usability scores were high as well, although the clinicians' assessment was significantly lower than the assessment of the KEs.

7.3.4.2 Guideline simulation

The GL simulation task is sometimes related to validation and testing tasks (de Clercq et al., 2004), aimed to determine that the structured elements of the GL are precise, unambiguous, and syntactically and semantically correct. The Gesher designers suggest testing the GL by using existing patient records, but they are not suggesting a methodology to perform this validation. In addition, patient records are not always available, especially during the phase of GL specification process. In fact, after or during the GL specification (or even during its development) there is a need to debug its quality by computational means, that is, to make sure that all the scenarios applied by the GL application engine are correct (i.e., all recommendations are correct) and complete (i.e., the engine does not misses any recommendations). The desired output of this phase is that the GL is valid and ready to be applied. An example for using GL simulation is the use the simulation engine developed by Freidman to test the technical assessment of the PICARD-CDSS engine (Freidman, 2012) (see Section 2.4.4.1.). This research involved using simulation methods to perform a technical evaluation in order to check the recommendations of the GL application engine by first generating all of the GL's possible scenarios, given its formal description, then creating a set of simulated patient records for each scenario, and finally applying key scenarios to the generated records, using the GL application engine. In addition, a functional evaluation is performed to test the GL's main scenarios manually by using human experts to check the quality of the GL modeling and the quality of the GL application engine.

7.3.4.3 Monitoring and alerting

The specification of the GL's declarative knowledge, although integrated with its procedural knowledge, is represented conceptually within a closely associated KB and therefore can be monitored once it is connected to patient data.

An example for this task is a CDSS client application that constantly monitors and reasons about a pattern that defines the declarative knowledge eligibility criteria for a particular GL, such as "moderate anemia for two weeks" (an abstraction that is derived by using the domain's declarative knowledge from a set of raw time-stamped hemoglobin values) and triggers an alert when the entry pattern is evaluated to a True value. This type of alerting is referred to as asynchronous, data-driven, or event-driven reasoning. Subscribers (typically, software modules) such as a DSS or even the patient's mobile device can subscribe to the patient's DB, given a suitable monitoring system, to get alerts. Another option to perform a monitoring task is through synchronous, query-driven (goal-driven) reasoning, which occurs when a specific client sends a request to the reasoning engine to calculate a given pattern (such as the one described above) and gets back the results of the evaluation

Fig. 7.6 displays the architecture of the IDAN temporal abstraction mediator (Boaz & Shahar, 2005). The mediator's controller effectively mediates a complex, knowledge-based query involving several domain-specific clinical abstractions by retrieving the relevant medical knowledge and clinical time-stamped data using the knowledge-based temporal abstraction (KBTA) ontology (Shahar, 1997); the temporal abstraction service then applies the appropriate context-sensitive knowledge to the relevant clinical data. The IDAN architecture is capable of accessing heterogeneous EMRs as well as providing sophisticated services for querying a patient's raw data and derived abstract concepts. Another important component of the IDAN architecture is the MEIDA system, which includes a vocabulary server and a standard term search engine (German, Leibowitz, & Shahar, 2009).

The use of standardized vocabularies and terms enables referral of queries by the GL runtime application system to the temporal abstraction mediator, such as the IDAN architecture, regardless of the terminology used in each local clinical database. Similarly, the MOMENTUM module is an active time-oriented database within the incremental temporal abstraction architecture for intelligent abstraction, exploration, and analysis of clinical data (Spokoiny & Shahar, 2007).

7.3.4.4 Quality assurance by guideline application

Quality assurance is a real-time task that involves the application of the procedural knowledge of the GL by the application engine, often by

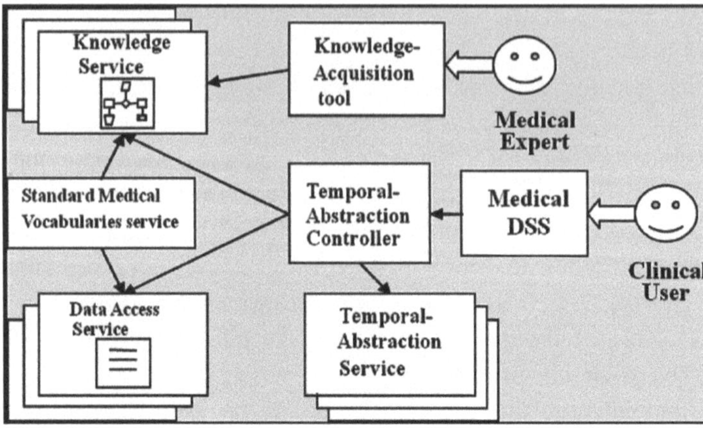

Figure 7.6 The architecture of the IDAN knowledge-based temporal abstraction mediator. A clinical user accesses a medical decision support system, such as for GL application or for intelligent exploration of patient data. The (abstract) query is answered by applying relevant temporal abstraction knowledge to appropriate time-oriented clinical data.

making recommendations to a healthcare provider at the point of care but also possibly remotely at the patient's home, directing the recommendations to the patient, the patient's family, or a nurse at a telemedicine call center. We are assuming that the GL is represented by using some specific machine-comprehensible GL representation language. The GL application decreases the variability of treatment and improves the quality of decisions. The GL application engine is usually domain-independent, so it can be used in multiple clinical domains, and it should support both a user-initiative synchronous mode, when for example a physician might initiate the GL application session and trigger the decision support process, and a data-driven asynchronous mode, when, for example, a new incoming data item or event might trigger a decision support session (e.g., a new laboratory result is added to the patient's record) (De Clercq et al., 2004).

7.3.4.4.1 A example of a guideline application in the case of preeclampsia/eclampsia/toxemia

In their work, Shalom et al. developed in a comprehensive, detailed, multidimensional framework and implemented it through a new GL application engine, the Picard Decision Support Framework, which is a flexible multiple-component framework that supports GL application (Shalom et al., 2015). At the core of that architecture is a multidimensional GL application engine, the PICARD-CDSS engine. This engine is implemented within a DeGeL framework. Within the study, an evaluation methodology was designed and evaluated to answer three specific research questions, defined in the context of the framework: (1) Is the overall multidimensional framework for GL application feasible? (2) Does the overall framework for GL application improve physician compliance to GLs? (3) Is the framework for GL application considered helpful by clinicians?

To address those three research questions, the study was performed by using the preeclampsia/eclampsia/toxemia GL. This included first performing a technical evaluation of the Picard CDSS by a new simulation engine that was developed in our laboratory, using 20 GL-based simulated scenarios. Then functional evaluation of the multidimensional framework was performed through the automated generation of patient records that simulate six clinical GL—based scenarios and a total of 60 decision points. Finally, a crossover in vitro clinical evaluation was performed with the help of 36 different clinicians at the OB/GYN department of the Soroka Hospital, Ben-Gurion University's academic medical center.

Each clinician managed half of the scenarios (a total of 30 decision points) manually without using the Picard CDSS, that is, in a non-CDSS mode, and half (for a total of another 30 decision points) were managed by using the Picard CDSS, that is, in a CDSS mode. Correctness and completeness of the actions relative to the GL were used as the main measures to assess the quality of management in both the CDSS mode and the non-CDSS mode by comparing them to a GL-based gold standard. A subjective questionnaire was also administered to the practitioners to assess the subjects' perceptions regarding the use of the CDSS.

The results of the evaluation were very encouraging: The total mean correctness and completeness in the technical evaluation were 1 ± 0.0 and 0.96 ± 0.03, respectively, meaning that all actions produced by the Picard CDSS GL application engine were correct and that almost all of the actions required by the GL were produced, when compared to a GL-based gold standard management. These results answer research question #1.

With respect to the in vitro functional clinical evaluation, we found that using the DSS significantly improved correctness and completeness and reduced the variability. Specifically, the mean completeness level was 0.9334 ± 0.06 in the CDSS mode versus 0.4725 ± 0.25 in the non-CDSS mode. Thus the completeness level when the CDSS mode was used increased by 46.32% compared to the manual, non-CDSS mode, with an accompanying decrease in the variance. With respect to correctness, in the CDSS mode the correctness was 0.9911 ± 0.01 versus 0.3274 ± 0.22 in the non-CDSS mode, an improvement of 66.37% while also reducing the variability. This effect was found to be valid across all the experiment dimensions, that is, for every scenario, for every clinician, for every expertise type, and for every decision type. Fig. 7.7 shows the mean completeness level of all decision points across all clinicians. Squares denote mean completeness for each decision point in the non-CDSS mode; triangles denote mean completeness for the same decision point in the CDSS mode. These results answer research question #2.

With respect to the subjective measures, we found that the mean general perception of the users of the CDSS mode was higher (5.25 ± 1.21) than the random mean of 4, on a scale of 1 to 7, where 1 is worst and 7 is best. These results answer research question #3.

The results showed that the GL-based CDSS plays the role of a big equalizer: it creates independence of the quality of the decision from any particular physician, any particular clinical scenario, and any particular decision type with the scenarios. The system thus ensures a high quality of clinical decision making (relative to a GL-based norm), owing to the increased adherence to the GL generated by the CDSS. Specifically, the Picard CDSS engine is potentially suitable for use in large-scale applications involving chronic patient monitoring and care in a continuous time frame. An example is the EU Mobiguide project (Peleg et al., 2017), which focuses on remote monitoring and care of chronic patients, in which the Picard CDSS served as the core CDSS and in which it is being evaluated.

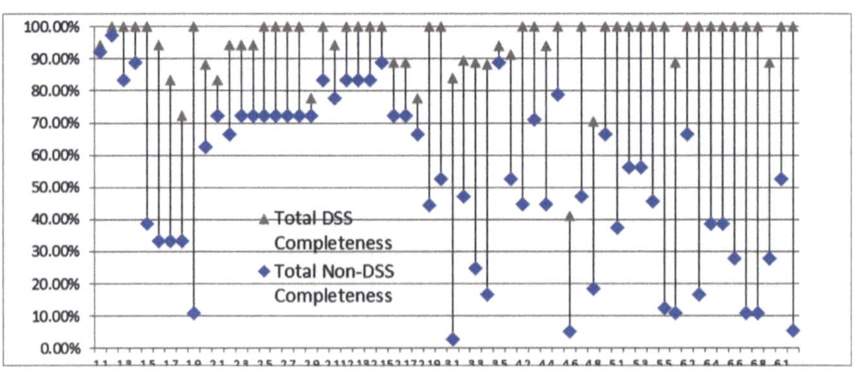

Figure 7.7 The mean completeness level of all decision points across all clinicians.

7.3.4.5 Visualization and exploration

In the context of the GL life cycle, since a unified medical procedural and a declarative knowledge base are used, this task includes tools for visualization and exploration of the time-oriented clinical data using declarative medical knowledge. The objective is to create GL-specific interpretations of the raw data and to display and browse them interactively and effectively to support better decisions.

Using GL-oriented context-sensitive knowledge can have a significant effect on the quality of decisions, since effective visualization and exploration tools can offer support at the point of care, enabling interpretation and browsing of the data of individual patients during their management (Klimov, Shahar, & Taieb-Maimon, 2010) as well as analysis and exploration of the data of multiple patients to gain more general insights that can affect organizational policy and support clinical research (e.g., noting associations across time for a medication and its effects or side effects).

Visual representation such as intelligent graphs and charts can reduce the time to search for information and the time to make complex decisions (Martins et al., 2008). Full support for visualization and exploration of high-level temporal abstractions (computed as needed by the KBTA method) at multiple temporal granularities (from seconds to decades) is provided through an ontology-driven interface that was developed previously at our research center, known as KNAVE-II project, and rigorously evaluated by clinicians in the oncology domain (Martins et al., 2008). The VISITORS project (Klimov, Shknevsky, & Shahar, 2014; Fig. 7.8) significantly extended the KNAVE-II system to enable visual display and exploration of multiple raw data and temporal abstraction concepts of patient populations at multiple temporal granularity levels, including the formation of complex queries for patient sets satisfying certain temporal and value constraints and the exploration of probabilistic temporal associations among pairs of concepts over time.

7.3.4.6 Retrospective quality assessment

This task involves GL quality assessment by retrospectively comparing a formally represented GL (e.g., a GL for treatment of hypertension) to one or more longitudinal records (e.g., a database of patients treated at an antihypertensive therapy clinic) of patients who might potentially benefit from the correct application of that GL. The output provides insights regarding the compliance or adherence of the healthcare provider or the patient to the GL. This task also has the potential to improve future care

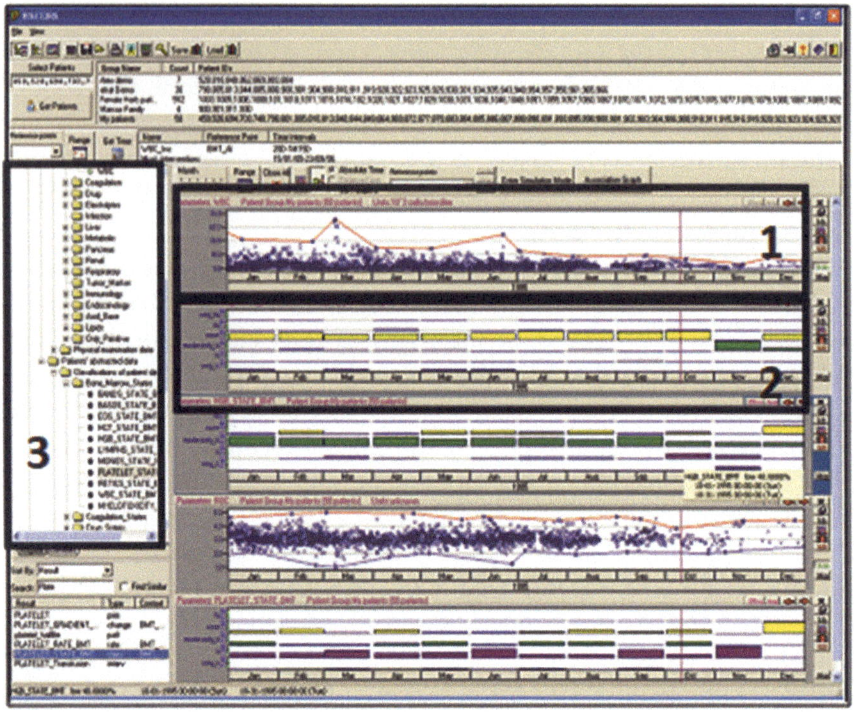

Figure 7.8 The VISITORS main interface, showing the hematological oncology domain. It shows the data for population for the white blood cell (WBC) count raw concept (1) and for the monthly distribution of the values of the WBC-state monthly distribution of the values of the WBC (2). The left panel (3) of the interface includes a knowledge-based browser showing the domain's ontology.

by affecting remodeling of the GL through an iterative specification (knowledge acquisition) process. Thus a complete cycle of GL specification and application is started again.

An example of a system performing the retrospective quality assessment task is the intelligent GL recognition framework (Boldo, 2007), which was developed to determine, given the patient's longitudinal record, which GL the patient was most likely to have been treated by and what the degree of adherence to the GL represented in a simplified version of Asbru is. The degree of a partial match between the patient record and the GL was determined by using fuzzy logic functions for values such as medication doses and temporal durations of administration of the drug. Another example is the DiscovErr system (Hatsek, 2014), which was designed, implemented, and evaluated as a comprehensive system for

GL-based critiquing and quality assessment. The DiscovErr system uses a formal representation of the procedural workflow knowledge inherent in clinical GLs and of the declarative domain-specific data interpretation knowledge they explicitly or implicitly use to perform quality assessment of the medical care by analyzing the longitudinal clinical data.

7.4 Computerized guidelines for decision support in heart failure

To illustrate an application of GLs in practice, we introduce a use case for heart failure application in home care. The presented work is based on the experience of the authors and their colleagues. The aim of this section is to introduce knowledge from GL modeling and implementation that can serve as the basis for further reading and research.

Home care settings are unique in comparison with inpatient care. The focus is mainly on chronic health conditions, most of the care is provided by nurses, and treatment is characterized by infrequent meetings with patients. The feasibility study described here is focused on evidence-based information systems with GLs that can support nurses in provision of home care for patients with heart failure (Topaz et al., 2013). Integration of these systems with home care agencies' electronic health records systems provides recommendations that can bridge the gaps in nurses' expertise and reduce potential negative effects on patient outcomes. Nursing GLs were extracted from the American Heart Association (Hunt et al., 2009) and Heart Failure Society of America (Lindenfeld, Albert, Boehmer, Collins, & Ezekowitz, 2010).

In this study, a modified knowledge acquisition methodology was used that had originally been developed and validated by Shalom and colleagues (Shalom et al., 2008). In the first step, an expert consensus had to be reached regarding the GLs to be used. The second step was focused on training the CE to formalize the GL into a computer-interpretable format.

The experts involved in the first step, which took 6 months, were two nurses from academic settings with PhD degrees and more than 20 years of experience in heart failure research and two experienced practice experts with clinical and managerial backgrounds. Nursing GLs were extracted from Hunt et al. and Lindenfeld et al. through a series of Delphi rounds until common agreement was reached on the final set of recommendations (Hunt et al., 2009; Lindenfeld et al., 2010). The resulting GL included 153 recommendations divided into 50 generic recommendations, 13 recommendations related to minority populations, 12 recommendations for normal ejection fraction, 63 recommendations for reduced ejection fraction, and 24 recommendations for comorbidities.

Formalization of GLs into computerized format was done by DeGeL and its tools that support several GL modeling languages. The CE was trained by the KE (E. Shalom) to use the DeGeL's graphical framework, called Gesher, for specification of clinical knowledge and generate computerized GL based on the Asbru language (Hatsek et al., 2010; Peleg et al., 2017).

Logic embedded in each of the recommendations was partially formalized using as a logical structure IF-THEN rules. For correct and understandable representation of GLs, its concepts had to be exactly defined, for example, explicit definition of hypertension as a concept with values for systolic blood pressure ≥ 140 mmHg and diastolic blood pressure ≥ 90 mmHg. This preparation phase took 2 months. Afterwards, Gesher was used to further specify the GL by generation of its semiformal representation with control structures (sequential or parallel ordering of subplans) and for specification of defined declarative GL concepts. In their study, the authors do not include information about how long this last phase took; they specified that the overall project duration was 11 months.

The resulting formalized GL included 167 recommendations because for clarity of knowledge representation, some of the original recommendations were specified into several formal parts. Quality assessment of the resulting computerized GL was based on evaluation of the level of similarity with free-text GL resulting from expert consensus and clarity of GL language in its computer-interpretable format. After expert review, it was concluded that the outcome is a comprehensive, hierarchical, and time-oriented nursing heart failure computerized GL with adequately presented knowledge. Eligibility criteria were specified for each of the recommendations in the GL, for example, based on the characteristics of target population that is, patients in New York Heart Association class III or class IV (severe heart failure).

Given the exploratory nature of the presented heart failure study, the authors recognized that a more detailed evaluation might be required by a group of experts with academic background, clinicians, and KEs or by a series of case studies focused on a broader range of clinical cases. Several limitations of the presented approach include bias introduced by expert consensus, few holistic concepts in creation of computerized nursing GLs, and not using the recognized standardized nursing terminologies.

7.5 Discussion: Benefits and contributions of using a guideline-based clinical decision support systems

In earlier sections of this chapter we introduced CDSSs and their specific use in the context of GL-based CDSSs through the life cycle of computerized GL-based CDSSs. In general, we can summarize the main effect of a GL-based CDSS,.

A GL-based CDSS can potentially lead to a higher quality of care for any scenario, for any particular clinical decision, by any physician.

Specifically, we can outline several main contributions:

1. *Contribution to physicians*: A GL-based CDSS has the potential to enhance physicians' adherence to clinical GLs, to enhance the team's competence in managing complicated medical situations, to improve dissemination of medical knowledge, to support training and education, and to create positive perceptions regarding the use of CDSSs.
2. *Contribution to healthcare organizations*: Use of CDSSs has the potential to enhance the quality of care by decreasing its variance, to enhance quality control, to improve risk management, and to enable better clinical outcomes while decreasing the costs of care.
3. *Contribution to the patient*: CDSSs have the potential to empower the patient at home through a mobile device or to provide support to a shared decision model, namely, a joint decision by the patient and the physician.
4. *Contribution for professional medical organizations and GL groups*: By using KA tools, CDSSs have the potential for support in the specification phase by assisting professional medical organizations in the maintenance of GL-based knowledge in every domain.
5. *Contribution to medical KEs and researchers*: CDSSs have the potential to assist a KE in the GL specification process and to assist researchers in defining research questions.

To demonstrate these benefit and contributions, the Picard CDSS served as the backbone of the MOBIGUDE project in the European Union, which is monitoring chronic patients at home (Peleg et al., 2017). The Picard CDSS sends the patient alerts as necessary and provides personalized GL-based recommendations to the patient's healthcare providers, using sensors on the patient or at the patient's home, and the patient's mobile devices. The interaction with the sensors, as well as the broadcasting of the data to the patient's medical record (thus implicitly to the Picard CDSS), was made through the patient's mobile device and a series of back end servers, with high compliance by both patients and physicians.

7.6 Conclusions

As this chapter illustrated, there exists sound methodology related to knowledge modeling and design of CDSSs based on clinical GLs. Despite this fact, CDSSs that use computerized GLs should not be seen as a silver bullet, ensuring their wide acceptance in clinical practice (Greenes et al., 2018). Factors impeding the wider implementation of CDSSs include physicians' belief that this technology might require their increased attention during patient encounters and influence their relationship with patients as a result of reduction of time devoted to communication with patients (Kilsdonk, Peute, & Jaspers, 2017). Therefore integration of the technology with preferences and varying workflows of clinical personnel is important. While some clinicians prefer support at the point of care, others require a preview of recommendations at the end of visit. To minimize differences in computer literacy, adequate educational materials and training should be available prior to deployment of a CDSS into daily practice. Therefore in considering design and implementation of a CDSS, it would be of benefit to address it through technological, human factors, and sociotechnical models (Kilsdonk et al., 2017).

For further reading, we would like to emphasize several active areas of research. Modeling computerized GLs for multimorbidity patients enables decision support for real-life conditions in which, for example, elderly patients often suffer from several comorbid diseases (Jafarpour, Raza Abidi, van Woensel, & Raza Abidi, 2019; Kogan, Tu, & Peleg, 2018). IT support is required to accommodate healthcare process variability and organizational processes in clinical workflow (Reichert Pryss, 2017; Shabo Shvo, Peleg, Parimbelli, Quaglini, & Napolitano, 2016). Other topics include evaluation of quality and safety of care flow systems, context-aware healthcare processes, process interoperability and standards in healthcare, and semantic interoperability in healthcare. As a starting point for further research, interested readers could use the proceedings of the workshop KR4HC-ProHealth 2019.

Acknowledgments

We would like to thank the Israeli Ministry of Science Office, the Gertner Institute for Epidemiology and Health Policy Research, and the EU MobiGuide FP7 project (FP7−287811) who supported this research.

This research has been supported by grant from Tatra banka Foundation (2018vs108).

References

Berner, S. E. (2016). *Clinical decision support systems*. Switzerland: Springer Cham.

Boaz, D., & Shahar, Y. (2005). A framework for distributed mediation of temporal-abstraction queries to clinical databases. *Artificial Intelligence in Medicine, 34*(1), 3−24.

Boldo, I. (2007). Knowledge-based recognition of clinical-guideline application in time-oriented medical records (Ph.D Thesis). Israel: Department of Industrial Engineering and Management, Technion.

Brown, M. A., Magee, L. A., Kenny, L. C., et al. (2018). On behalf of the International Society for the Study of Hypertension in pregnancy (ISSHP). The hypertensive disorders of pregnancy: ISSHP classification, diagnosis & management recommendation for international practice. *Pregnancy Hypertension, 13*, 291−310.

Combi, C., Keravnou-Papailiou, E., & Shahar, Y. (2010). *Temporal information systems in medicine*. Springer-Verlag New York Inc.

De Clercq, P. A., Blom, J. A., Korsten, H. H. M., & Hasman, A. (2004). Approaches for creating computer-interpretable guidelines that facilitate decision support. *Artificial Intelligence in Medicine, 31*(1), 1−27.

ESC Guidelines for the diagnosis and treatment of acute and chronic heart failure. (2016). *European Heart Journal, 37*(27), 2129−2200.

Freidman, I. (2012). Evaluation of guideline-application engines by longitudinal simulation (Master thesis). Beer-Sheva, Israel: Ben-Gurion University of the Negev.

Furberg, R. D., Williams, P., Bagwell, J., & LaBresh, K. (2017). A mobile clinical decision support tool for pediatric cardiovascular risk-reduction clinical practice guidelines: Development and description. *JMIR Mhealth Uhealth, 5*(3), e29.

German, E., Leibowitz, A., & Shahar, Y. (2009). An architecture for linking medical decision-support applications to clinical databases and its evaluation. *Journal of Biomedical Informatics, 42*(2), 203−218.

Greenes, R. A., Bates, D. W., Kawamoto, K., Middleton, B., Osheroff, J., & Shahar, Y. (2018). Clinical decision support models and frameworks: Seeking to address research issues underlying implementation successes and failures. *Journal of Biomedical Informatics, 78*, 134−143.

Hansen, D., Rovelo Ruiz, G., Doherty, P., Iliou, M. C., Vromen, T., Hinton, S., ... Ambrosetti, M. (2018). Do clinicians prescribe exercise similarly in patients with different cardiovascular diseases? Findings from the EAPC EXPERT working group survey. *European Journal of Preventive Cardiology, 25*(7), 682−691.

Hatsek, A., 2014. A knowledge-based assessment of compliance to the longitudinal application of clinical guidelines. Ben-Gurion University of the Negev, Engineering, Department of Information System Engineering.

Hatsek, A., Shahar, Y., Taieb-Maimon, M., Shalom, E., Klimov, D., & Lunenfeld, E. (2010). A scalable architecture for incremental specification and maintenance of procedural and declarative clinical decision-support knowledge. *The Open Medical Informatics Journal, 4*, 255.

Hunt, S. A., Abraham, W. T., Chin, M. H., Feldman, A. M., Francis, G. S., Ganiats, T. G., et al. (2009). Focused update incorporated into the ACC/AHA 2005 guidelines for the diagnosis and management of heart failure in adults: A report of the American College of Cardiology Foundation/American Heart Association Task Force on practice guidelines: Developed in collaboration with the International Society for Heart and Lung Transplantation. *Circulation, 119*, e391–e479.

Isern, D., & Moreno, A. (2008). Computer-based execution of clinical guidelines: A review. *International Journal of Medical Informatics*, 77(12), 787–808.

Jafarpour, B., Raza Abidi, S., van Woensel, W., & Raza Abidi, S. S. (2019). Execution-time integration of clinical practice guidelines to provide decision support for comorbid conditions. *Artificial Intelligence in Medicine, 94*, 117–137.

Kilsdonk, E., Peute, L., & Jaspers, M. W. (2017). Factors influencing implementation success of guideline-based clinical decision support systems: A systematic review and gaps analysis. *International Journal of Medical Informatics, 98*(2017), 56–64.

Klimov, D., Shahar, Y., & Taieb-Maimon, M. (2010). Intelligent visualization and exploration of time-oriented data of multiple patients. *Artificial Intelligence in Medicine, 49*(1), 11–31.

Klimov, D., Shknevsky, A., & Shahar, Y. (2014). Exploration of patterns predicting renal damage in patients with diabetes type II using a visual temporal analysis laboratory. *Journal of the American Medical Informatics Association, 22*(2), 275–289.

Kogan, A., Tu, S.W., & Peleg, M. (2018). Goal-driven management of interacting clinical guidelines for multimorbidity patients. AMIA... Annual Symposium proceedings. AMIA Symposium, 2018, 690–699.

Kongwattanakul, K., Saksiriwuttho, P., Chaiyarach, S., et al. (2018). Incidence, characteristics, maternal complications, and perinatal outcomes associated with preeclampsia with severe features and HELLP syndrome. *International Journal of Women's Health* (10), 371–377.

Levinson, D.R., & General, I. (2010). Adverse events in hospitals: National incidence among medicare beneficiaries. Department of Health and Human Services Office of the Inspector General.

Lindenfeld, J., Albert, N. M., Boehmer, J. P., Collins, S. P., Ezekowitz, J. A., et al. (2010). Heart Failure Society of America, HFSA 2010 comprehensive heart failure practice guideline. *Journal of Cardiac Failure, 16*, e1–194.

Makary, M. A., & Daniel, M. (2016). Medical error—The third leading cause of death in the United States. *BMJ, 353*, i2139.

Martins, S. B., Shahar, Y., Goren-Bar, D., Galperin, M., Kaizer, H., Basso, L. V., ... Goldstein, M. K. (2008). Evaluation of an architecture for intelligent query and exploration of time-oriented clinical data. *Artificial Intelligence in Medicine, 43*(1), 17–34.

Musen, M. A., Fagan, L. M., Combs, D. M., & Shortliffe, E. H. (1987). Use of a domain model to drive an interactive knowledge-editing tool. *International Journal of Man-Machine Studies, 26*(1), 105–121.

Peleg, M., & González-Ferrer, A. (2014). In R. Greenes (Ed.), *Clinical decision support – The road ahead* (pp. 435–465). Elsevier.

Peleg, M., Shahar, Y., Quaglini, S., Fux, A., García-Sáez, G., Goldstein, A., ... Parimbelli, E. (2017). MobiGuide: A personalized and patient-centric decision-support system and its evaluation in the atrial fibrillation and gestational diabetes domains. *User Modeling and User-Adapted Interaction, 27*(2), 159–213.

Reichert, M., & Pryss, R. (2017). Flexible support of healthcare processes. In C. Combi, G. Pozzi, & P. Veltri (Eds.), *Process modeling and management for healthcare* (pp. 35–66). London: Taylor & Francis Group.

Shabo Shvo, A., Peleg, M., Parimbelli, E., Quaglini, S., & Napolitano, C. (2016). Interplay between clinical guidelines and organizational workflow systems: Experience from the mobiguide project. *Methods of Information in Medicine, 55*(6), 488–494.

Shahar, Y. (1997). A framework for knowledge-based temporal abstraction. *Artificial Intelligence, 90*(1–2), 79–133.

Shalom, E., Shahar, Y., & Lunenfeld, E. (2016). An architecture for a continuous, user-driven, and data-driven application of clinical guidelines and its evaluation. *Journal of Biomedical Informatics, 59*, 130–148.

Shalom, E., Shahar, Y., Lunenfeld, E., Taieb-Maimon, M., Young, O., Goren-Bar, D., ... Yarkoni, A. (2006). The importance of creating an ontology-specific consensus before a markup-based specification of clinical guidelines. Paper presented at the Proceeding of the Biennial European Conference on Artificial Intelligence (ECAI).

Shalom, E., Shahar, Y., Parmet, Y., & Lunenfeld, E. (2015). A multiple-scenario assessment of the effect of a continuous-care, guideline-based decision support system on clinicians' compliance to clinical guidelines. *International journal of medical informatics, 84*(4), 248–262.

Shalom, E., Shahar, Y., Taieb-Maimon, M., Bar, G., Yarkoni, A., Young, O., ... Liel, Y. (2008). A quantitative assessment of a methodology for collaborative specification and evaluation of clinical guidelines. *Journal of Biomedical Informatics, 41*(6), 889–903.

Shalom, E., Shahar, Y., Taieb-Maimon, M., Martins, S. B., Vaszar, L. T., Goldstein, M. K., ... Lunenfeld, E. (2009). Ability of expert physicians to structure clinical guidelines: Reality vs perception. *Journal of Evaluation in Clinical Practice, 15*(6), 1043–1053.

Spokoiny, A., & Shahar, Y. (2007). An active database architecture for knowledge-based incremental abstraction of complex concepts from continuously arriving time-oriented raw data. *Journal of Intelligent Information Systems, 28*(3), 199–231.

The American College of Obstetricians and Gynecologist (ACOG, 2013). Retrieved from http://www.acog.org/. Accessed 25.06.19.

The European Society of Cardiology (ESC Guidelines, 2013). Retrieved from https://www.escardio.org/Guidelines/Clinical-Practice-Guidelines/Arterial-Hypertension-Management-of. Accessed 25.06.19.

Topaz, M., Shalom, E., Masterson-Creber, R., Rhadakrishnan, K., Monsen, K. A., & Bowles, K. H. (2013). Developing nursing computer interpretable guidelines: A feasibility study of heart failure guidelines in homecare. *AMIA Annual Symposium Proceedings, 2013*, 1353–1361, Published 2013 Nov 16.

Tso, G.J., Tu, S.W., Oshiro, C., Martins, S., Ashcraft, M., Yuen, K.W., ... Goldstein, M. K. (2017). Automating guidelines for clinical decision support: Knowledge engineering and implementation. AMIA... Annual Symposium proceedings. AMIA Symposium, 2016, 1189–1198.

CHAPTER 8

Digital coaching for personalized healthcare of cardiovascular diseases

Enrique Dorronzoro-Zubiete[1], Octavio Rivera-Romero[1], Francisco J. Nuñez-Benjumea[2], and Sergio Cervera-Torres[2]
[1]Participatory Health Informatics and Personalization Research Group, Universidad de Sevilla, Seville, Spain
[2]Adhera Heath Inc, Seville, Spain

8.1 Introduction

Cardiovascular diseases (CVDs) comprise a wide range of diseases affecting the heart, vascular diseases of the brain, and diseases of blood vessels. A common taxonomy of the different types of CVDs classifies them into two major groups: (1) CVDs due to atherosclerosis, including ischemic heart disease (IHD) and coronary artery disease (e.g., heart attack), cerebrovascular disease (CBD) (e.g., stroke), and diseases of the aorta and arteries, including hypertension and peripheral vascular disease, and (2) other CVDs, including congenital heart disease, rheumatic heart disease, cardiomyopathies, and cardiac arrhythmias (Mendis et al., 2011).

According to the World Health Organization, 17.9 million people die each year from CVDs, that is, an estimated 31% of all deaths worldwide, and CVD is the leading cause of mortality globally (World Health Organization (WHO), 2017). IHDs and CBDs are responsible for the vast majority of overall deaths from CVD in both men (80%) and women (75%), followed by hypertensive heart diseases (6% in men, 7% in women) (Mendis et al., 2011). To better understand the incidence, prevalence, and mortality associated with CVDs, the 2015 Global Burden of Disease (GBD) study (Roth et al., 2017) pooled information from a wide range of data sources and methods to produce age-, sex-, and country-specific results for the years 1990–2015. The research found an estimated prevalence of 422.7 million cases of CVD worldwide and an alarming finding that trends in CVD mortality have plateaued and are no longer declining in high-income regions.

Personalized Health Systems for Cardiovascular Disease
DOI: https://doi.org/10.1016/B978-0-12-818950-4.00013-6

Risk factors for atherosclerotic diseases such as IHD and CBD are well identified and include behavioral risk factors, such as tobacco use, physical inactivity, unhealthy diet, and alcohol abuse; metabolic risk factors, such as hypertension, diabetes, high cholesterol levels, and overweight/obesity; and other risk factors, such as poverty, gender, genetic disposition, and psychological factors (e.g., stress, depression) (Mendis et al., 2011). Moreover, most of these risk factors are commonly intertwined, further affecting health outcomes related to CVD, which poses the challenge of delivering multicomponent interventions to better manage this condition (Goodie, Wilfong, & Kroke, 2019). CVD is usually identified as an aging-related disease. However, the increase in the prevalence of risk factors of CVD among young adults (age 18–50 years) seems to be reversing this trend in developed countries, potentially leading to a new epidemic in this young segment of the population as they age (Andersson & Vasan, 2018).

Nonetheless, most of the identified risk factors of CVD are linked to individual lifestyles and therefore are potentially preventable by means of personalized behavioral interventions. A recent review of the evidence carried out by the U.S. Preventive Services Task Force (Krist et al., 2020) concluded with moderate certainty that behavioral counseling interventions promoting a healthy diet and physical activity have a moderate net benefit on CVD risk in adults who are at increased risk for CVD. A systematic review focusing on theory-based psychological approaches to promote a Mediterranean-style diet found that the use of the social cognitive theory and self-determination theory can help to increase understanding and promote diet adherence for reducing CVD risk and events (Willis, Brown, & Greene, 2019). Cognitive behavioral therapy has also been shown to improve health behaviors including diet (e.g., reduced sugar, increased intake of fruits and vegetables), physical activity, and smoking cessation in some studies of healthy adults and those with or at risk for CVD (Kaar, Luberto, Campbell, & Huffman, 2017). With a focus on the psychological risk factors for CVD, Scott-Sheldon et al. (2020) examined the effects of mindfulness-based interventions in adults with CVD through a systematic review and metaanalysis. Their findings suggest that such interventions have demonstrated favorable effects on both psychological and physiological outcomes in this population.

The delivery of personalized behavioral interventions, especially through digital means (e.g., web-based platforms, mobile applications), has shown promising potential regarding efficacy in tackling specific health behaviors such as weight, body mass index, and blood pressure control

(Lau, Chee, Chow, Cheng, & Wong, 2020; Ma, Cheng, Cheng, & Sit, 2019); smoking cessation (Carrasco-Hernandez et al., 2020); and management of stress and anxiety (Eze, Mateus, & Hashiguchi, 2020). In this regard, digital technologies seem to be a suitable intervention means, as they can leverage the potential scalability and cost-effectiveness that personalized digital health solutions offer. However, personalized behavioral digital interventions still need to tackle several usability and human factors—related barriers to become a feasible tool to be included in clinical practice (Li et al., 2019; Seo, Kim, Sheen, & Cha, 2020; Wattanapisit, Tuangratananon, & Wattanapisit, 2020).

Against this background, the objectives of this chapter are twofold: First, we review and summarize some of the most relevant patients' and healthcare professionals' needs, preferences, and attitudes toward the use of digital solutions for CVD prevention and self-management reported in the scientific literature. Second, we provide an overview of the current state of the art in personal health coaching systems, analyzing relevant issues such as types of technological solution, theoretical foundations, personalization techniques used, included motivational elements, and conducted evaluations and main outcomes. Following this approach, we identify successful features, the design lessons that were learned, unmet needs, and research gaps to provide a basis for further research.

8.2 Needs, preferences, and attitudes

This section highlights psychological processes in terms of attitudes, affective responses, needs, and preferences associated with the use of CVD e-health solutions. These solutions are mainly focused on CVD prevention or rehabilitation (e.g., congestive heart failure or stroke) either at home or at the hospital.

Here, opinions about solutions including educational CVD contents, activity-monitoring systems, and promotion of exercise, mostly directed to middle-aged and elderly people are overviewed. To be more precise, attitudes, preferences, and needs have been structured around different thematic areas wherein motivational barriers and facilitators for engaging with CVD digital solutions can be identified, together with unmet needs.

8.2.1 Illness perceptions and health beliefs

Illness perceptions and health beliefs constitute one of the most important factors influencing decision making for engaging with a health solution. Two different categories have been differentiated.

8.2.1.1 Emotional receptiveness of risk information

Being confronted with health information that does not match one's self-perceived health status can trigger different type of psychological reactions. For example, some people at high risk for CVD resist accepting the importance to CVD prevention, assigning the risk to, for example, family antecedents. Moreover, some people who have already suffered myocardial infarction and/or did not exercise before a CVD incident believe that exercising is not important for their rehabilitation (Ottaviano, Vera-Muñoz, Arredondo, & Salvi, 2010). This type of reactions is dangerous in the sense that it denotes a very inaccurate perception of the person's health risk, potentially hindering implementation of preventive health behaviors and use of digital solutions for reducing risks of CVD. Optimism bias, a belief in one's positive health status, usually when compared to peers of same age and gender (Clarke, Lovegrove, Williams, & Machperson, 2000), might be a psychological mechanism at work in those cases.

Other people may experience either intensified feelings of vulnerability accompanied by emotional reactions (e.g., fear, anxiety, worry, irritation) and perceptions of fatalistic health future or, by contrast, increased interest in their own risk profiles. For example, they may be motivated to increase their knowledge about the underlying causes of the disease or to learn about self-management of stress, physical activity, and symptom monitoring.

All these different psychological reactions denote strong interindividual differences in sensitivity to health risk and coping mechanisms concerning perceived risk for CVD (e.g., emotion-focused vs solution-focused (Lazarus, 1999)). Being able to acknowledge this information might be very relevant to increase the potential success of a digital CVD intervention.

8.2.1.2 Confidence in self-managed exercise

Self-efficacy is defined as the perception of feeling capable or confident to implement a course of action, which is pivotal in health behavior change (Jeng & Braun, 1994). Low self-efficacy can lead some people to feel insecure about exercising at home via a guided digital intervention without close supervision. Factors contributing to that feeling are, for example, prior sedentary lifestyle (lack of knowledge about how to exercise), perceptions of inadequacy of exercises (e.g., age-appropriateness or the perception that gamification as a methodology does not match the person's idea of "serious" exercising), and especially doubts about acceptable physical reactions to particular exercises (e.g., heart rate).

When included in the solution, contacting with a professional health coach can transmit feelings of reassurance and boosted confidence about the health solution (Rawstorn et al., 2018). Therefore to reduce uncertainty, information needs to be facilitated so that expectations about physical symptoms during exercise are foreseen, especially concerning symptoms preceding an adverse event and false alarms, an aspect that is strongly addressed by health care professionals.

8.2.2 Relationship with technology

In general, the literature reports the prevalence of positive attitudes toward digital technologies for CVD prevention, rehabilitation, and support of quality of life. This is particularly important in considering elderly people, who typically face problems adapting to new technologies and processing digital information (e.g., some may want to be able to print materials). Indeed, digital literacy, that is, the ability to use and understand digital technologies still emerges as an important factor to account for engagement with CVD solutions.

Users typically remark on the need for technologies that have been made easy to use by making solutions flexible enough to be included in technologies they already know without the requirement to learn about new devices and enhancing familiarization with the system. Face-to-face coaching seems to be preferred followed by phone support, emails, and videos or even quick manuals with diagrams and pictures. Including an introductory video has been considered especially valuable. Integration of music and incorporation of mind-training exercises have also been suggested as features that potentially improve engagement with the system.

Two aspects deserve special mention for engagement with the systems:

- The integration of activities in daily life schedules to diminish lack of time as a reason making it difficult to log into the system.
- Increase in the "meaningful value" of digital solutions by integrating them into the course of primary care structure so that self-managed care becomes part of the health routine.

8.2.3 Digital coaching features

In terms of coaching features and techniques, preferences for personalization of feedback and goal setting are two of the most mentioned.

8.2.3.1 Personalized feedback

In general, people seem to prefer clear and easy visual feedback, such as progress bars and performance indicators. Personalized prompts have also been seen as important for initiation and maintenance of lifestyle change. Appropriate feedback might be critical to increase self-awareness and self-reflection about the user's own health.

If included in the system, real-time coaching from specialists can boost confidence and motivation to adhere to the health CVD program. In this regard, a trustworthiness atmosphere provided by the coach might be a pivotal element to achieve sustained engagement with the system.

Health care professionals (HCPs) have also noted that progress feedback regarding key outcomes is essential. For example, body mass, height, weight, cholesterol levels, alcohol consumption, smoking cessation, medication adherence, blood pressure, steps, physical activity (frequency, intensity, type, and time), nutrition, well-being, general mental health, quality of life, satisfaction, self-efficacy, engagement, social support, and social interaction are preferred to be summarized in a format comprising no more than one page (e.g., a sort of indicators dashboard).

8.2.3.2 Personalized goal setting

Adapting goals to one's own specific needs can lead to an increased sense of commitment. However, it still appears necessary to account for contextual factors (e.g., living in a city or the country or goal functionality in terms of "why") and deeper analysis of the person's current lifestyle. HCPs point out as well the need to focus on health promotion rather than disease.

8.2.3.3 Opportunity for social interaction

Including functionalities for social interaction is an aspect that is recurrently addressed not only by users but also by healthcare providers. Different levels of socialization have been proposed:

- Making family members active agents of the intervention, particularly if relatives are also primary caregivers. Facilitating family connections is considered as an advantage to potentially leveraged health-related behavior commitment. Of course, that requires a more detailed evaluation of the user context and interaction with different agents.
- HCPs also suggest that digital solutions have the capacity to bridge hospital-generated social connections during rehabilitation (e.g., after a heart attack) and new community social networks, thus supporting a

richer social ecosystem, including connections with HCPs themselves (Walsh et al., 2018).

- The idea that patients can become mentors of other patients can be considered another source of social motivation to strength health habit forming. This is especially the case because some people find that connecting with peers' experiences and emotions makes CVD content more emphatic and credible (Oosterom-Calo, te Velde, Stut, & Brug, 2015).

8.3 Study cases of coaching systems for cardiovascular diseases in the literature

In this section we present several study cases of personalized health coaching systems designed for CVD management found in the scientific literature. Aligned with our objectives, in this chapter we focus on studies reporting the design process or results of an evaluation of a personalized digital coaching system for CVDs.

8.3.1 Description of study cases

Bartlett et al. (2014) presented the SMART Personalized Self-Management System (PSMS), which provides support to people with congestive heart failure, chronic pain, or stroke. The PSMS allows users to monitor their symptoms and incorporates aspects of rehabilitation, behavior change and education. The PSMS consists of a mobile app and desktop software designed according to a user-centered design methodology. Regarding the functionalities integrated into the PSMS, the user can create a daily plan of activities; input blood pressure and weight measurements; review his or her daily walk; get graphical feedback on weight, blood pressure, symptoms, and activities level; and get access to heart failure–related information. The authors conducted a realistic evaluation of PSMS through a nonexperimental study involving seven participants for 4 weeks. The use of the system and the monitor devices, usability, changes in knowledge about congestive heart failure, and levels of activities were analyzed in this study.

The Text4Health program is delivered by using mobile health devices and a website (Dale et al., 2015). This program is intended for adults with coronary heart disease and is based on the use of a supporting website and automated daily short message service text messages. The Text4Health program aims for patient education through short videos and recommendations. This program was developed by using the mHealth Development and Evaluation Framework. The effectiveness of Text4Health and adherence to it were evaluated through a two-arm, parallel randomized control trial involving 123 participants for 24 weeks.

Davies et al. (2016) developed a personalized self-management rehabilitation system for monitoring of stroke survivors. The system consists of a mobile phone app, a home hub, and a professional platform. The main functionalities of this system are data collection regarding rehabilitation monitoring, visual feedback, and instructional videos. The gathered information is used to personalize the exercise programs. The development process involved three cycles. The authors conducted a realistic evaluation through a nonexperimental study involving five participants for 7 weeks to analyze the effectiveness of the system in gait rehabilitation.

The study presented by Engelen et al. (2020) used a web-based self-management program that contains six modules (coping with CVD, setting boundaries, lifestyle, healthy nutrition, being physically active, and interaction with health professionals) aiming to increase self-management behavior. This program was designed by following the user-centered design methodology. The authors evaluated the effectiveness of this program through an explorative randomized control trial involving 208 participants for 12 weeks.

Goyal et al. (2016) used a mobile app for their intervention. The app aims to empower users to easily and effectively manage their heart health on a daily basis. First, the user completed an assessment of risk factors. Then the user prioritizes his or her modifiable risk factors. The mobile app suggested simple daily activities based on identified risk factors, provided resources and encouragement, and tailored content to the individual's risk profile. The mobile app was designed by following the user-centered design methodology. The authors conducted a retrospective nonexperimental study to analyze the engagement and effect of incentives on the overall uptake and usage behaviors.

Jongstra et al. (2017) used the interactive HATICE platform intended for older adults. HATICE is a web platform aimed at CVD prevention. It is focused on seven modifiable cardiovascular risk factors (hypertension, dyslipidemia, diabetes mellitus, overweight, lack of physical exercise, smoking, and unhealthy nutrition). HATICE integrates several interesting functionalities, such as interactive information, goal setting, reminders, automated positive feedback, the cognitive training programs. The design of HATICE consisted of five phases: (1) conceptual framework design, (2) platform concept and functional design, (3) platform implementation (software and content), (4) testing and pilot study, and (5) final product development. Participatory methods were used in some of those phases. The authors conducted two nonexperimental studies to evaluate the usability and the acceptability and feasibility of HATICE.

Khanji et al. (2019) conducted a digital coaching lifestyle intervention for CVD prevention among individuals who are at increased risk of developing CVD. The intervention was conducted by using the Happy London tool. This system is a web-based tool that provides a personalized score for the user's lifestyle and a 10-year CVD risk score. Once scores have been calculated, the system provides advice and information tailored specifically for those suboptimal factors, recommendations about ideal targets for each individual based on his or her scores, dynamic tailoring, and reminders sent by email. The authors evaluated the effectiveness of the intervention through a single-center two-arm randomized control trial involving 402 participants for 6 months.

eMate is a behavior change support system that uses a computational model based on multiple psychological theories of behavior change (Klein, Mogles, & van Wissen, 2014). This system consists of a phone app and an online lifestyle diary for self-management. It is intended for use by chronic patients with type 2 diabetes, HIV, or CVD. eMate allows determination of the stage of change of the user, monitors the user's behaviors to estimate the level of adherence, supports changes in the user's perception of specific psychological aspects, and updates the user's beliefs. The system was validated by using a nonexperimental study involving 17 participants with chronic illness.

Lin et al. (2015) presented a mobile app for CVD prevention intended for people with obesity. The app integrates tutorials, a food tracker, a weight tracker, a buddy system, physical activity, goal setting, countdown, challenge games, rewards, and feedback. It was developed by using user-centered methodology involving stakeholders in the different stages of the process.

CardioFit, the system used by Reid et al., is an Internet-based expert system that was designed to promote physical activity in patients with coronary heart disease who were not participating in cardiac rehabilitation (Reid et al., 2012). This web-based system implements several functionalities, such as online tutorials, a physical activity plan, and email feedback. The effectiveness of CardioFit was evaluated through an experimental study that was based on a randomized control trials involving 223 participants for 12 months.

Van Den Brekel-Dijkstra, Rengers, Niessen, De Wit, and Kraaijenhagen (2016) used a web-based health risk assessment based on a questionnaire that covered sociodemographic variables, family and personal medical history, lifestyle behavior, and psychological variables. Using this risk assessment tool, a personalized prevention intervention was designed. The feasibility and effectiveness of the risk assessment tool were evaluated through an experimental study involving 230 participants who were at high risk of developing CVD.

Finally, Yousuf et al. (2019) defined an intervention using MyCLIC. MyCLIC is an e-coaching lifestyle intervention tool that consists of a mobile app and a website. This system provides personalized health plans and calculates the user's risk factors based on his or her body mass index. The authors validated the risk estimation compared to the 10-year CVD risk scores in a nonexperimental study. They also evaluated the effectiveness of the intervention by using an experimental study involving a randomized control trial.

8.3.2 Theoretical foundations of study cases

Coaching systems aim to affect the user's behavior so that the user adopts a healthier lifestyle. To reach this objective, including a strong theoretical basis considering different aspects of behavior change is crucial. Several studies have showed that digital interventions tend to be more effective when relying on behavior change theories and models (Fanning, Mullen, & Mcauley, 2012).

Among the study cases, there is a prevalence of those that explicitly report behavior change theories as theoretical foundations of the described system. There are two different approaches: using a single theory or model or using a combination of two or more theories or models. We can find examples of both approaches in the study cases. Although a wide range of different theories or models are frequently mentioned in the literature, the most common theory is the social cognitive theory. Other popular theories are the transtheoretical model and the theory of planned behavior. Table 8.1 presents the behavior change theories that were implemented in the study cases.

Michie et al. (2013) proposed a behavior change technique taxonomy that it is commonly used to code techniques implemented in digital

Table 8.1 Behavior change theories used in the study cases.

Study	AFT	COMBI	CSM	CT	HBM	ICM	PMT	RPM	SCT	SRT	TTM	TPB	TRA	PMT
Bartlett et al. (2014)				•										
Dale et al. (2015)			•						•					
Engelen et al. (2020)						•								
Goyal et al. (2016)												•		
Jongstra et al. (2017)									•					
Klein et al. (2014)	•	•			•			•	•	•	•	•	•	
Lin et al. (2015)									•		•			
Van Den Brekel-Dijkstra et al. (2016)							•		•		•			

AFT, Attitude formation theory; *COMBI*, computerized behavior intervention; *CSM*, common sense model; *CT*, control theory; *HBM*, health belief model; *PMT*, protection motivation theory; *RPM*, relapse prevention model; *SCT*, social cognitive theory; *SRT*, self-regulation theories; *TPB*, theory of planned behavior; *TRA*, theory of reasoned action; *TTM*, transtheoretical model.

interventions. We used this taxonomy to identify and code techniques that were implemented in the study cases. Most of the study cases include a combination of several behavior change techniques. Goal setting, feedback, self-monitoring, and action planning are the most commonly used behavior change techniques in the study cases. Although social interaction has been reported as a desired feature to be integrated into digital coaching systems, it is relevant that behavior change techniques related to social issues such as social support, "information about other approval," or social comparison are not commonly implemented. Regarding techniques related to health literacy, "instructions on how to perform the behavior" is a technique that is frequently implemented in these systems, while "information about health consequences" is not usually implemented. Table 8.2 presents the behavior change techniques implemented in the study cases.

8.3.3 Personalization

As was mentioned earlier in the chapter, personalization is key in the coaching systems, since each person is unique and his or her condition, needs, and preferences may change over time. We have analyzed the personalization features included in the study cases by using the tailoring model defined by Op den Akker, Jones, and Hermens (2014).

It is interesting that all analyzed study cases include a combination of personalization techniques. The most frequently used techniques are feedback and goal setting. It is difficult to find studies that implement context aware or self-learning. Table 8.3 shows the personalization techniques that were implemented in the study cases.

8.3.4 Gamification

Lack of enjoyment in the use of digital health solutions is commonly reported as a big demotivator among target users (Giunti, Kool, Rivera Romero, & Dorronzoro Zubiete, 2018; Monteiro-Guerra, Signorelli, Rivera-Romero, Dorronzoro-Zubiete, & Caulfield, 2020). Including game elements to digital health solutions, especially in coaching systems promoting healthy lifestyles, is potentially a positive and desirable feature. Gamification is defined as "the use of game design elements in nongame contexts" (Deterding et al., 2011). Gamification has become a popular strategy to increase the users' enjoyment of and engagement with

Table 8.2 Behavior change techniques implemented in the study cases.

Study	Behavior change techniques		
Bartlett et al. (2014)	Self-monitoring Goal setting Action planning	Feedback Biofeedback	
Dale et al. (2015)	Self-monitoring Monitoring of behavior by others Instruction on how to perform the behavior Identification of self as role model	Prompts/cues Reduce Prompts/cues Feedback Imaginary reward	Goal setting Social support Incentives
Davies et al. (2016)	Demonstration of the behavior Instruction on how to perform the behavior Monitoring the behavior by others without feedback	Biofeedback Goal setting Self-monitoring	
Engelen et al. (2020)	Action planning Information about other approval Self-monitoring Demonstration of the behavior	Goal setting Review goal behavior Review outcome goal Graded task	Social comparison Self-beliefs Problem solving Feedback
Goyal et al. (2016)	Goal setting Action planning	Review behavior goal Feedback	
Jongstra et al. (2017)	Goal setting Action planning	Instruction of how to perform the behavior Feedback	Review behavior goal Social support

(*Continued*)

Table 8.2 (Continued)

Study	Behavior change techniques		
Khanji et al. (2019)	Goal setting		
Klein et al. (2014)	Feedback	Instruction on how to perform the behavior	Self-monitoring
	Goal setting	Information about other approval Discrepancy between current behavior and goal	Pros and cons Habit formation
Lin et al. (2015)	Self-monitoring Goal setting Feedback	Review behavior goal Information about health consequences	Social support Prompts/cues
Reid et al. (2012)	Action planning Self-monitoring	Biofeedback Feedback	Goal setting Social support
Van Den Brekel-Dijkstra et al. (2016)	Biofeedback Feedback Action planning	Information about antecedents Information about health consequences	
Yousuf et al. (2019)	Feedback	Information on how to perform the behavior Review behavior goal	Action planning
	Goal setting Reward		Self-monitoring

Table 8.3 Personalization techniques implemented in the study cases.

Study	CA	Ad	GS	UT	IHI	FB	SL
Bartlett et al. (2014)		•	•			•	
Dale et al. (2015)				•	•	•	
Davies et al. (2016)		•	•	•	•	•	
Engelen et al. (2020)		•	•	•		•	
Goyal et al. (2016)		•	•	•		•	
Jongstra et al. (2017)		•	•		•	•	
Khanji et al. (2019)		•	•	•			
Klein et al. (2014)		•	•	•		•	
Lin et al. (2015)			•		•	•	
Reid et al. (2012)			•		•	•	
Van Den Brekel-Dijkstra et al. (2016)		•				•	
Yousuf et al. (2019)			•	•		•	

Ad, Adaptation; *CA*, context awareness; *FB*, feedback; *GS*, goal settings; *IHI*, inter-human interaction; *SL*, self-learning; *UT*, user targeting.

technological solutions in the digital health domain. However, gamification elements are rarely included in coaching systems for CVD management.

8.4 Matching users' needs and preferences with features implemented in study cases

We have analyzed several study cases reported in the scientific literature that describe personalized coaching systems for self-management of CVDs. The analyzed systems offer a wide set of solutions for people who suffer from CVDs or are at risk of suffering from them in the future. The technologies that were used for the interventions are well known and widely used, which may make their acceptance easier among the target population. However, despite evidence of positive effects on adoption, engagement, and adherence of involving target users in the design process (Dabbs et al., 2009; Giunti, 2018), some systems have been developed with limited or no user involvement. A participatory design approach would probably identify barriers and needs that were not considered in these solutions. Thus the involvement of the final users, whether patients, caregivers, or professionals, is strongly recommended.

It is remarkable that most of coaching systems include a wide spectrum of different types of personalization, which is a great addition, as personalization can contribute to maintaining the user's interest and thus preventing abandonment by the user (Monteiro-Guerra et al., 2020). On the other hand, few coaching systems include gamification, which is another element to increase the user's interest and satisfaction. It is also important to point that although most systems evaluate some variables, such as acceptance, usability, feasibility, or effectiveness, only a small number of those conduct experimental studies. Therefore there is need for further research to evaluate the effectiveness of these personalized coaching systems. Additionally, deeper analysis of the independent effect of the different components may help in better understanding how they directly affect the user's motivation and satisfaction and finally the desired behavior change.

8.4.1 Illness perceptions and health beliefs

One of the problems that is, commonly identified among people who suffer from CVDs is the low-risk perception. This need for information is aligned with actual systems, as most of the study cases provide this type of information. Coaching systems include video and text about risks and lifestyle habits. On the other hand, just a few provide information about how to perform properly the exercises that are included in the exercise program. One of the concerns of people who are at risk of CVD is confidence in self-managed exercises. Some systems include instructional videos (Dale et al., 2015), and others also include direct contact with professionals. In this way, the professionals can provide personalized feedback to patients (Engelen et al., 2020), which makes users more confident about the right way to perform the exercise (Table 8.4).

8.4.2 Relationship with technology

One of the identified needs is easy-to-use technologies. The actual coaching systems use familiar technologies in that all the systems are web-based and/or involve mobile apps. However, although some of the systems found in the literature provide direct communication with professionals (Engelen et al., 2020), there is no mention of any tutorial through text, diagrams, or videos about how to use the applications.

Engagement is also an important aspect of these types of systems. User engagement is a key factor in determining the success of an app, as it is related to the user's intention to continue using the app (Holdener, Gut, & Angerer, 2020). However, relevant data such as the attrition rate of the

Table 8.4 Information about exercises and confidence in exercises in study cases.

Study	Information	Confidence in exercises
Bartlett et al. (2014)	No	No
Dale et al. (2015)	Yes	Yes (short videos)
Davies et al. (2016)	Yes	Yes (monitoring, instructional videos, personalized exercise programs)
Engelen et al. (2020)	Yes (awareness, habits, etc.)	Yes (interaction with health professionals)
Goyal et al. (2016)	Yes	No
Jongstra et al. (2017)	Yes	No
Khanji et al. (2019)	Yes	No
Klein et al. (2014)	Yes (information portal)	No
Lin et al. (2015)	Yes	Yes (videos)
Reid et al. (2012)	No	Yes (professional feedback by email, online tutorials)
Van Den Brekel-Dijkstra et al. (2016)	Yes	No
Yousuf et al. (2019)	Yes	No

intervention are not commonly reported. From the two demanded functionalities that were identified aiming to increase the engagement, only one of the study cases provides an integration of the activities with the daily life (Goyal et al., 2016), and there is no mention of the integration with the primary structure.

8.4.3 Digital coaching features

As was previously stated, engagement is an important aspect to consider in designing a coaching app. One of the specific needs for users to be engaged is personalized feedback, which is present in most of the study cases as the prevalent engagement feature. One of the most relevant needs is the possibility of creating personalized goals that can be adapted to the user context; this feature is also included in most of the systems.

Even though these two features are aligned with the user's needs, the demand for real-time coaching is not included in any of the analyzed systems. This demand is related to the confidence in self-managed exercises, but the system designers decided to provide this support through asynchronous feedback from specialists, probably because of the difficulties of implementing a real-time coaching feature.

8.4.4 Opportunity for social interaction

There is a lack of social interaction features in general in the coaching systems reported in the literature. Any kind of social interaction is rarely included among study cases. The social features that were included in the study cases basically consisted of email contact with professionals (Engelen et al., 2020; Reid et al., 2012). Efforts should be made to offer users the social interactions that they are demanding. It would be of great value for these coaching systems to include family members as an active agent in the intervention, as other health-related studies have shown that family care is beneficial for the patient's physical and mental health (Chesla, 2010).

Peer-mentoring interventions are intended to support individuals in managing their conditions by connecting them with peers who have similar health conditions. The users and peers may share ideas for improving and managing their health. Interventions with peer-monitoring support have proven to improve outcomes for patients in low-resource settings (Knox et al., 2015). None of the study cases implement peer support, which can be seen as a lost opportunity to evaluate and incorporate an element that may have a positive effect on patients' emotional and social well-being.

8.5 Conclusions

International literature reports many examples of personalized coaching systems for CVD self-management. From our findings, it is clear that there is a need for further research and considerations in designing these systems. We summarize them in the following list:

- Personalized coaching systems should be designed by using a participatory approach to identify potential barriers and facilitators to be considered in the design process.
- There is still limited evidence of the effectiveness of personalized coaching systems in engagement in healthy lifestyles by people with CVDs.
- There is a need to conduct studies to analyze the independent effect of each system components and their combinations.

- More complex personalization strategies and techniques, such as self-learning and context awareness, should be explored. Also, further research and design of personalized coaching systems should include real-time personalization strategies.
- Gamification could positively affect user engagement. Therefore studies analyzing the potential impact of including game elements as motivational features on the overall effectiveness of the system should be conducted.
- System trustworthiness, particularly in information contained in the system, should be considered.
- Social issues should be analyzed as behavior change techniques and/or as personalization strategies, including optional social features in coaching systems that meet the needs and preferences of people with CVDs.

Acknowledgment

Enrique Dorronzoro-Zubiete is supported by the "V Plan Propio de Investigación" of the Universidad de Sevilla.

References

Andersson, C., & Vasan, R. S. (2018). Epidemiology of cardiovascular disease in young individuals. *Nature Reviews Cardiology*, *15*(4), 230–240. Available from https://doi.org/10.1038/nrcardio.2017.154.

Bartlett, Y. K., Haywood, A., Bentley, C. L., Parker, J., Hawley, M. S., Mountain, G. A., & Mawson, S. (2014). The SMART personalised self-management system for congestive heart failure: Results of a realist evaluation. *BMC Medical Informatics and Decision Making*, *14*(1). Available from https://doi.org/10.1186/s12911-014-0109-3.

Carrasco-Hernandez, L., Jódar-Sánchez, F., Conde, J. M., Conde, F., González, M. M., Civit-Balcells, A., ... Ortega-Ruiz, F. (2020). A mobile health solution complementing psychopharmacology-supported smoking cessation: Randomized controlled trial. *Journal of Medical Internet Research*, *22*(4), e17530. Available from https://doi.org/10.2196/17530.

Chesla, C. A. (2010). Do family interventions improve health? *Journal of Family Nursing*, *16*(4), 355–377. Available from https://doi.org/10.1177/1074840710383145.

Clarke, V. A., Lovegrove, H., Williams, A., & Machperson, M. (2000). Unrealistic optimism and the health belief model. *Journal of Behavioral Medicine*, *23*(4), 367–376. Available from https://doi.org/10.1023/A:1005500917875.

Dabbs, A. D. V., Myers, B. A., Dunbar-Jacob, J., Curry, K. R. M., Hawkins, R. P., Begey, A., & Dew, M. A. (2009). User-centered design and interactive health technologies for patients. *CIN: Computers, Informatics, Nursing*, *27*(3), 175–183. Available from https://doi.org/10.1097/NCN.0b013e31819f7c7c.

Dale, L. P., Whittaker, R., Jiang, Y., Stewart, R., Rolleston, A., & Maddison, R. (2015). Text message and internet support for coronary heart disease self-management: Results from the text4heart randomized controlled trial. *Journal of Medical Internet Research*, *17*(10). Available from https://doi.org/10.2196/jmir.4944.

Davies, R. J., Parker, J., McCullagh, P., Zheng, H., Nugent, C., Black, N. D., & Mawson, S. (2016). A personalized self-management rehabilitation system for stroke survivors: A quantitative gait analysis using a smart insole. *JMIR Rehabilitation and Assistive Technologies*, *3*(2), e11. Available from https://doi.org/10.2196/rehab.5449.

Deterding, S., Dixon, D., Khaled, R., Nacke, L., Sicart, M., & O'Hara, K. (2011). Gamification: Using game design elements in non-game contexts. *Proceeding of 2011 Annual Conference Extended Abstracts Human Factors Computing Systems (CHI 2011)*, 2425–2428. Available from https://doi.org/10.1145/1979742.1979575.

Engelen, M. M., Van Dulmen, S., Puijk-Hekman, S., Vermeulen, H., Nijhuis-van der Sanden, M. W. G., Bredie, S. J. H., & van Gaal, B. G. I. (2020). Evaluation of a web-based self-management program for patients with cardiovascular disease: Explorative randomized controlled trial. *Journal of Medical Internet Research*, *22*(7). Available from https://doi.org/10.2196/17422.

Eze, N. D., Mateus, C., & Hashiguchi, T. C. O. (2020). Telemedicine in the OECD: An umbrella review of clinical and cost-effectiveness, patient experience and implementation. *PLoS One*, *15*, e0237585. Available from https://doi.org/10.1371/journal.pone.0237585.

Fanning, J., Mullen, S. P., & Mcauley, E. (2012). Increasing physical activity with mobile devices: A *meta*-analysis. *Journal of Medical Internet Research*, *14*(6). Available from https://doi.org/10.2196/jmir.2171.

Giunti, G. (2018). 3MD for chronic conditions, a model for motivational mHealth design: Embedded case study. *Journal of Medical Internet Research*, *20*(8), e11631. Available from https://doi.org/10.2196/11631.

Giunti, G., Kool, J., Rivera Romero, O., & Dorronzoro Zubiete, E. (2018). Exploring the specific needs of persons with multiple sclerosis for mHealth solutions for physical activity: Mixed-methods study. *JMIR mHealth uHealth*, *6*(2), e37. Available from https://doi.org/10.2196/mhealth.8996.

Goodie, J. L., Wilfong, K., & Kroke, P. (2019). *The influence of health behaviors upon the association between stress and depression and cardiovascular disease. Cardiovascular implications of stress and depression* (pp. 225–264). Elsevier. Available from http://doi.org/10.1016/B978-0-12-815015-3.00010-6.

Goyal, S., Morita, P. P., Picton, P., Seto, E., Zbib, A., & Cafazzo, J. A. (2016). Uptake of a consumer-focused mhealth application for the assessment and prevention of heart disease: The <30 days study. *JMIR mHealth uHealth*, *4*(1), e32. Available from https://doi.org/10.2196/mhealth.4730.

Holdener, M., Gut, A., & Angerer, A. (2020). Applicability of the user engagement scale to mobile health: A survey-based quantitative study. *Journal of Medical Internet Research*, *22*(1), e13244. Available from https://doi.org/10.2196/13244.

Jeng, C., & Braun, L. T. (1994). Bandura's self-efficacy theory: A guide for cardiac rehabilitation nursing practice. *Journal of Holistic Nursing: Official Journal of the American Holistic Nurses' Association*, *12*(4), 425–436. Available from https://doi.org/10.1177/089801019401200411.

Jongstra, S., Beishuizen, C., Andrieu, S., Barbera, M., van Dorp, M., van de Groep, B., ... Richard, E. (2017). Development and validation of an interactive internet platform for older people: The healthy ageing through internet counselling in the elderly study. *Telemed e-Health*, *23*(2), 96–104. Available from https://doi.org/10.1089/tmj.2016.0066.

Kaar, J. L., Luberto, C. M., Campbell, K. A., & Huffman, J. C. (2017). Sleep, health behaviors, and behavioral interventions: Reducing the risk of cardiovascular disease in adults. *World Journal of Cardiology*, *9*(5), 396. Available from https://doi.org/10.4330/wjc.v9.i5.396.

Khanji, M. Y., Balawon, A., Boubertakh, R., Hofstra, L., Narula, J., Hunink, M., ... Petersen, S. E. (2019). Personalized e-coaching in cardiovascular risk reduction: A randomized controlled trial. *Annals of Global Health, 85*(1). Available from https://doi.org/10.5334/aogh.2496.

Klein, M., Mogles, N., & van Wissen, A. (2014). Intelligent mobile support for therapy adherence and behavior change. *Journal of Biomedical Informatics, 51*, 137–151. Available from https://doi.org/10.1016/j.jbi.2014.05.005.

Knox, L., Huff, J., Graham, D., Henry, M., Bracho, A., Henderson, C., & Emsermann, C. (2015). What peer mentoring adds to already good patient care: Implementing the Carpeta Roja peer mentoring program in a well-resourced health care system. *Annals of Family Medicine, 13*(Suppl. 1), S59–S65. Available from https://doi.org/10.1370/afm.1804.

Krist, A. H., Davidson, K. W., Mangione, C. M., Barry, M. J., Cabana, M., Caughey, A., & Wong, J. B. (2020). Behavioral counseling interventions to promote a healthy diet and physical activity for cardiovascular disease prevention in adults with cardiovascular risk factors: United States preventive services task force recommendation statement. *JAMA: The Journal of the American Medical Association, 324*(20), 2069–2075. Available from https://doi.org/10.1001/jama.2020.21749.

Lau, Y., Chee, D. G. H., Chow, X. P., Cheng, L. J., & Wong, S. N. (2020). Personalised eHealth interventions in adults with overweight and obesity: A systematic review and *meta*-analysis of randomised controlled trials. *Preventive Medicine (Baltim), 132*, 106001. Available from https://doi.org/10.1016/j.ypmed.2020.106001.

Lazarus, R. S. (1999). *Stress and emotion: A new synthesis. Company*. New York: Springer Publishing.

Li, D. H., Brown, C. H., Gallo, C., Morgan, E., Sullivan, P. S., Young, S. D., & Mustanski, B. (2019). Design considerations for implementing eHealth behavioral interventions for HIV prevention in evolving sociotechnical landscapes. *Current HIV/AIDS Reports, 16*(4), 335–348. Available from https://doi.org/10.1007/s11904-019-00455-4.

Lin, P.-H., Intille, S., Bennett, G., Bosworth, H. B., Corsino, L., Voils, C., ... Svetkey, L. P. (2015). Adaptive intervention design in mobile health: Intervention design and development in the cell phone intervention for you trial. *Clinical Trials (London, England), 12*(6), 634–645. Available from https://doi.org/10.1177/1740774515597222.

Ma, Y., Cheng, H. Y., Cheng, L., & Sit, J. W. H. (2019). The effectiveness of electronic health interventions on blood pressure control, self-care behavioural outcomes and psychosocial well-being in patients with hypertension: A systematic review and *meta*-analysis. *International Journal of Nursing Studies, 92*, 27–46. Available from https://doi.org/10.1016/j.ijnurstu.2018.11.007.

Mendis, S., Puska, P., Norrving, B., Organization, W. H., Federation, W. H., & Organization, W. S. (2011). In Shanthi Mendis, et al. (Eds.), *Global atlas on cardiovascular disease prevention and control*. World Health Organization in Coll.

Michie, S., Richardson, M., Johnston, M., Abraham, C., Francis, J., Hardeman, W., ... Wood, C. E. (2013). The behavior change technique taxonomy (v1) of 93 hierarchically clustered techniques: Building an international consensus for the reporting of behavior change interventions. *Annals of Behavioral Medicine: A Publication of the Society of Behavioral Medicine, 46*(1), 81–95. Available from https://doi.org/10.1007/s12160-013-9486-6.

Monteiro-Guerra, F., Signorelli, G. R., Rivera-Romero, O., Dorronzoro-Zubiete, E., & Caulfield, B. (2020). Breast cancer survivors' perspectives on motivational and personalization strategies in mobile app-based physical activity coaching interventions: Qualitative study. *JMIR mHealth uHealth, 8*(9). Available from https://doi.org/10.2196/18867.

Oosterom-Calo, R., te Velde, S. J., Stut, W., & Brug, J. (2015). Development of motivate4change Using the intervention mapping protocol: An interactive technology physical activity and medication adherence promotion program for hospitalized heart failure patients. *JMIR Research Protocols*, *4*(3), e88. Available from https://doi.org/10.2196/resprot.4282.

Op den Akker, H., Jones, V. M., & Hermens, H. J. (2014). Tailoring real-time physical activity coaching systems: A literature survey and model. *User Modeling and User-adapted Interaction*, *24*(5), 351–392. Available from https://doi.org/10.1007/s11257-014-9146-y.

Ottaviano, M., Vera-Muñoz, C., Arredondo, M. T., & Salvi, D. (2010). A system to promote self-behaviors of patients with coronary heart disease. In *2010 Annual International Conference of the IEEE Engineering in Medicine and Biology Society, EMBC'10* (Vol. 2010, pp. 3843–3846). doi: 10.1109/IEMBS.2010.5627694.

Rawstorn, J. C., Gant, N., Rolleston, A., Whittaker, R., Stewart, R., Benatar, J., … Maddison, R. (2018). End users want alternative intervention delivery models: Usability and acceptability of the REMOTE-CR exercise-based cardiac telerehabilitation program. *Archives of Physical Medicine and Rehabilitation*, *99*(11), 2373–2377. Available from https://doi.org/10.1016/j.apmr.2018.06.027.

Reid, R. D., Morrin, L. I., Beaton, L. J., Papadakis, S., Kocourek, J., McDonnell, L., & Pipe, A. l. (2012). Randomized trial of an internet-based computer-tailored expert system for physical activity in patients with heart disease. *European Journal of Preventive Cardiology*, *19* (6), 1357–1364. Available from https://doi.org/10.1177/1741826711422988.

Roth, G. A., Johnson, C., Abajobir, A., Abd-Allah, F., Abera, S. F., Abyu, G., … Murray, C. (2017). Global, regional, and national burden of cardiovascular diseases for 10 causes, 1990 to 2015. *Journal of the American College of Cardiology*, *70*(1), 1–25. Available from https://doi.org/10.1016/j.jacc.2017.04.052.

Scott-Sheldon, L. A. J., Gathright, E. C., Donahue, M. L., Balletto, B., Feulner, M. M., DeCosta, J., … Salmoirago-Blotcher, E. (2020). Mindfulness-based interventions for adults with cardiovascular disease: A systematic review and *meta*-analysis. *Annals of Behavioral Medicine: A Publication of the Society of Behavioral Medicine*, *54*(1), 67–73. Available from https://doi.org/10.1093/abm/kaz020.

Seo, H.-J., Kim, S. Y., Sheen, S.-S., & Cha, Y. (2020). e-Health interventions for community-dwelling type 2 diabetes: A scoping review. *Telemedicine and e-Health, 27*. Available from https://doi.org/10.1089/tmj.2019.0263.

Van Den Brekel-Dijkstra, K., Rengers, A. H., Niessen, M. A. J., De Wit, N. J., & Kraaijenhagen, R. A. (2016). Personalized prevention approach with use of a web-based cardiovascular risk assessment with tailored lifestyle follow-up in primary care practice—A pilot study. *European Journal of Preventive Cardiology*, *23*(5), 544–551. Available from https://doi.org/10.1177/2047487315591441.

Walsh, D. M. J., Moran, K., Cornelissen, V., Buys, R., Cornelis, N., & Woods, C. (2018). Electronic health physical activity behavior change intervention to self-manage cardiovascular disease: Qualitative exploration of patient and health professional requirements. *Journal of Medical Internet Research*, *20*(5). Available from https://doi.org/10.2196/jmir.9181.

Wattanapisit, A., Tuangratananon, T., & Wattanapisit, S. (2020). Usability and utility of eHealth for physical activity counselling in primary health care: A scoping review. *BMC Family Practice*, *21*(1), 229. Available from https://doi.org/10.1186/s12875-020-01304-9.

Willis, A. W., Brown, O. N., & Greene, M. W. (2019). The use of psychological methodologies in cardiovascular disease interventions promoting a Mediterranean style diet: A systematic review. *Nutrition, Metabolism, and Cardiovascular Diseases: NMCD*, *29*(4), 325–333. Available from https://doi.org/10.1016/j.numecd.2018.12.011.

World Health Organization (WHO). (2017). *Cardiovascular diseases (CVDs). Cardiovascular diseases (CVDs) fact sheet.* https://www.who.int/news-room/fact-sheets/detail/cardio-vascular-diseases-(cvds). Accessed December 17, 2020.

Yousuf, H., Reintjens, R., Slipszenko, E., Blok, S., Somsen, G. A., Tulevski, I. I., & Hofstra, L. (2019). Effectiveness of web-based personalised e-coaching lifestyle interventions. *Netherlands Heart Journal*, *27*(1), 24–29. Available from https://doi.org/10.1007/s12471-018-1200-7.

CHAPTER 9

Methods for app development in p-health

Antonio Martinez-Millana[1], Gunnar Hartvigsen[2], and Vicente Traver Salcedo[3]
[1]Instituto ITACA, Universitat Politècnica de València, Valencia, Spain
[2]Department of Computer Science, Arctic University of Tromsø, Tromsø, Norway
[3]Department of Electronic Engineering, Universitat Politècnica de València, Valencia, Spain

9.1 Introduction

This chapter addresses the mobile health paradigm from the perspective of the development and regulation of personal health (p-health) systems. The emergence of mobile technologies has led to the proliferation of health and wellness apps as a tool to manage the health of many people, especially patients suffering from chronic conditions (Chomutare, Fernandez-Luque, Arsand, & Hartvigsen, 2011; Marcolino et al., 2018; Martinez-Millana, Jarones, Fernandez-Llatas, Hartvigsen, & Traver, 2018). This chapter aims to provide a general view of the complex context for apps in p-health, including the regulatory framework, privacy issues, the market, and stakeholders. The chapter describes the components that make up a mobile health system and the criteria for the classification of apps. The chapter concludes with current initiatives in mobile health interoperability for p-health.

Technology has evolved at a dizzying pace, influencing the evolution of society as we know it today. Every day, more people have access to a smartphone, fueling what is sometimes referred to as the digital revolution (Koutroumpis, 2019). The digital revolution is a reality that is changing the way we live, work, and enjoy. It has been experiencing a progressive transformation at all levels. In reality, mobile technologies are very recent; the first smartphone appeared on the market in 2007 and tablets were introduced in 2010.

The use of mobile phones (which evolved into today's smartphones) as an instrument for medical practice and for public health is known as mobile health or mHealth (Gagnon, Ngangue, Payne-Gagnon, & Desmartis, 2015). The term is not exclusive to mobile phones; it also refers to the use of mobile communication for healthcare services through

Personalized Health Systems for Cardiovascular Disease
DOI: https://doi.org/10.1016/B978-0-12-818950-4.00006-9

devices such as phones, tablets, smart watches, and other gadgets under the umbrella of "Internet of things," mainly wearables.

The mHealth field has emerged as a subsegment of e-health, which is characterized by the use of information and communication technologies for the provision of healthcare services (Boogerd, Arts, Engelen, & van De Belt, 2015). MHealth applications include the use of community and clinical healthcare devices; access and delivery of health-related information to professionals, researchers, and patients; real-time monitoring of physiological signals; and provision of medical care (on the border with home telemedicine).

Specifically, the term mHealth as we use it address in this chapter refers to the applications (or apps) that can be connected to medical devices or sensors (e.g., wrist bands or smart watches) and display health data, those that serve to monitor the person's lifestyle, and those with intelligent therapy recommendation systems and medication reminders.

9.2 Apps for p-health

The scientific literature lacks solid evidence demonstrating the positive impact that mHealth solutions have had on reducing healthcare costs (Agarwal et al., 2016). However, there are numerous scientists and politicians who firmly believe that there is consistent evidence that mHealth solutions can have a positive impact on healthcare delivery processes.

Results of pilot studies have shown that the use of apps has led to fewer emergency admissions, hospitalizations, and bed days per intervention, as well as reducing mortality (Coorey, Neubeck, Mulley, & Redfern, 2018). However, despite the potential benefits to healthcare systems, the adoption of mHealth remains limited in Europe. This is due to the lack of simple business models that support the mass adoption of mHealth services and applications. The solutions that have been implemented to date have been adapted and developed for specific regional or local authorities, each with different requirements, for specific use cases and situations. This has led to the current status of numerous pilot programs but no massive adoption of mHealth, owing to lack of interoperability and economies of scale.

9.2.1 App markets

The app market faces an entry barrier in the healthcare sector that is currently insurmountable. Research and innovation promotion programs such as Horizon 2020 of the European Commission have the potential to create tools and standards that will help to overcome these barriers.

In the United States, mHealth solutions enjoy greater penetration in the healthcare market, largely owing to the involvement of risk capital and the way in which healthcare has evolved in the United States. However, regardless of financing and business models, the lack of existing interoperable standards remains a major obstacle to market entry. This is undoubtedly the most serious obstacle for mHealth solutions to enter the health market and grow the developer's business. The adoption in the European Union of the global standards and specifications that are already available will be key to creating better market entry conditions in this regard.

In 2018 more than 300,000 health apps were found on the top app stores worldwide (twice the number that were available in 2015) (Balapour, Reychav, Sabherwal, & Azuri, 2019; Ramachandran et al., 2013). While the vast majority of these apps belong to the Health and Wellness categories in the two main app markets, the Apple Store for iOS and the Google Play for Android applications, there are important differences between Fitness and Health apps. Moreover, the number of users of mobile health apps increased by 10% in the period 2016–18, accounting for 46% of consumers who manage their health using technology.

There are two main types of applications:

- Apps that facilitate general well-being, such as exercise and diet apps.
- Apps that focus specifically on the management of a disease through the implementation of treatment protocols, such as medication reminders, dose calculation, and sending data to the doctor.

MHealth applications that include wellness make up two-thirds of the mHealth application space. This includes the areas of fitness, lifestyle and stress, and diet and nutrition. The areas of disease management and treatment account for approximately one-quarter of mHealth applications, with a small part of them dedicated to a particular disease (the orange sector in Fig. 9.1).

The official way to access apps is through virtual stores (also known as app markets). App markets allow customers and developers to distribute mobile applications worldwide. There are specific markets depending on the mobile operating system: Google Play Store for Android and the App Store for iOS, which are the most commonly used operation systems. Nevertheless, there are also alternative virtual markets to download apps such as the Amazon App Store, which is the main alternative; F-Droid, an

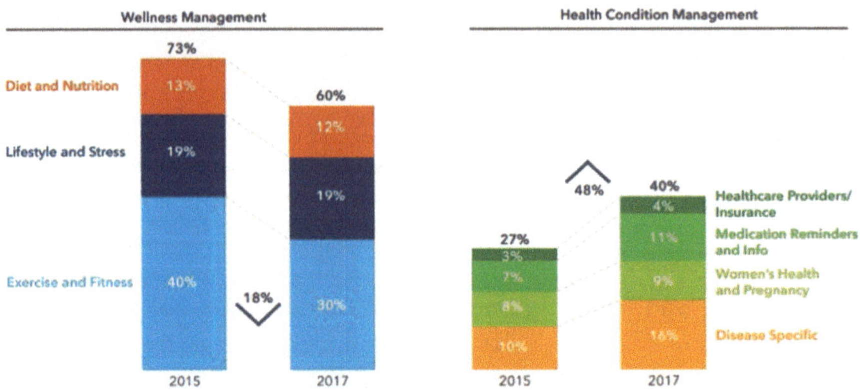

Figure 9.1 Distribution of the type of applications related to health. *Data from H. Health. (2017, November). The growing value of digital health.*

Apache 2.0 license-based market; GetJar, which is a multiplatform store for Android, iOS, Windows Mobile apps; and Microsoft Store, which is the official Microsoft store.

Google Play is the official store of Google, Inc.; it sells ebooks, music, movies, apps, and games. The specific section for mobile apps, called Google Play Store, contained more than 2.9 million apps[1] in December 2019, organized in different categories. To publish an application on Google Play Store, it is imperative to comply with the policies of the program for developers and accept the distribution agreement for developers. The company offers tips to follow to fulfill these requirements. These policies relate to the contents of the app, impersonation, intellectual property, privacy, security and deception, obtaining of income, and presence of advertising.

The App Store is the distribution platform from Apple, Inc. This market offered more than 1.8 million apps in the fourth quarter of 2019 (https://financesonline.com/number-of-apps-in-apple-app-store-in-2019-2020-demographics-statistics-and-predictions/). The apps in the App Store are organized by categories such as Health and Fitness. All applications that are published in the App Store are prereviewed by an expert at Apple, but the requirements that must be fulfilled are very similar to those indicated for publication in the Google Play Store. Apple has set

[1] https://www.statista.com/statistics/266210/number-of-available-applications-in-the-google-play-store/ (Last visit January 2020).

recommendations and good practices that are specified on the App Store website, related to the review of applications, user interface, or marketing.

9.2.2 Apps in p-health systems

The most characteristic feature of an mHealth application is its general objective. Based on this general objective, the application will present a specific design and a pattern of use that adapts to the type of user and target disease. Listed below are five of the most widespread purposes of the apps that are available in the virtual repositories.

9.2.2.1 Empowerment of patients

It is important for the patient to take an active role in the treatment of a disease and follow-up. Within the paradigm of an empowered patient, the application will propose an action-reaction model based on continuous training in which the patient will learn to be aware of the consequences of their decisions and the importance of adequate control to avoid acute episodes and/or comorbidities.

The application must allow the patient to make decisions (previously agreed with the healthcare professional) based on the analyses that are performed on the patient's data and evolution so that the system responds to the real needs of its context.

9.2.2.2 Remote tracking

Mobile health applications are intended to be a direct data gateway from the patient's environment to the healthcare professional. Data transmission is done by existing mobile (3G/4G) and WiFi communication networks. The applications incorporate logical connection interfaces over physical interfaces to store the data locally and then send the data to a dedicated server or to a cloud-based system, in which they are structured for later review by analysis algorithms and eventually a healthcare professional.

In general, mobile phones need peripheral sensors to capture data. However, the latest innovations are capable of obtaining heart rate and oxygen saturation by near-infrared analysis (present in most mobile phone cameras). The data reported by the patient through questionnaires also represent a valuable source of information about their health status and evolution.

9.2.2.3 Lifestyle change

The purpose of applications that promote lifestyle change is to modify the behavior and habits of a patient that have been identified as risk factors (e.g., smoking, sedentary lifestyle, unbalanced diet). The mechanism of these apps is based on the observation and personalized recommendation in a certain area through persuasive messages and scenarios of the "what would happen if . . ." type.

Numerous scientists are analyzing the opportunities offered by gamified environments to motivate users to modify their lifestyle, either individually or within a user community.

9.2.2.4 Personal management and reminders

The purpose of mHealth apps is to support the patient in the management of a disease through reminders, annotations, data plotting, and access to specialized information. Smartphones and tablets are an indispensable tools in the day-to-day life of many professionals, and this should be the case for patients, since it allows the information related to the evolution of symptoms and treatments to be concentrated in a single point. With this type of apps, patients have an electronic diary in which to record relevant information for the diagnosis and, from the information, prepare useful reports and statistics for healthcare professionals.

Some regional healthcare systems have started publishing apps for administrative procedures, such as requesting appointments, making copayments, printing electronic prescriptions, and making general inquiries.

9.2.2.5 Sentry in the shadow

The purpose of "sentry in the shadow" apps is controversial. Such apps use the mobile support (with all its components) to perform complete user monitoring in the background. Always having the legislative framework for data protection and preserving the right to privacy, the smartphone is an endless source of data that reveals the behavior of patients.

By using accelerometer sensors, analyzing the trace of applications used (type of app and runtime), triangulating positions, mapping GPS, and even observing the time of use of the mobile, a lot of valuable information can be obtained for the early detection of mental states such as anxiety and depression.

These are some of the main purposes of mHealth applications. There are many different purposes, including access to medical databases, forums, social networks, and encyclopedias. The fundamental lever to boost the popularization of the mHealth paradigm is the elimination of communication barriers between the patient and the healthcare provider in any context. Thus this paradigm presents a great opportunity for developing countries, allowing expansion of the use of health apps in parts of the world where traditional technology has not been deployed.

Mobile devices allow access to health resources even in the most desolate and remote areas. The apps facilitate remote and/or face-to-face diagnosis of a wide variety of pathologies. Within the remote health paradigm introduced by telemedicine, apps facilitate remote care and emergency intervention. That is, they work both if the doctor has been able to move to the area, supporting their work, and when it is necessary to provide a specialized remote intervention.

In the case of Africa, for example, the growth of mobile connections with 3G and the increasing coverage, even in the sub-Saharan region, are enabling the transmission of high-quality images from isolated communities to specialists in medical centers with greater potential for analysis. The latest Pricewaterhouse Coopers report points out that mobile applications could save more than one million lives in sub-Saharan Africa over the next 5 years (https://www.pwc.com/gx/en/healthcare/mhealth/assets/pwc-emerging-mhealth-full.pdf).

9.2.3 Architecture of an mHealth system

An mHealth system is based on the integration and interaction of three main components:

- An app managed by a patient or caregiver
- An application (mobile, web, or desktop) managed by a healthcare provider
- A server that offers data synchronization services between the first two components.

In some systems the professional supervision component is omitted, which is valid for the mHealth concept focused on well-being. However, in this section we will analyze a system that integrates all three components.

Fig. 9.2 shows a diagram of an mHealth system with the three integrated components. The communications flow follows a consecutive order according to the segments numbered in the figure and explained in the following list:

(1) Remote storage of the event log

The app used in this example is a remote monitoring app based on questionnaires that the patient must fill out. The diary allows recording of data such as mood, general condition of the patient, symptoms, and measurements made with sensors. These data are processed and displayed in the form of event logs, charts, and aggregated indicators back to the patient. The mobile application combines two modes of operation: ONLINE when there is a connection to the server, and OFFLINE, when the mobile does not have a connection or the server is not accessible. During OFFLINE operation, all measurements are stored in a local database. As soon as the ONLINE mode is activated, all data are synchronized, also remaining in the local database for the generation of graphs and statistics.

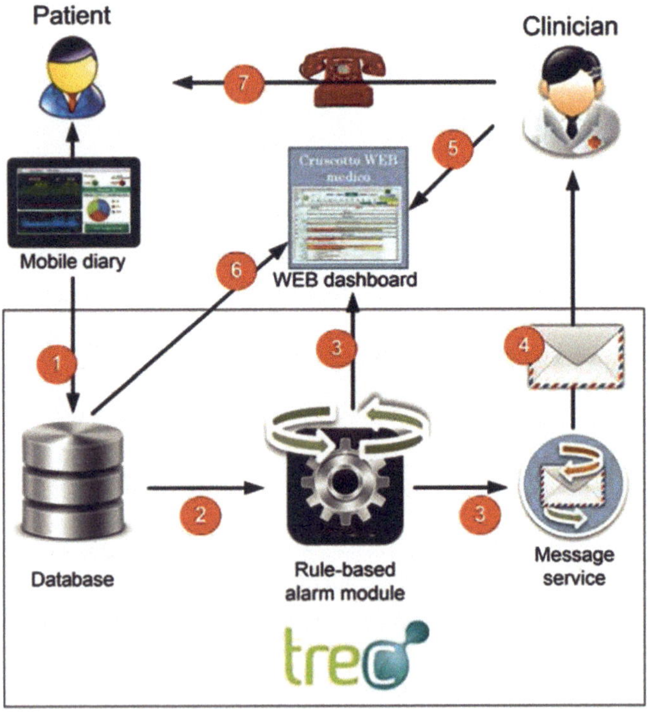

Figure 9.2 Communications diagram of an mHealth system. *Galligioni, E., et al. (2015). Integrating mHealth in oncology: Experience in the province of Trento.* Journal of Medical Internet Research, 17*(5), e114.*

(2) Real-time analysis

Once synchronized, the data are analyzed by rule-based models and with time series trend analysis methods to detect whether there is any abnormality or worrying trend in the data that the patient has reported.

(3) Message generator module

(4) If the analysis detects anomalous or worrisome trends, the alarm generator sends a specific message based on the reason for the alarm to the application of the healthcare professional. Professional communication service.

The healthcare provider can use a web application, a desktop application, a mobile application, or even a corporate application. The purpose of the communication service is to transmit the alarm to the corresponding application that the healthcare professional is using.

(5) **(6)** **(7)** Professional application

The application used by the healthcare professional to monitor the patient is a critical point of the system, since it is very rare to find systems that have this level of integration. Most commonly, an application external to the corporate health network is used, and communications with the patient are carried out by conventional means (a landline telephone in this example).

9.3 Directive for p-health app development

The problem related to the integration of apps as part of the health system requires an analysis to be carried out to determine the design principles that guarantee the use of a health app.

The mHealth sector remains a niche market in all countries of the European Union, and although these solutions are not part of any health system, each country has its own starting position. In general, companies that want to invest in the mHealth business or simply want to market their mHealth solution in one or more of the EU countries should pay special attention to the six dimensions that some analysts have identified. As part of their strategy for entering the EU market, mHealth companies must do the following:

- **Identify the institutions** that support mHealth businesses in each country.
- **Understand the criteria and conditions of the environment** that have an impact on the business model of a mobile application, including the regulatory framework, certifications, and the like.

- Have a clear **vision** and a deep understanding of **how the healthcare system works** in each country.
- **Prioritize countries** with more developed health information systems, such as Denmark, Finland, the Netherlands, Sweden, and the United Kingdom.
- Make use of the **experience of professionals** from the countries of interest and consult at least 10 of them before entering the market
- **Check the willingness of doctors and patients** to use the service in the country before launch.

The country's institutions must understand that they are competing with each other for the best talents and solutions to make mHealth work in their healthcare systems and must realize the potential benefits of mHealth to improve patient outcomes and reduce spending on healthcare in the country.

An analysis conducted in 2014 by Pricewaterhouse Coopers reveals that, with some exceptions such as Denmark and Spain, government institutions have not taken on the challenge of making their countries attractive to mHealth (Coopers, 2014). This means that by formulating the country's mHealth roadmap and guidelines, the country could gain a competitive advantage and compensate for market conditions that are not favorable for starting an mHealth business.

One of the most important factors in planning the development of an app is the software framework. Depending on the selected framework, the app will be tailored for one or many mobile operative systems. Moreover, this selection affects many different aspects related to the target user, usability, and costs (e.g., licenses, qualified developers, designers). Software frameworks can be classified in two general groups: native applications and cross-platform applications.

Native applications are developed specifically for a particular operating system. These apps are generally developed by using an integrated development environment that contains the reference libraries of the mobile operating system, allowing the developer to benefit from all the resources of the device at the software and hardware levels (e.g., accelerometers, GPS, camera). The integrated development environment usually allows developing apps in one (or many) programming languages, depending on the software level (interfaces, executable, low-level libraries). Native applications are optimal with respect to resource management. Native applications are recommended for developing apps that require high performance and use of hardware resources. Examples of native applications are Android apps, which are to be developed in Android Studio[2] and the java/xaml programming language, and iOS apps, which are to be developed in the XCode[3] and Objective-C/Swift programming languages.

Cross-platform applications are developed for use with many operating systems. These applications are developed by using a high-level programming language (a web language such as JavaScript, HTML5, Node.js, etc.) that can be executed by the majority of web browsers. This type of applications allows limited access to hardware resources and feature high consumption of the device's random-access memory (RAM). Among the relevant factors to be considered in developing of a cross-platform app, the two most important are the capacity of the different mobile operating system to execute web applications and the responsiveness of the app to fit into the layout of the device (different sizes, resolutions, etc.). One of the main drawbacks is the limitation of using the hardware elements of the device or other options, such as native notifications. Examples of cross-platform development environments are ReactNative,[4] which involves efficient use of GPU and CPU with intelligent debugging tools, and Ionic,[5] which involves difficult access to native libraries and formatting of layouts and does not feature runtime debugging.

9.4 Interoperability for apps in p-health

The penetration of mobile technologies and the extensive use of health sensors are driving mHealth to a higher level of acceptance, although the interoperability barrier persists and hinders massive adoption of such solutions.

The current problems are based on the lack of reference models for infrastructure and messaging; security, reliability, and privacy issues; and the number of nonscalable solutions (adapted to a specific environment). That is why several working groups in the orbit of international standardization organizations (IEEE, ISO, HL7) are promoting the generation of standards for interoperability with mobile applications. This section describes four cases of emerging standards in the field of mHealth.

[2] https://developer.android.com/studio.
[3] https://developer.apple.com/xcode/.
[4] http://www.reactnative.com/.
[5] https://ionicframework.com/.

9.4.1 mFHAST

mFHAST is focused on standardizing brief communications between health services through telephone networks (e.g., SMS) and other types of networks over the Internet (e.g., Twitter). According to the promoters, the term "short communications" encompasses communications in natural language between 140 and 160 characters, and it is necessary to implement a low-cost infrastructure to support the sending and processing of approximately 200,000 messages per second.

9.4.2 MH2F

MH2F is focused on aspects that refer to security, privacy, and control by the user (patient). The acronym in English comes from the term "mobile health application functional framework." This standard will allow creation of applications that monitor patients, integrate sensitive information, and ensure the quality of the data that are collected.

9.4.3 HL7-FHIR

HL7-FHIR is focused on the standardization of tools for interoperability of mobile applications and hospital information systems. The objective is to develop interfaces (APIs) that allow a fast and efficient use of the FHIR standard (Fig. 9.3). With this, mobile devices will be able to capture peripheral sensor data and send the data to the electronic medical record as if the mobile device were another medical device. Similarly, mobile applications can access the medical history of a particular patient. FHIR v4.0.1 is currently standard with a significant number of deployment tests. FHIR is an upgrade of previous HL7 family standards messaging and documentation directives. FHIR specifications are defined on a REST architecture (representational state transfer) to synchronize mobile devices and data servers, and the message exchange formatting is usually implemented in JSON. The FHIR community has two main APIs: HAPI[6] in J2EE and Firely[7] in the .Net platform. These APIs also allow the creation of a server based on FHIR, specifically prepared for store data structures from mobile apps and sensors. Every observation or descriptor of a resource has a defined type and cardinality.

[6] https://hapifhir.io/.

[7] https://fire.ly/.

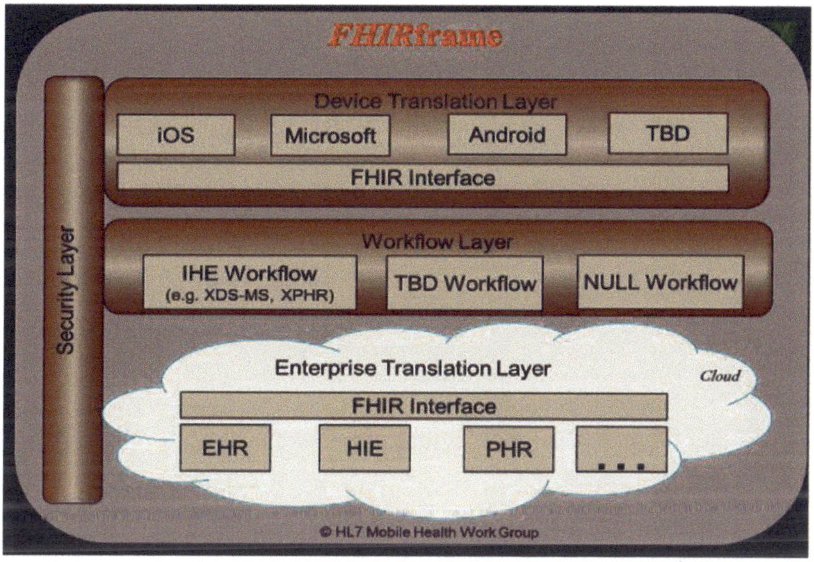

Figure 9.3 Concept framework of the FHIR standard for mobile. *Data from HL7 Mobile Health Working Group.*

SMART on FHIR is a universal API to interoperate electronic health records (EHRs) with health apps. The SMART on FHIR API was developed as an open, free, and standards-based API.[8]

9.4.4 Open mHealth

Open mHealth is a nonprofit initiative supported by many prestigious universities and companies worldwide to define the rules and design principles for the development and interoperability of mobile health apps. The architecture of Open mHealth is focused in the interface of data sources (e.g., sensors, data providers, cloud services) of any nature and granularity (e.g., personal health records, wearables, laboratory tests) and high-level applications (e.g., electronic medical systems, EHRs, and billing systems). This intermediate layer contains four processing units: APIs, data storage, data processing, and data visualization, which allow app developers to provide functionalities to the apps. Open mHealth has defined more than 50 schemas for atomic observations in the form of JSON messages (Fig. 9.4) containing descriptors that allow identification of the type of object it represents. These schemas aim to offer an ideal format and

[8] https://smarthealthit.org/.

```
{
    "body_temperature": {
        "value": 96.5,
        "unit": "F"
    },
    "effective_time_frame": {
        "time_interval": {
            "start_date_time": "2015-02-05T06:00:00Z",
            "end_date_time": "2015-02-06T06:00:00Z"
        }
    },
    "measurement_location": "oral",
    "descriptive_statistic": "maximum"
}
```


Figure 9.4 Example of the JSON object for representing body temperature according to open mHealth.

description of digital health data for supporting clinical care and self-care. When possible, these schemas are linked to standard clinical vocabularies that are being used for EHR data (e.g., SNOMED for diagnoses, LOINC or SNOMED for lab tests, and RxNORM for medications).

9.4.5 SNOMED CT

SNOMED CT is a dictionary of clinical terms that is accepted worldwide and implemented in many languages, allowing standardization of clinical concepts such as diseases, diagnoses, and treatments. These components are represented into a hierarchy of organized concepts, including synonyms (different descriptions), which are connected between them through relationships.

9.5 Regulatory framework for health apps

A medical device is any instrument, apparatus, appliance, software, material, or other article, whether used alone or in combination, including software, that is, intended by its manufacturer to be used specifically for diagnostic and/or therapeutic purposes and necessary for its proper application to be used for human beings for the following purposes:

- Diagnosis, prevention, monitoring, treatment, or alleviation of disease

- Diagnosis, monitoring, treatment, alleviation, or compensation for an injury or handicap
- Investigation, replacement, or modification of part of the anatomy or of a physiological process.

The definition and legal framework of a medical device depend on the market and geographic area. In the European Union the 2007/47/EC directive provides the aforementioned definition but delegates to the corresponding office for each member state the responsibility of transposing medical device directives into national law to apply them. In the United States the U.S. Food and Drug Administration (FDA) is the regulatory body in charge of defining laws, procedures, and penalties for medical devices, defining them as any medical machine, implant, other similar or related article or component intended for use in the diagnosis of disease or other conditions or in the cure, mitigation, treatment, or prevention of disease in humans or other animals.

Is a medical app a medical device? Regulated definitions state very clearly the features that characterize an app as a medical app and thus a medical device that, according to law, should be certified be official bodies.

The mobile health paradigm turns the smartphone into a medical device, capable of executing applications that directly influence the user's health. The regulatory framework for medical devices is no stranger to this reality and is currently developing a regulatory framework on which to evaluate the technological innovations of the mHealth paradigm. The 2007 revision of the framework explicitly introduced software, including applications, in the regulatory field and sufficiently clear definitions and guidelines (e.g., MEDDEV in stand-alone software) to determine whether a given application is intended to be used specifically for diagnosis and/or therapeutic purposes.

While concerns about the treatment of health data are often raised in the context of mHealth, the current EU data protection framework, as specified in Directive 95/46/EC, establishes a complete and coherent set of rules that protect the personal data of citizens on all technology platforms, including mobile devices, with specific provisions for special categories of data, such as health data.

This framework has resulted in strict legislation of the member states regarding the processing of health data, which prohibits any unwanted exchange with third parties (with exceptions allowed only for reasons of public interest). These provisions are complemented by the Electronic Privacy Directive, which prescribes that clear and complete consent and information to the user are necessary to place the data and retrieve it from the devices.

Regarding the development and consumption of mHealth applications, there are principles to minimize the risks of handling and storing high sensitivity information. The guiding principles currently in force are based on the following:

- Data minimization, meaning not storing data that do not serve the purpose of the app
- Data protection by design to ensure that data protection is carefully considered in the design and implementation of the app
- The default data protection assumes data privacy and security for any interface or system node.

The European Commission and the FDA have established a regulatory framework for the certification of health apps. To identify in the design phase whether a mobile application is considered to be a medical device is fundamental, since in the case of medical devices the applicable legislation must be complied with. Fig. 9.5 depicts a simplified schema for the classification of risk that leads to the type of regulation that affects medical apps. Conformity assessment procedures for Class I products should generally be carried out under the sole responsibility of the manufacturer, given the low degree of vulnerability associated with these products. In the case of products of Classes IIa and IIb, an appropriate level of intervention by a notified body must be mandatory.

The CE marking for EU countries is based on conformity to the following documents:

- General Data Protection Regulation (GDPR)
- ISO 13485: Medical devices—Quality management systems—Requirements for regulatory purposes
- Risk Management Plan
- IEC 62304: Medical device software—Software life cycle processes.

The GDPR defines personal data as any information related to an identifiable person that can be identified directly or indirectly by reference of an identifier. Examples of personal data are the person's name, postal address, GPS location, health information, and income. Within the personal data, the GDPR differentiates those that are considered sensitive and therefore require the maximum security measures. The GDPR prohibits the processing of any type of sensitive data unless there is explicit consent. Data processing (or treatment) covers a broad range of operations on personal data, whether manual or automatic, including collection, recording, organization, structuring, storage,

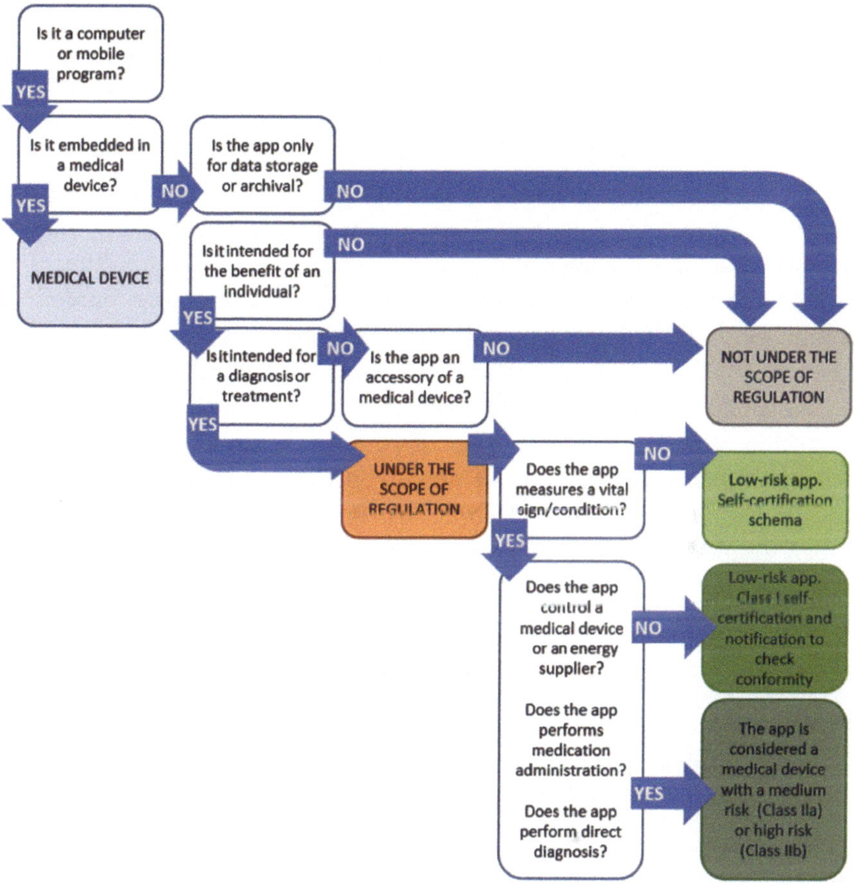

Figure 9.5 Decision workflow for the classification of regulated health apps as medical devices.

adaptation or alteration, recovery, consultation, use, transmission, or dissemination. The GDPR establishes that appropriate measures must be taken to grant the proper use of personal data, considering the current technologies for security; the costs of implementation; the nature, the scope, context and objective of the processing; and as the risks and severity of these rights and freedoms of people.

9.6 Conclusions

This chapter provided a general introduction to the ecosystem of apps in the p-health context. The rapid adoption of mobile health apps in healthcare management has been led by the individual contributions of app developers and patients who want to manage their own health using new information and communication technologies. Nevertheless, the development of health apps is constrained by a complex context involving regulatory issues, technical considerations, and usability aspects. Even though the number of available apps is extensive, their use is not a central part of healthcare management. Reasons for this lack of maturity may be based on the lack of evidence on the apps' usability and health efficacy to achieve the goals of maintaining health and reducing the burden of healthcare. The chapter has described the use scenarios for mHealth, which should be taken into consideration in designing new interventions to adequately evaluate all the involved dimensions.

In conclusion, the factors that affect the adoption of mobile health apps in the p-health paradigm are heterogeneous and need strong collaboration between engineers and clinicians. Regulatory and interoperability aspects should be taken into account from the early design stages to ensure a successful transference of the results from research to market environments.

References

Agarwal, S., LeFevre, A. E., Lee, J., L'Engle, K., Mehl, G., Sinha, C., et al. (2016). Guidelines for reporting of health interventions using mobile phones: Mobile health (mHealth) evidence reporting and assessment (mERA) checklist. *BMJ (Clinical Research Ed.), 352*, i1174.

Balapour, A., Reychav, I., Sabherwal, R., & Azuri, J. (2019). Mobile technology identity and self-efficacy: Implications for the adoption of clinically supported mobile health apps. *International Journal of Information Management, 49*, 58–68.

Boogerd, E. A., Arts, T., Engelen, L. J., & van De Belt, T. H. (2015). 'What is eHealth': Time for an update? *JMIR Research Protocols, 4*(1), e29.

Chomutare, T., Fernandez-Luque, L., Arsand, E., & Hartvigsen, G. (2011). Features of mobile diabetes applications: Review of the literature and analysis of current applications compared against evidence-based guidelines. *Journal of Medical Internet Research, 13*(3), e65.

Coopers, P. (2014). Emerging mHealth: Paths for growth.

Coorey, G. M., Neubeck, L., Mulley, J., & Redfern, J. (2018). Effectiveness, acceptability and usefulness of mobile applications for cardiovascular disease self-management: Systematic review with *meta*-synthesis of quantitative and qualitative data. *European Journal of Preventive Cardiology, 25*(5), 505–521.

Gagnon, M.-P., Ngangue, P., Payne-Gagnon, J., & Desmartis, M. (2015). m-Health adoption by healthcare professionals: A systematic review. *Journal of the American Medical Informatics Association, 23*(1), 212–220.

Galligioni, E., Piras, E. M., Galvagni, M., Eccher, C., Caramatti, S., Zanolli, D., et al. (2015). Integrating mHealth in oncology: Experience in the province of Trento. *Journal of Medical Internet Research, 17*(5), e114.

H. Health. (2017, November). The growing value of digital health.
Koutroumpis, P. (2019). The economic impact of broadband: Evidence from OECD countries. *Technological Forecasting and Social Change*, *148*, 119719.
Marcolino, M. S., Oliveira, J. A. Q., D'Agostino, M., Ribeiro, A. L., Alkmim, M. B. M., & Novillo-Ortiz, D. (2018). The impact of mHealth interventions: Systematic review of systematic reviews. *JMIR mHealth uHealth*, *6*(1), e23.
Martinez-Millana, A., Jarones, E., Fernandez-Llatas, C., Hartvigsen, G., & Traver, V. (2018). App features for type 1 diabetes support and patient empowerment: Systematic literature review and benchmark comparison. *JMIR mHealth uHealth*, *6*(11), e12237.
Ramachandran, A., Snehalatha, C., Ram, J., Selvam, S., Simon, M., Nanditha, A., et al. (2013). Effectiveness of mobile phone messaging in prevention of type 2 diabetes by lifestyle modification in men in India: a prospective, parallel-group, randomised controlled trial. *Lancet. Diabetes & Endocrinology*, *1*(3), 191–198.

CHAPTER 10

Devices for p-health: Which regulations in Europe?

Dario Pirovano
Pirovano Management, Waterloo, Belgium

10.1 Introduction

Products that are used for p-health can be either medical devices or in vitro diagnostic devices (IVDDs). From May 2021, in Europe, medical devices can exclusively be placed on the market and put into service only if they comply with Regulation 2017/745. Similarly, IVDDs will be allowed to be placed on the market and put into service only if, from May 2022, they comply with Regulation 2017/746.

Article 2 (1) of the Medical Devices Regulation 2017/745 (MDR) defines a medical devices as "any instrument, apparatus, appliance, software, implant, reagent, material or other article intended by the manufacturer to be used, alone or in combination, for human beings for one or more of the following specific medical purposes:

- diagnosis, prevention, monitoring, prediction, prognosis, treatment or alleviation of disease,
- diagnosis, monitoring, treatment, alleviation of, or compensation for, an injury or disability,
- investigation, replacement or modification of the anatomy or of a physiological or pathological process or state,
- providing information by means of in vitro examination of specimens derived from the human body, including organ, blood and tissue donations, and which does not achieve its principal intended action by pharmacological, immunological or metabolic means, in or on the human body, but which may be assisted in its function by such means."

The following products shall also be deemed to be medical devices:

- Devices for the control or support of conception;

Personalized Health Systems for Cardiovascular Disease
DOI: https://doi.org/10.1016/B978-0-12-818950-4.00008-2

- Products specifically intended for the cleaning, disinfection or sterilization of devices as referred to in Article 1(4) and of those referred to in the first paragraph of this point.

Article 2(2) of the In Vitro Diagnostic Devices Regulation 2017/746 defines IVDD as "any medical device which is a reagent, reagent product, calibrator, control material, kit, instrument, apparatus, piece of equipment, software or system, whether used alone or in combination, intended by the manufacturer to be used in vitro for the examination of specimens, including blood and tissue donations, derived from the human body, solely or principally for the purpose of providing information on one or more of the following:

- concerning a physiological or pathological process or state;
- concerning congenital physical or mental impairments;
- concerning the predisposition to a medical condition or a disease;
- to determine the safety and compatibility with potential recipients;
- to predict treatment response or reactions;
- to define or monitoring therapeutic measures."

Specimen receptacles shall also be deemed to be in vitro diagnostic medical devices.

Regulation 2017/745 replaces Directives 90/385/EEC on Active Implantable Medical Devices and 93/42/EEC on Medical Devices, while Regulation 2017/746 replaces Directive 98/79/EEC on In Vitro Diagnostic Medical Devices.

The two regulations have similar structures, although some features are obviously different, owing to the different impact the devices have on the human body. In the following sections the main principles on which the regulations are based will be listed and described.

10.2 Principles of the regulations

The principles constituting the regulations are basically as follows:

1. Devices can be placed on the market and put into service only if their manufacturers are in the position to show that they have complied with all the requirements of the Regulations which apply to them (CE marking). This applies also for devices made available via Internet.
2. Manufacturers that are not based in the European Union (EU) shall nominate an authorized representative (AR) having its place of business within the EU.

3. Manufacturers and, if appropriate, their AR shall jointly be liable for damages caused by defective devices.
4. Importers and distributors are also covered by relevant requirements of the regulation.
5. Devices are divided into four classes, depending on their level of impact on patients and their health.
6. All devices shall show conformity to the so-called general safety and performance requirements (GSPR).
7. To show conformity to the GSPR, manufacturers can use standards that have been judged appropriate at the EU level.
8. All manufacturers shall demonstrate that their devices have collected, before marketing, a sufficient level of clinical evidence.
9. All devices shall be covered by an appropriate quality management system (QMS).
10. Notified bodies (NBs) shall be identified and evaluated jointly by member states and the EU Commission.
11. Devices shall be subject to an evaluation by a third party (the NB) at different levels of depth depending upon the class into which they fall.
12. Manufacturers are responsible for the conduct of appropriate post-marketing vigilance activities, the results of which need to be taken into account in the constant updating of the documentation related to each product.
13. Manufacturers are responsible for the traceability of the products they place on the market.
14. Transparency toward users and general public of critical information shall be ensured.

Guidance on the implementation of the regulations has been (and will be) issued by the Medical Devices Coordination Group (MDCG), which is constituted of nominated representatives of the EU member states. This group is helped in its tasks by 11 subgroups. In nine of them the presence of stakeholders (manufacturers, patients, health care professionals, etc.) is allowed.

The MDCG publishes regularly new guidance on the Commission's website: https://ec.europa.eu/docsroom/documents?locale = en&keywords = medical%20device

In the following, each of the principles constituting the regulations is thoroughly described and discussed.

1. **Devices can be placed on the EU market and put into service only if their manufacturers are in the position to show that they have complied with all the requirements of the regulations that apply to them (CE marking).**

   This is the application to medical devices of the general rules that cover industrial products in the EU. It allows products that have undergone an appropriate conformity assessment procedure to be available throughout the EU without the need for further national evaluations. Currently, this is done via conformity to Directive 90/385/EEC on active implantable medical devices or Directive 93/42/EEC on medical devices (MDD). These directives were developed in the 1990s and have been replaced by Regulation 2017/745. This chapter will concentrate on the medical devices regulation: there is no grandfathering clause, so devices that are on the market today (even for several years) will have to be reassessed to show conformity to the regulations.

   The transition period of the MDR, when both regimes (i.e., directives and regulation) were both applicable, ended in May 2021, although it will still be possible for devices that are still covered by valid directives certificates to be made available to users or patients until May 2025 (Article 120).

   The need for a CE marking applies to all devices, with the exception of devices that are manufactured specifically for a named patient according to a specific request from a health care professional that defines the specific characteristics of the device. Devices that are intended to be used during premarket clinical investigations are also not required to bear the CE marking.

   It is worth remembering that devices that are made available via Internet have to comply with the regulation, independently of whether these are physical products or, for example, apps that can be downloaded from the Internet. This latter situation opens a series of questions on the effective implementation of the regulation with regard to apps. At the time of writing this chapter, there is no specific guideline; however, a guidance document on the legal status of app providers is in preparation.

2. **Manufacturers that are not based in the EU shall nominate an authorized representative (AR) having its place of business within the EU.**

Manufacturers outside the EU have several duties related to contacts with national and European authorities. These duties can be better complied with if the authorities can contact an entity within the EU that can act as a liaison between the non-EU manufacturer and the authorities. Language, time zones, and proximity are obvious advantages of this situation.

The AR, while having the duty to ensure that the manufacturer it represents has complied with the administrative requirements of the regulations, is not responsible for the placing on the market of the products; nor must it verify the appropriateness of the technical or scientific means used by the manufacturer to show compliance with the regulation. It nevertheless has the obligation to terminate the contract with the manufacturer if the manufacturer fails to comply with the premarket and postmarketing obligations of the regulations.

3. **Manufacturers and, if appropriate, their AR shall jointly be liable for damages caused by defective devices.**

   As has been noted, the AR is not responsible for the conformity of the device to the regulation. However, to protect the patients, if the manufacturer has not put into place some financial mechanism (insurance or other means) to cover damages caused by a defective product as defined in Directive 85/374/EEC,[1] then the AR is "legally liable for defective devices on the same basis as, and jointly and severally with, the manufacturer" (Article 11.5).

4. **Importers and distributors are also covered by relevant requirements of the regulation.**

   The previous directives left the management of importers (i.e., the entities that bring into the EU market devices manufactured outside the EU) and distributors to the legal requirements of the various member states. The new regulation envisages a set of rules and obligations to both economic operators that involve, in particular, in the traceability of devices and in the postmarketing vigilance system. Importers have to be registered in the central database Eudamed (https://ec.europa.eu/health/md_eudamed/overview_it) and shall be identified on the label or other document accompanying the device.

[1] Council Directive 85/374/EEC of July 25, 1985 on the approximation of the laws, regulations and administrative provisions of the Member States concerning liability for defective products.

5. **Devices are divided into four classes, depending on their level of impact on patients and their health.**

   From the definition of medical device, it is evident that each product that fits such a definition has a different risk profile when used on humans. The potential harm caused by a faulty tongue depressor is different from that caused by a faulty pacemaker. This has brought the regulators to subdivide the family of medical devices, differently from what happens with medicinal products, into four risk classes: I, IIa, IIb, and III. To each class corresponds a different level of control of the effectiveness of manufacturers in ensuring that their devices are safe and perform as intended. Such control is delegated to an entity that has been evaluated at the EU level and approved for the evaluation of the technology utilized: the NB (see points 10 and 11).

   This concept was already one of the pillars of the previous directives, but it has been further developed in the new regulation to take into account the scientific and technical developments in this field that have occurred since the 1990s, when the directives were conceived.

   In particular, the increased role of software and the increased number of remote applications that could be used directly by patients have driven the regulators to increase the classification of these products. The issue of artificial intelligence has also been taken into account by assigning to the highest class those devices that perform directly a medical action on patients on the basis of a "diagnosis" made by another device without the intervention of a health care professional. These are the so-called closed-loop devices, which play a relevant role in home monitoring and p-health systems.
6. **All devices shall show conformity to the General Safety and Performance Requirements (GSPR).**
7. **Use of standards**

   The GSPR are a set of general requirements that guide the manufacturer to put together sufficient evidence that its product is safe, that it performs as intended by its manufacturer, and that such performance is able to deliver a clinical benefit to the patient.

   The GSPR evolved from the essential requirements contained in the previous directives. Their origin goes back to the 1980s, when the Commission developed the so-called new approach to technical regulations, subsequently developed in the "new legislative framework" at the beginning of this century. Both legislative techniques recognized that in the technical field, innovation and developments occur much faster than any legislation or standard. This is even more true for the field of medical devices, in which the upgrading of a device happens on average every 18 months.

For this reason, instead of making reference to standards or embedding in the legislative text specific technical requirements, it was decided to list points that shall be analyzed and taken into account in the determination of safety and performance of devices. These points cover the following:

- General requirements, which basically require that all means be put into place by the manufacturer to reduce to the minimum achievable the residual risks that are inevitably connected with the intrusion of a medical device into the human body environment. This reduced residual risk shall be outweighed by the benefits that the manufacturer predicts
- This reduction shall be analyzed, described, and kept up to date during the entire life of the device through an appropriate risk management system, which shall be constantly updated on the basis of data collected during the postmarketing phase
- Chemical physical and biological properties
- Infection and microbial contamination
- Devices that incorporate substances that are considered to be medicinal products
- Devices that are composed of substances or a combination of substances that are absorbed by or locally dispersed in the human body
- Devices that incorporate materials of biological origin
- Construction of devices and interaction with their environment
- Devices with diagnostic or measuring function
- Protection against radiation
- Electronic programmable systems: devices that incorporate electronic programmable systems and software that are devices themselves (this includes requirements for cybersecurity, which is the scope of a newly produced guidance document: https://ec.europa.eu/docsroom/documents/38941?locale = en)
- Active devices and devices that are connected to them
- Particular requirements for active implantable devices
- Protection against mechanical and thermal risks
- Protection against the risk posed to patients or users by devices that supply energy or substances
- Protection against the risks posed by medical devices that are intended by their manufacturers for use by laypeople

- Requirements regarding the information that is, supplied with the device

For all of these points, the manufacturer shall indicate whether they are applicable to its device and specify the methodologies that have been adopted to show conformity. The use of standards is encouraged to show compliance with the GSPR. In particular, conformity to those European standards, the references of which are published in the *Official Journal of the European Union*, give the so-called presumption of conformity of the methods that are used to comply with specifically identified GSPR. Nevertheless, the use of standards is not mandatory.

When standards do not exist or when the standards do not cover some GSPR for some products, the MDCG might produce guidance documents, called common specifications, which cover, in particular, clinical aspects for identified categories of devices. Whenever such common specifications exist, manufacturers are expected to comply with them unless appropriate justification for not using them is provided by the manufacturer.

Manufacturers and the AR shall have at their disposal continuously a person who is responsible for regulatory compliance (PRRC). The PRRC shall be responsible to check that all the relevant provisions of the regulation have been complied with. The PRRC shall suffer no disadvantage with the manufacturer or AR organization in relation to the proper fulfillment of his or her duties, whether or not he or she is an employee of the organization.

8. **All manufacturers shall demonstrate that their devices have collected, before marketing, a sufficient level of clinical evidence.**

   A sufficient amount of clinical evidence means that clinical data and clinical evaluation results pertaining to a device have to be of a sufficient amount and quality to allow a qualified assessment of whether the device is safe and achieves the intended clinical benefit(s) when used as intended by the manufacturer. Clinical data consists of information concerning safety or performance that is generated from the use of a device and is sourced from the following:

- Clinical investigation(s) of the device concerned
- Clinical investigation(s) or other studies reported in scientific literature of a device for which equivalence to the device in question can be demonstrated

- Reports published in peer-reviewed scientific literature on other clinical experience of either the device in question or a device for which equivalence to the device in question can be demonstrated
- Clinically relevant information coming from postmarketing surveillance, in particular the postmarketing clinical follow-up

The manufacturer shall collect this clinical evidence, before placing the device on the market, by a combination of the following, as applicable:

(a) a critical evaluation of the relevant scientific literature currently available relating to the safety, performance, design characteristics, and intended purpose of the device, where the following conditions are satisfied:
  - it has been demonstrated that the device subject to clinical evaluation for the intended purpose is equivalent to the device to which the data relate, in accordance with Section 3 of Annex XIV, and
  - the data adequately demonstrate compliance with the relevant general safety and performance requirements;

(b) a critical evaluation of the results of all available clinical investigations, taking duly into consideration whether the investigations were performed under Articles 62–80, any acts adopted pursuant to Article 81, and Annex XV; and

(c) a consideration of currently available alternative treatment options for that purpose, if any.

This evidence is requested for all devices of all classes. However, for the most critical devices (Class III and implantable Class IIb devices) the conducting of a premarket clinical investigation is compulsory, although some exceptions are envisaged. When implantable Class III devices and Class IIb devices that are intended to administer a medicinal product represent a novelty or where evidence from the field shows a particular increase of incidents with similar products, the evaluation of the clinical evidence made by the notified body may be analyzed by a further check by a panel of independent experts. It is possible to refer to clinical experience gathered with devices that are considered equivalent to the one under evaluation; however, the conditions under which such equivalence can be claimed have been rendered stricter than those in the directives.

Guidance was made available during 2020.

It is worth remembering that clinical evidence shall be kept updated constantly on the basis of the data collected during the postmarketing phase.

9. All devices shall be covered by an appropriate QMS.

The new regulation requires that all devices be made within an appropriate QMS.

With the exception of class I devices, all the others shall have the QMS approved and maintained under the supervision of a notified body. Notwithstanding the voluntary nature of standards, this means in practice that manufacturers should apply standard ISO 13485.

10. **NBs shall be identified and evaluated jointly by member states and the Commission.**

    This concept is derived from the "new legislative framework" (see points 6 and 7). Since the concept of CE marking allows commercialization of devices throughout the EU without the need to apply for approval in each of the 27 member states, it was deemed appropriate to give the possibility to each manufacturer to apply, if required by the regulation (see point 11), to a conformity assessment body close to its premises. This is even more appropriate for medium and small companies (95% of the total number of manufacturers). The complexity and variety of technologies and the number of items that are covered by the definition of "medical device" (500,000) suggested that it would not have been feasible to concentrate the evaluation of these products in one single agency, as has been done for pharmaceutical products.

    Under the directives, NBs were evaluated and notified to the Commission and the other member states under the sole responsibility of the member state in which they operate. Some discrepancies in this process caused varied levels of performance among NBs. This triggered the need to change the system, and the regulation now requires that these conformity assessment bodies be evaluated by a pool of experts from three different member states backed by a representative of the Commission. In addition, each NB is now notified for identified groups of devices for which it has been demonstrated to have a sufficient level of knowledge.

11. **Devices shall be subject to an evaluation by a third party (the NB) at different levels of depth depending upon the class into which they fall.**

As was mentioned in point 5, devices are classified into four classes: I, IIa, IIb, and III. The reason for this unusual way of numbering the classes is part of the legends surrounding the early days of the development of the directives and does not have a place here, but I will be happy to discuss it with any of you who are interested.

Class I devices have to comply with the GSPR and the requirements related to the needs of:

- Registering in the central database, Eudamed
- Producing and keeping up to date the technical documentation
- Being able to produce and maintain appropriate clinical evidence
- Working within an appropriate QMS
- Performing an appropriate postmarketing surveillance and, if necessary, providing notification of serious incidents related to the use of the device (see point 12)

Manufacturers of Class I devices are not required to apply to a NB to be able to affix the CE marking. A sort of self-certification is sufficient.

Exceptions to this rule are Class I devices that are placed on the market in a sterile state, or that have a measuring function, or—and this is a novelty of the regulation—are reusable surgical instruments. For these devices the manufacturer needs to seek the advice of a NB for the sterilization process, the way the accuracy of the measurements are made, and the methods suggested for the decontamination, cleaning, and reconditioning, respectively.

For devices of higher classes, in addition to the aforementioned requirements, manufacturers have to seek approval from a NB of their QMS and have their technical documentation evaluated as follows:

- For Class IIa: at least one representative device for each category of devices
- For Class IIb nonimplantable: at least one representative device per generic device group, that is, a set of devices having the same or similar intended purposes or a commonality of technology allowing them to be classified in a generic manner not reflecting specific characteristics
- For Class III and implantable Class IIb: every device

If a Class III device contains, as an integral part, a substance that, if used alone, could be defined as a medicinal product or a substance derived from tissues and cells of animal or human origin that acts in an ancillary way to support the intended purpose of the device, the NB shall request an additional evaluation of the relevant part of the technical documentation by either the relevant national authority responsible for the relevant substance or the European Medicine Agency.

As was mentioned in point 8, a review by a panel of independent experts of the clinical evidence assessment report for implantable class III devices and for Class IIb devices that are intended to deliver a medicinal product is envisaged according to some conditions.

12. **Manufacturers are responsible for the conduct of appropriate postmarketing vigilance activities, the results of which need to be taken into account in the constant updating of the documentation related to each product.**

    Manufacturers must have in place a proactive procedure to collect information from the field on the use of their devices. They must pay particular attention to incidents involving their products. If the incident is considered serious, that is, has caused death or serious deterioration of the state of health of the patient or user, then the regulation envisages a set of procedures for investigating the causes and implementing the appropriate corrective actions.

    Manufacturers are requested to produce and maintain several documents related to this activity: the postmarketing surveillance report, the periodic safety update report, the trend report (related to nonserious incidents), the field corrective action, the field safety notice, and so on.

13. **Manufacturers are responsible for the traceability of the products they place on the market.**

    The traceability of medical devices has to be assumed by the various economic operators, depending on their role in the distribution chain. As a general principle, each economic operator shall be able to trace where and when it has delivered the device to the next operator. To facilitate this, the regulation introduced the obligation to assign a unique device identifier (UDI) that will have to accompany each device. The obligation to assign a basic UDI will start on the date of application of the regulation. The obligation to affix a bar code to the device will start at different times, depending on the classification.

14. **Transparency toward users and general public of critical information shall be ensured.**

One of the most debated issues during negotiation of the regulation was how to render publicly available some data related to the devices while protecting intellectual property rights. The tool to render these data available is the centralized database called Eudamed. This database is managed by the EU Commission and is constituted of several modules related, for example, to the notification of economic operators and devices, clinical aspects, and vigilance.

The regulation specifies who is responsible for uploading the data and who has access to the various parts of it. Access to the full Eudamed content will be given to competent authorities and NBs, while only selected sections will be accessible to the general public.

The most important document that will be available to the general public will be the Summary of Safety and Clinical Performance (SSCP), which shall be prepared by the manufacturer of implantable and Class III devices. The SSCP shall contain abridged information about the safety of each product, including data related to the postmarketing activities of the manufacturer as well as the clinical profile of the device. The SSCP is part of the documentation that is supplied to the NB in the conformity assessment procedure. Once the SSCP evaluated by the NB, the NB will upload it to Eudamed.

At the time of writing this chapter, the availability of Eudamed has been postponed to May 2022, owing to unpredicted difficulties in the finalization of its various modules.

The MDCG is evaluating and drafting guidance on how to render the SSCP available in the absence of Eudamed.

10.3 Conclusions

The views expressed in this chapter are exclusively those of the author and cannot be considered as those of the companies or associations with which the author has working relations.

This chapter has provided the overall requirements to comply with applicable legislative requirements in the EU, and which have to be applied also for p-health solutions. The subject is complex and requires a careful analysis of all the mentioned items to guarantee safety for the user and correct performance of the device. It is important to keep in mind that regulations and related guidance are always evolving, and this chapter was developed on the basis of the information that was available at the time of writing. It was worth noting that the regulations mentioned in the chapter were intended to have dates of application of May 2021 for the medical devices regulation and May 2022 for the in vitro diagnostic devices.

Both regulations require a certain number of tools in order to ensure their correct implementation. Several of these tools are not ready yet, in spite of the enormous amount of work that both the EU Commission and the member states have been devoting to their preparation. The author has tried to include in each section an indication of where we stand with the developments. It is possible that some of these indications will have become obsolete between the final drafting of the chapter and the effective publication of this book. It is important to keep in mind that the purpose of the chapter was to provide a general view and the main principles behind regulations. The recommendation is always to refer to updated documentation, which is always made available by the Commission at https://ec.europa.eu/docsroom/documents?locale = en&keywords = medical%20device.

CHAPTER 11

Remote management of heart failure patients: A p-health example

Anna Maria Bianchi[1], Jorge Henriques[2], and Vicente Traver Salcedo[3]
[1]Department of Electronics, Information and Bioengineering, Politecnico di Milano, Milan, Italy
[2]Center for Informatics and Systems of the University of Coimbra, Department of Informatics Engineering, University of Coimbra, Coimbra, Portugal
[3]Department of Electronic Engineering, Universitat Politècnica de València, Valencia, Spain

11.1 Introduction

In the previous chapters, many aspects related to p-health (personal health) and m-Health (mobile health) solutions were discussed, and different strategies for the management of sensors, signals, and systems were described.

As fundamental motivation these applications aim to improve healthcare provided to patients and citizens, improving their quality of life and contributing to decreased occurrence of hard outcomes, such as hospitalization rates and long-term drug treatments. Additionally, the use of these technologies plays a significant role in reducing healthcare- associated expenses, as this is a significant burden in modern societies, in particular due to the increasing in life expectancy and the incidence of cardiovascular chronic diseases.

In practical terms, the described technologies and solutions allow moving toward a different concept of healthcare services, not only concentrated inside the hospital (where highly specialized activities are available), but also distributed among the population, allowing a more friendly management of the disease and a better quality of life for patients, as reflected in concepts such as high-value care or patient-reported outcomes measurements.

In this chapter we summarize the main concepts described in the book and illustrate a procedural example involving a concrete use case: the management of heart failure (HF).

11.2 Heart failure and management strategies

In the following sections we describe the main considerations for the design and the use of a p-health solution focused on the use case of HF.

Personalized Health Systems for Cardiovascular Disease
DOI: https://doi.org/10.1016/B978-0-12-818950-4.00010-0

The main aspects that must be taken into consideration are (1) specific and properly defined clinical needs, (2) available technological solutions, (3) benefit for the patient and caregivers, and (4) communication between the patient and physicians.

HF is a common, serious syndrome with a prevalence of 1%–2% in the adult population rising to 10% in the elderly (Ambrosy et al., 2014; Bergethon et al., 2016; Ponikowski et al., 2014). Globally, 26 million adults have been diagnosed with HF, and 3.6 million are newly diagnosed every year (Ponikowski et al., 2014). Although the mortality rate has improved in recent years, HF is still a leading cause of mortality worldwide (Ambrosy et al., 2014; Centers for Medicare and Medicaid Services; Cook, Cole, Asaria, Jabbour, & Francis, 2014), and it has been recognized as a major and increasing public health problem. Although associated with a short survival time, it still causes considerable disability and morbidity. This in turn is very costly because of the need for complex pharmacotherapy, community care, and, most of all, frequent hospital admissions.

Clinically, HF is a cardiovascular condition in which the heart cannot pump enough oxygenated blood to meet the needs of the body's organs. Initially, symptoms may occur only when the patient is exercising. However, over time, breathing problems and other symptoms may occur even when the patient is at rest. Common symptoms are fatigue, weakness, faintness, a fast or irregular pulse rate, a sensation of feeling the heartbeat (palpitations), shortness of breath during activity, swollen feet and ankles, and weight gain (Triposkiadis et al., 2009). Therefore the identification of the associated measurements and biosignals that should be collected in the context of telemonitoring systems and their significance and connection with the clinical outcomes are of major importance. Typical vital signs that can be recorded at home include blood pressure, body weight, heart rate, photoplethysmogram (PPG), ballistocardiogram (BCG), and electrocardiogram (ECG); the latter is of particular use in detecting the presence of arrhythmias (Joseph, Cedars, Ewald, Geltman, & Mann, 2009).

These raw biosignals, continuously acquired during a period of time (e.g., the ECG or the PPG) or collected periodically during the day (e.g., blood pressure or body weight), are not straightforward to interpret and normally present a high dimensionality, especially if they are acquired during long periods of time (e.g., months). Therefore proper procedures, including preprocessing, feature extraction, and modeling, are of primary relevance. The goal of the preprocessing and feature extraction phases is to map high-dimensional vectors (e.g., temporal biosignals such as an ECG) into lower-dimensional ones (e.g., features or parameters such as the heart rate extracted from an ECG), mainly to make readable and interpretable the clinical information and to simplify the decision-making process at the point of care. Moreover, the obtained features, through proper interpretative models, may reveal an additional understanding of the data, which can be valuable for decision making by professionals (Bellos, Papadopoulos, Rosso, & Fotiadis, 2010). Among the numerous methods that have been proposed, three main groups of preprocessing and feature extraction approaches can be identified: time-domain or signal-based methods, transform-based methods, which includes frequency-domain methods; and nonlinear methods, including information domain techniques.

At the first level, the biosignals that are collected periodically can be locally processed (at home) to infer patient's health status and for the detection and classification of specific clinical events. A possible outcome is the generation of alarms when there is any clinical significant alteration in the patient's physiological condition. Further, data can be sent to clinical medical back-end systems (at hospitals or care centers) for further analysis, where more sophisticated algorithms are used to analyze the patient's data. A general schema of the described architecture is shown in Fig. 11.1.

By taking advantage of the historical information that is routinely collected by telemonitoring systems, the conception of early prevention methodologies, able to detect not only the occurrence of a specific event but also its progression, is possible. In addition, multivariable algorithms based on several sources of information typically stored in the electronic health record, such as historical information, collected vital signals, laboratory results, and symptom questionnaires, can offer valuable tools to integrate clinical decision support systems (DSS).

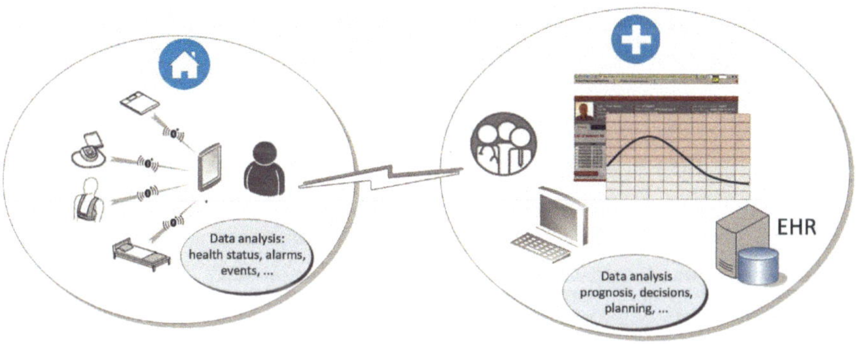

Figure 11.1 A general schema of a p-health system for remote monitoring of heart failure patients.

11.3 Success and potential of home monitoring and self-care in heart failure

HF patients are prone to sudden worsening and frequent hospital readmissions. They need constant monitoring of their condition and treatment adaptation with frequent physician's interventions. The correct management of the patient at home may contribute to prevent worsening and rehospitalization. When the patient is discharged from hospital, he or she is given many recommendations about monitoring vital signs, lifestyle, and treatment, and the patient can greatly benefit from proper tools and support for the correct management of his or her health. In practice, patients strongly benefit from p-health solutions that are tailored to their specific needs and can support them in better self-management.

Clinical guidelines provide recommendations for the management of the HF patient that include a continuum of care with constant involvement of the entire healthcare system (hospital, community, home assistance, etc.) in which a fundamental role is also played by the patient herself or himself through proper and aware self-management. The goal is to provide a high-quality standard of care (Lainscak et al., 2011), which requires a multidisciplinary approach with the expertise of cardiologists, primary care physicians, nurses, pharmacists, physiotherapists, dietitians, psychologists (Feltner et al., 2014; McAlister, Stewart, Ferrua, & McMurray, 2004; Ponikowski et al., 2016), and others according to the specific needs of the patients and the possible presence of comorbidities. It has been demonstrated that the application of these strategies can reduce the need for rehospitalization and the mortality rate. In this view, p-health can provide valuable tools assisting the physician and caregivers in identifying classes of patients and the associated risk and implementing methodologies that help in the correct management and self-management through proper sensors, data analysis, and supporting software and apps.

Home monitoring systems integrated into p-health solutions have the potential to contribute to this new healthcare systems paradigm. In effect, home monitoring systems offer several advantages and may provide added value for the reorientation of the healthcare process. Several studies have demonstrated that telemonitoring is an effective, efficient, and practical tool for treating patients with chronic illness when compared with standard care (Hasan and Paul, 2011; Willemse, Adriaenssens, Dilles, & Remmen, 2014). However, despite its potential and the significant developments that have been observed in last decades, from the commercial and mass consumption perspective home telemonitoring is not yet a standard in chronic disease management, even though the COVID-19 pandemic has strongly increased the adoption of such technologies. In effect, systematic reviews on chronic disease management and telemonitoring, while acknowledging the potential benefit of telemonitoring, highlight the need for further research (Chaudhry et al., 2007; Paré, Jaana, & Sicotte, 2007). Among others, more studies are still required to clearly identify the clinical effects of telemonitoring solutions, their cost effectiveness, their impact on the utilization of health services, and their acceptance by the participants. Additionally, more rigorous research will build stronger evidence for changes in the practice and management of chronic illnesses and therefore to the acceptance of home monitoring and its integration into the overall process of care. Finally, there are some issues involving regulatory aspects that need to be solved.

Nevertheless, the importance of self-care for HF patients is clear. The clinical guidelines strongly insist on the importance of making the patient aware and educating him or her on the need for full adherence to treatment, changing one's lifestyle, keeping vital parameters and symptoms monitored, and responding adequately to any change that suggests a worsening of the clinical condition.

As is shown in Fig. 11.2, self-care leans on three main pillars (Jaarsma et al., 2020):

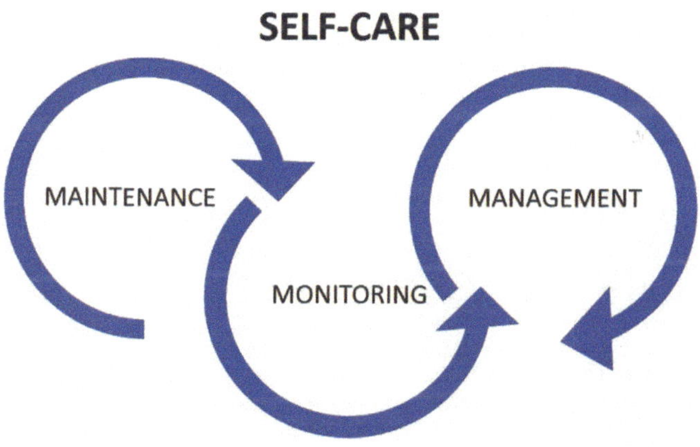

Figure 11.2 Self-care is of paramount importance for heart failure patients. It is sustained by three main pillars: maintenance, monitoring, and management. *Adapted from Jaarsma, T., Hill, L., Bayes-Genis, A., La Rocca, H.B., Castiello, T., Čelutkienė, J., … Strömberg, A. (2020). Self-care of heart failure patients: Practical management recommendations from the Heart Failure Association of the European Society of Cardiology.* European Journal of Heart Failure: Journal of the Working Group on Heart Failure of the European Society of Cardiology, *ejhf.2008. https://doi.org/10.1002/ejhf.2008.*

- Maintenance, that is, the ability to adopt (change and keep) all the behaviors that lead to maintaining stable clinical conditions
- Monitoring, that is, the careful observation of one's state and the ability to recognize changes in vital parameters and symptoms
- Management, that is, the ability to modify one's therapies when a change in status is recognized or forecasted

11.4 Steps toward personalized solutions

Adequate self-care has beneficial effects over time with respect to hospitalization and quality of life in general, and p-health systems, such as those described in this book, can constitute a valid support for each of the three pillars (maintenance, monitoring, and management) by intervening with different and multidisciplinary tools.

The personalization process of the p-health system refers to different steps starting at the patients' discharge and continuing with supporting proper home monitoring and treatment management (Fig. 11.3).

Let us now consider the patient who, after an acute episode of decompensation and the ensuing hospitalization, returns to daily life with a series of recommendations and therapies that need to be followed with precision and continuity. In practice, the patient has to face various changes in his or her lifestyle and also has to be able to promptly recognize any signs or symptoms of deterioration in her or his health in order to adequately modify the therapy or to contact the healthcare provider. The

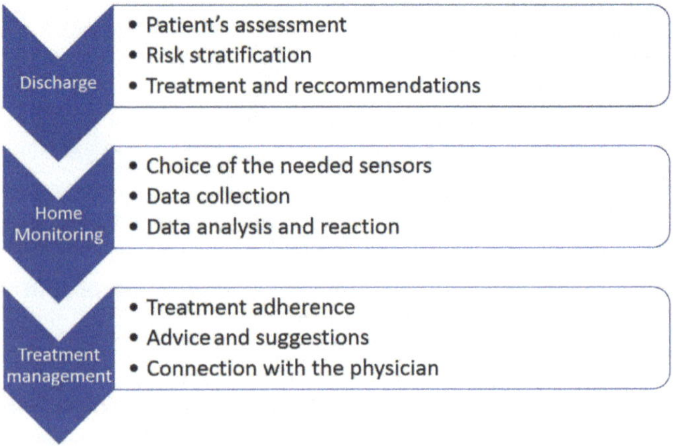

Figure 11.3 Personalization process for a p-health system.

methodologies and systems described in the previous chapters provide the necessary support in various stages, as illustrated in Fig. 11.3.

11.4.1 When discharged from the hospital

When discharge from the hospital, the patient is clinically evaluated and is provided with therapy and a series of recommendations for new habits and lifestyles in accordance with clinical guidelines and the experience of the treating physician. Risk stratification models and DSS make it possible to better phenotype patients on the basis of their characteristics and any comorbidities, which guide suggestions for the most appropriate choices of therapies and self-care and monitoring strategies.

Discharge is a key point. Early readmission after hospital discharge is common in HF patients. As a result, preventing readmissions has become an increasing priority for clinicians, researchers, and various stakeholders. Numerous studies have addressed the efficacy of different programs and approaches for reducing readmissions for HF patients (Centers for Medicare and Medicaid Services; Cook et al., 2014; Lee et al., 2003). These may be addressed through proper discharge planning (Ponikowski et al., 2016), which must take into account the specific patient's characteristics and needs. Different predictive models have been developed to identify patients who are at high risk for hospital readmissions and to enable addressing specific interventions for the patients who are likely to benefit most (Eapen et al., 2013; Kansagara et al., 2011; Lagu et al., 2016; Levy et al., 2006; O'Connor et al., 2012; Peterson et al., 2010; Pocock et al., 2013; Ponikowski et al., 2016; Rahimi et al., 2014; Senni et al., 2013; Sun, Hu, Azorin-Peris, Kalawsky, & Greenwald, 2012; Van Walraven et al., 2010).

Prediction models are naturally linked with the concept of clinical prognosis, aiming to predict the future of a specific variable, a clinical condition, or, ultimately, the health status of the patient (Henriques et al., 2015; Rocha, Paredes, Carvalho, Morais, & Henriques, 2015). In this context, data-mining techniques that can discover patterns, trends, rules, and correlations enclosed within the data have been successfully applied for prognosis tasks. A particular useful application of artificial intelligence techniques is the risk assessment for HF patients (Awan, Bennamoun, Sohel, Sanfilippo, & Dwivedi, 2019; Tripoliti, Papadopoulos, Karanasiou, Naka, & Fotiadis, 2017), with respect to the prognosis of some specific events, such as a new decompensation event or death (Marques et al., 2015; Paredes et al., 2011). Typically, these methodologies make use of fusion techniques to combine information coming from populations with the historical data as well as symptoms and laboratory exams from individual patients. Moreover, DSS and predictive data mining can be applied to help in the planning and adjusting of treatments by forecasting the effectiveness of the therapy in the future.

11.4.2 While at home

When the patient returns home, he or she starts the monitoring plan, performing a regular acquisition of a set of biosignals using adequate devices as well as the prescribed therapy in accordance with the plan that was established at discharge from the hospital.

In addition to pharmacological treatment, lifestyle adjustments are of paramount importance. Awareness and self-management are fundamental for the patient at home in order to decrease readmissions. Starting from the hospital stay, patients must be provided with the correct information and education to promote self-care and a lifestyle that may improve their quality of life and prognosis. Practical recommendations can be found in the work of Lainscak and colleagues (Lainscak et al., 2011).

However, changes in habits and following new rules as well as the adherence to a specific therapeutic plan may prove difficult for many patients once they are at home.

Apps and other software tools can be the means to convey proper up-to-date information and education and may provide support to make decisions on lifestyle adjustment and self-care.

Coaching systems are able to support long-term adherence to therapies by helping the patient to adopt a new lifestyle, providing reminders of daily deadlines, and highlighting omissions.

It is fundamental to identify a series of clinical parameters that must be monitored through the proper devices and sensors. The data and signals will be collected automatically, and appropriate software will be able to operate the following functions:

- Extracting from the collected data the parameters of clinical interest
- Comparing these parameters with the patient's typical trends or with appropriate alarm thresholds
- Inserting the measured values into the patient's health condition assessment templates to highlight changes in the clinical states

Periodic evaluation must make use of devices and instruments other than those available in a clinical setting and are intended not so much for diagnosis as for the early identification of any deviation from a stable state of the patient.

Devices and instrumentation as well as the associated software must be noninvasive and user friendly, and both the patient and the caregivers should be able to use them with no mistakes or stress.

As a practical example, let us consider some of the physiological parameters that are recommended for the daily assessment of an HF patient:

- Blood pressure
- Heart rate
- Presence of arrhythmias
- Sleep quality
- Weight

Recently, in an EU-funded project (HeartCycle, FP7), a bed sensor was proposed for the measurement of the BCG signal during the night (https://www.digitalhealthnews.eu/research-and-development/fp7-projects/1013-heartcycle). Proper software was developed that allows to extract the following clinical parameters from the sensor:

- Heart rate and heart rate variability throughout the whole night
- Presence of cardiac arrhythmias
- Sleep staging and sleep related parameters
- Breathing disorders (sleep apneas)

Fig. 11.4 shows an example of the physiological and clinical parameters coming from the bed sensor.

This approach has many advantages. It is not intrusive and does not affect the daily life of the patient. In addition, the resting conditions during the night guarantee a better quality of the recorded signals, and the long time duration of the recordings leads to more reliable estimation of the clinical data and more robust statistical evaluation. The patient is monitored, night after night, in replicable conditions with no interference caused by daytime activities (which may be different from one day to another), thus guaranteeing more reliable trends and comparisons. Data and features are automatically uploaded and collected on the electronic support, and the analysis is completely automatic. Other data, such as blood pressure, daily activity, and weight, are also collected through different devices and integrated into interpretative models for assessing the risk level, while DSS and coaching systems suggest behavioral changes or treatment adjustments. This is not an available device yet, on the other hand, it is an example of a possible solution able to provide many of the required measurements, also taking into consideration low intrusiveness and quality of life.

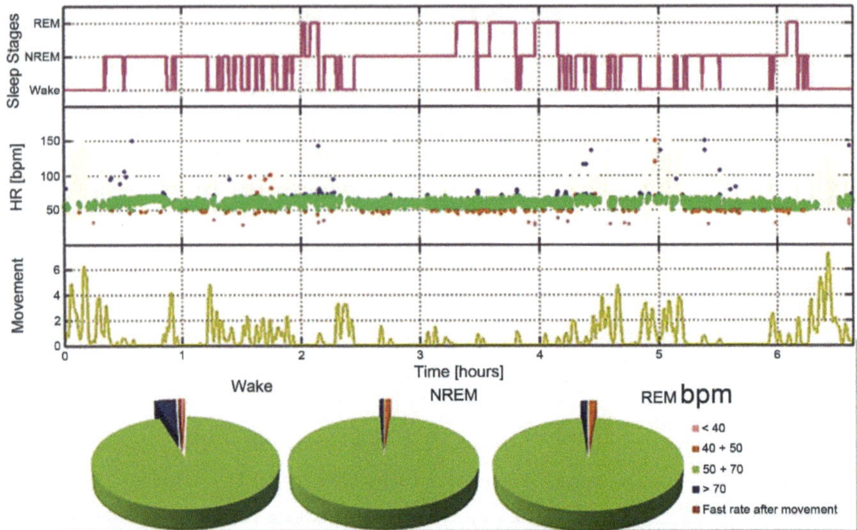

Sleep parameters from hypnogram
TIB: Time spent in bed with the intention of sleep.
SOL: Sleep onset latency.
WASO: Wake after sleep onset
TST: Total sleep time = TIB-TWT
SE: Sleep efficiency = (TST/TIB)*100

Figure 11.4 Example of the output of a bed sensor for monitoring heart failure patients. From the BCG signal beat-to-beat, respiration and motions are obtained. From the interbeat signal extracted from BCG, the hypnogram (sleep stages) is estimated, and the heart rate and arrhythmias are detected and reported related to the different sleep stages.

11.4.3 P-health: An integrated care system centered on the patient

The patients and their home are the center of an ecosystem, including technologies and experts, that aims to guarantee both adequate healthcare and good quality of life (see Fig. 11.5).

Moreover, personalization can be achieved by using p-health solutions through an optimal monitoring system based on the possibility of adapting to the patient's characteristics. Such a system includes the following:

- A personalized set of sensors (standard devices, wearable, included into the environment or implanted)

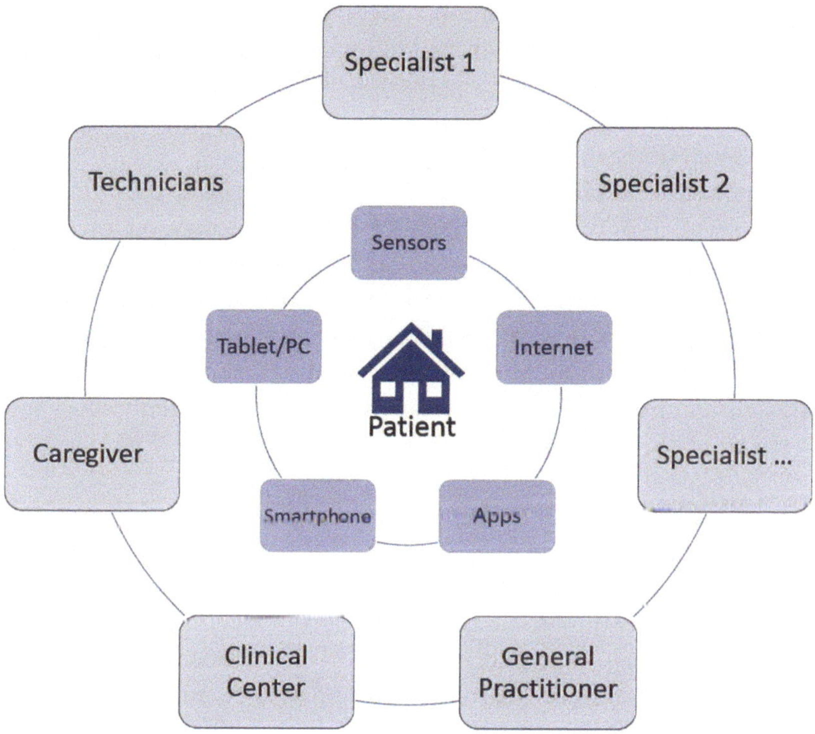

Figure 11.5 The heart failure patient is the center of a complex and multidisciplinary ecosystem.

- Personalized software that implements the model for the patient's assessment and predicts changes in the patient's clinical condition
- Apps and software that provide advice in lifestyle changes and therapy adjustments, based on acquired data and clinical guidelines
- Connection with the healthcare provider, who will be able to intervene in case of need

It is worth mentioning that periodic measurements will make use of devices and instrumentation other than those available in a clinical setting that are not finalized for diagnosis but rather are intended for the early identification of any deviation from a stable state of the patient.

On the other hand, biosignals and other information that are collected at home can be sent for further analysis to clinical medical back-end applications at hospitals or treatment centers, where more advanced algorithms are used to interpret patient data. As a result, permanent care of patients is possible, assisting clinical professionals in the remote management of patients and the implementation of prompt corrective intervention, thereby achieving an immediate clinical outcome in the patient's health.

According to the patient's needs, other sets of sensors could be required. These may be more specific or more intrusive.

Different studies and systematic reviews have been published (Athilingam and Jenkins, 2018; Masterson Creber et al., 2016) about the use of apps to support management of HF and promotion of self-care. Even though most such studies were heterogeneous, having different bias or quality problems in the assessment, they proved the impact and potential cost effectiveness of such mobile health solutions. Common features of such good practice solutions are remote monitoring and patient empowerment in their own home care by personalized feedback.

11.5 Conclusions

P-health solutions provide the possibility of implementing platforms for continuity of care at home through the support of innovative technologies. For patients with chronic illnesses, it becomes of fundamental importance to identify structured, integrated, continuous, care pathways complemented by proper sets of sensors and analysis tools that allow the necessary customization through interoperable and scalable modules. These systems are intended to connect, motivate, and support the patient and caregivers to adopt care at an optimal level of efficiency and engagement with respect to the clinical goals and that will be measured and validated by health professionals.

A fundamental aspect concerns the multidisciplinary integration in the provision of integrated care services, which is essential in the management of chronic diseases such as HF. Thanks to digital technology, it is possible to implement efficient clinic-home communication through a double-loop model that includes all the key actions—assessment, monitoring, clinical decision, and feedback to the patient and to the clinical professional—in a way that can be synchronous or asynchronous. The collected data provide the clinician with required information for monitoring the progress of the patient's clinical path through specific indicators and quantitative parameters.

The use of p-health solutions, such as the one presented in the example, can have numerous impacts from several points of view. First of all, according to the perspective on the patient's well-being, they provide assistance that is tailored to the patient's needs without social detachment.

One of the consequences deriving from the COVID-19 pandemic has been the feeling of isolation with respect to both health and emotional care by caregivers and family members. This feeling greatly threatens the patient's vulnerability in addition to causing both physical and mental deterioration. In this sense, the use of technological devices allows a greater guarantee of adherence to the continuity of care at home based on specific individual needs, also reducing the experiences of loneliness, stress, and fear.

Another impacting factor is preserving the autonomy of chronic patients. Other positive aspects are linked to an improvement in the connection processes among cooperating professionals and operating units.

A negative aspect may be linked to acceptance of the technology by patients and caregivers. However, as learning increases, the degree of acceptability also improves.

Health services that make use of platforms such as those described can be associated with a general increase in accessibility to the service. In fact, thanks to the lower cost that the health system could experience following the introduction of the p-health ecosystem, there may be sufficient economic savings to make it possible to treat a wider segment of the population that requires such services.

A further advantage linked to the innovative system is of an organizational nature, since moving the rehabilitation setting from hospital to home makes it possible to save healthcare resources that could potentially be destined for other uses.

References

Ambrosy, A. P., Fonarow, G. C., Butler, J., Chioncel, O., Greene, S. J., Vaduganathan, M., . . . Gheorghiade, M. (2014). The global health and economic burden of hospitalizations for heart failure: Lessons learned from hospitalized heart failure registries. *Journal of the American College of Cardiology*. Available from https://doi.org/10.1016/j.jacc.2013.11.053.

Athilingam, P., & Jenkins, B. (2018). Mobile phone apps to support heart failure self-care management: Integrative review. *JMIR Cardio, 2*, e10057. Available from https://doi.org/10.2196/10057.

Awan, S. E., Bennamoun, M., Sohel, F., Sanfilippo, F. M., & Dwivedi, G. (2019). Machine learning- based prediction of heart failure readmission or death: Implications of choosing the right model and the right metrics. *ESC Heart Failure*. Available from https://doi.org/10.1002/ehf2.12419.

Bellos, C. C., Papadopoulos, A., & Rosso Fotiadis, R. (2010). *Extraction and analysis of features acquired by wearable sensors network. Proceedings of the 10th IEEE international conference on Information Technology Applications in Biomedicine* (pp. 1–4). IEEE. Available from https://doi.org/10.1109/ITAB.2010.5687761.

Bergethon, K. E., Ju, C., DeVore, A. D., Chantelle Hardy, N., Fonarow, G. C., Yancy, C. W., ... Hernandez, A. F. (2016). Trends in 30-day readmission rates for patients hospitalized with heart failure: Findings from the get with the guidelines-heart failure registry. *Circulation: Heart Failure.* Available from https://doi.org/10.1161/CIRCHEARTFAILURE.115.002594.

Centers for Medicare and Medicaid Services. Readmission Reduction Program, (n.d.). https://www.cms.gov/Medicare/Medicare-Fee-for-Service-Payment/AcuteInpatientPPS/Readmissions-Reduction-Program.

Chaudhry, S. I., Phillips, C. O., Stewart, S. S., Riegel, B., Mattera, J. A., Jerant, A. F., ... Krumholz, H. M. (2007). Telemonitoring for patients with chronic heart failure: A systematic review. *Journal of Cardiac Failure, 13*, 56–62. Available from https://doi.org/10.1016/j.cardfail.2006.09.001.

Cook, C., Cole, G., Asaria, P., Jabbour, R., & Francis, D. P. (2014). The annual global economic burden of heart failure. *International Journal of Cardiology.* Available from https://doi.org/10.1016/j.ijcard.2013.12.028.

Eapen, Z. J., Liang, L., Fonarow, G. C., Heidenreich, P. A., Curtis, L. H., Peterson, E. D., ... Hernandez, A. F. (2013). Validated, electronic health record deployable prediction models for assessing patient risk of 30-day rehospitalization and mortality in older heart failure patients. *JACC Heart Failure.* Available from https://doi.org/10.1016/j.jchf.2013.01.008.

Feltner, C., Jones, C. D., Cené, C. W., Zheng, Z. J., Sueta, C. A., Coker-Schwimmer, E. J. L., ... Jonas, D. E. (2014). Transitional care interventions to prevent readmissions for persons with heart failure: A systematic review and meta-analysis. *Annals of Internal Medicine.* Available from https://doi.org/10.7326/M14-0083.

Hasan, A., & Paul, V. (2011). Telemonitoring in chronic heart failure. *European Heart Journal, 32*, 1457–1464. Available from https://doi.org/10.1093/eurheartj/ehr005.

Henriques, J., Carvalho, P., Paredes, S., Rocha, T., Habetha, J., Antunes, M., ... Morais, J. (2015). Prediction of heart failure decompensation events by trend analysis of telemonitoring data. *IEEE Journal of Biomedical and Health Informatics.* Available from https://doi.org/10.1109/JBHI.2014.2358715.

Jaarsma, T., Hill, L., Bayes-Genis, A., La Rocca, H. B., Castiello, T., Čelutkienė, J., ... Strömberg, A. (2020). Self-care of heart failure patients: Practical management recommendations from the Heart Failure Association of the European Society of Cardiology. *European Journal of Heart Failure: Journal of the Working Group on Heart Failure of the European Society of Cardiology*, ejhf.2008. Available from https://doi.org/10.1002/ejhf.2008.

Joseph, S. M., Cedars, A. M., Ewald, G. A., Geltman, E. M., & Mann, D. L. (2009). Acute decompensated heart failure: Contemporary medical management. *Texas Heart Institute Journal.*

Kansagara, D., Englander, H., Salanitro, A., Kagen, D., Theobald, C., Freeman, M., ... Kripalani, S. (2011). Risk prediction models for hospital readmission: A systematic review. *JAMA: Journal of the American Medical Association.* Available from https://doi.org/10.1001/jama.2011.1515.

Lagu, T., Pekow, P. S., Shieh, M. S., Stefan, M., Pack, Q. R., Kashef, M. A., ... Lindenauer, P. K. (2016). Validation and comparison of seven mortality prediction models for hospitalized patients with acute decompensated heart failure. *Circulation: Heart Failure.* Available from https://doi.org/10.1161/CIRCHEARTFAILURE.115.002912.

Lainscak, M., Blue, L., Clark, A. L., Dahlström, U., Dickstein, K., Ekman, I., ... Jaarsma, T. (2011). Self-care management of heart failure: Practical recommendations from the patient care committee of the heart failure association of the European society of cardiology. *European Journal of Heart Failure: Journal of the Working Group on Heart Failure of the European Society of Cardiology.* Available from https://doi.org/10.1093/eurjhf/hfq219.

Lee, D. S., Austin, P. C., Rouleau, J. L., Liu, P. P., Naimark, D., & Tu, J. V. (2003). Predicting mortality among patients hospitalized for heart failure: Derivation and validation of a clinical model. *Journal of the American Medical Association*. Available from https://doi.org/10.1001/jama.290.19.2581.

Levy, W. C., Mozaffarian, D., Linker, D. T., Sutradhar, S. C., Anker, S. D., Cropp, A. B., ... Packer, M. (2006). The seattle heart failure model: Prediction of survival in heart failure. *Circulation*. Available from https://doi.org/10.1161/CIRCULATIONAHA.105.584102.

Marques, T., Henriques, J., de Carvalho, P., Paredes, S., Rocha, T., & Morais, J. (2015). Personalization based on grouping strategies for short-term cardiovascular event risk assessment. *Cardiovascular Engineering and Technology*, *6*, 392–399. Available from https://doi.org/10.1007/s13239-015-0228-8.

Masterson Creber, R. M., Maurer, M. S., Reading, M., Hiraldo, G., Hickey, K. T., & Iribarren, S. (2016). Review and analysis of existing mobile phone apps to support heart failure symptom monitoring and self-care management using the mobile application rating scale (MARS). *JMIR MHealth UHealth*, *4*, e74. Available from https://doi.org/10.2196/mhealth.5882.

McAlister, F. A., Stewart, S., Ferrua, S., & McMurray, J. J. J. V. (2004). Multidisciplinary strategies for the management of heart failure patients at high risk for admission: A systematic review of randomized trials. *Journal of the American College of Cardiology*. Available from https://doi.org/10.1016/j.jacc.2004.05.055.

O'Connor, C. M., Whellan, D. J., Wojdyla, D., Leifer, E., Clare, R. M., Ellis, S. J., ... Lee, K. L. (2012). Factors related to morbidity and mortality in patients with chronic heart failure with systolic dysfunction the HF-ACTION predictive risk score model. *Circulation: Heart Failure*. Available from https://doi.org/10.1161/CIRCHEARTFAILURE.111.963462.

Paré, G., Jaana, M., & Sicotte, C. (2007). Systematic review of home telemonitoring for chronic diseases: The evidence base. *Journal of the American Medical Informatics Association*. Available from https://doi.org/10.1197/jamia.M2270.

Paredes, S., Rocha, T., de Carvalho, P., Henriques, J., Harris, M., & Morais, J. (2011). Long term cardiovascular risk models' combination. *Computer Methods and Programs in Biomedicine*. Available from https://doi.org/10.1016/j.cmpb.2010.12.015.

Peterson, P. N., Rumsfeld, J. S., Liang, L., Albert, N. M., Hernandez, A. F., Peterson, E. D., ... Masoudi, F. A. (2010). A validated risk score for in-hospital mortality in patients with heart failure from the American heart association get with the guidelines program. *Circulation: Cardiovascular Quality and Outcomes*. Available from https://doi.org/10.1161/CIRCOUTCOMES.109.854877.

Pocock, S. J., Ariti, C. A., McMurray, J. J. V., Maggioni, A., Køber, L., Squire, I. B., ... Doughty, R. N. (2013). Predicting survival in heart failure: A risk score based on 39 372 patients from 30 studies. *European Heart Journal*. Available from https://doi.org/10.1093/eurheartj/ehs337.

Ponikowski, P., Anker, S. D., AlHabib, K. F., Cowie, M. R., Force, T. L., Hu, S., ... Filippatos, G. (2014). Heart failure: Preventing disease and death worldwide. *ESC Heart Failure*. Available from https://doi.org/10.1002/ehf2.12005.

Ponikowski, P., Voors, A. A., Anker, S. D., Bueno, H., Cleland, J. G. F., Coats, A. J. S., ... Zamorano, J. L. (2016). ESC Guidelines for the diagnosis and treatment of acute and chronic heart failure: The Task Force for the diagnosis and treatment of acute and chronic heart failure of the European Society of Cardiology (ESC). Developed with the special contribution. *European Journal of Heart Failure: Journal of the Working Group on Heart Failure of the European Society of Cardiology*. Available from https://doi.org/10.1002/ejhf.592.

Rahimi, K., Bennett, D., Conrad, N., Williams, T. M., Basu, J., Dwight, J., ... MacMahon, S. (2014). Risk prediction in patients with heart failure: A systematic review and analysis. *JACC Heart Failure*. Available from https://doi.org/10.1016/j.jchf.2014.04.008.

Rocha, T., Paredes, S., Carvalho, P., Morais, J., & Henriques, J. (2015). Trend analysis of telemonitoring for the prediction of heart failure decompensation events. *IFMBE Proceedings*. Available from https://doi.org/10.1007/978-3-319-11128-5_168.

Senni, M., Parrella, P., De Maria, R., Cottini, C., Böhm, M., Ponikowski, P., ... Gavazzi, A. (2013). Predicting heart failure outcome from cardiac and comorbid conditions: The 3C-HF score. *International Journal of Cardiology*. Available from https://doi.org/10.1016/j.ijcard.2011.10.071.

Sun, Y., Hu, S., Azorin-Peris, V., Kalawsky, R., & Greenwald, S. (2012). Noncontact imaging photoplethysmography to effectively access pulse rate variability. *Journal of Biomedical Optics*, *18*, 061205. Available from https://doi.org/10.1117/1.jbo.18.6.061205.

Tripoliti, E. E., Papadopoulos, T. G., Karanasiou, G. S., Naka, K. K., & Fotiadis, D. I. (2017). Heart failure: Diagnosis, severity estimation and prediction of adverse events through machine learning techniques. *Computational and Structural Biotechnology Journal*. Available from https://doi.org/10.1016/j.csbj.2016.11.001.

Triposkiadis, F., Karayannis, G., Giamouzis, G., Skoularigis, J., Louridas, G., & Butler, J. (2009). The sympathetic nervous system in heart failure. Physiology, pathophysiology, and clinical implications. *Journal of the American College of Cardiology*. Available from https://doi.org/10.1016/j.jacc.2009.05.015.

Van Walraven, C., Dhalla, I. A., Bell, C., Etchells, E., Stiell, I. G., Zarnke, K., ... Forster, A. J. (2010). Derivation and validation of an index to predict early death or unplanned readmission after discharge from hospital to the community. *CMAJ: Canadian Medical Association Journal = Journal de l'Association Medicale Canadienne*. Available from https://doi.org/10.1503/cmaj.091117.

Willemse, E., Adriaenssens, J., Dilles, T., & Remmen, R. (2014). Do telemonitoring projects of heart failure fit the chronic care model? *International Journal of Integrated Care*, *14*. Available from https://doi.org/10.5334/ijic.1178.

Index

Note: Page numbers followed by "*f*" and "*t*" refer to figures and tables, respectively.

D

E

F

G

U

V

W

X

FSC
www.fsc.org
MIX
Papier | Fördert gute Waldnutzung
FSC® C083411

Kolibri 360 GmbH
Ferdinand-Jühlke-Straße 7
99095 Erfurt, Deutschland
produktsicherheit@kolibri360.de